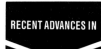

RECENT ADVANCES IN

Haematology

RECENT ADVANCES IN HAEMATOLOGY

Contents of Number 6
Edited by A. V. Hoffbrand, M. K. Brenner

ISBN 0443 043809

You can place your order by contacting your local medical bookseller or the Sales Promotion Department, Robert Stevenson House, 1–3 Baxter's Place, Leith Walk, Edinburgh EH1 3AF, UK

Tel: (031) 556 2424; Telex: 727511 LONGMN G; Fax: (031) 558 1278

Look out for *Recent Advances in Haematology 8* in September 1995

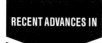

Haematology

Edited by

M. K. Brenner MA MB PhD FRCP MRCPath
Director, Division of Bone Marrow Transplantation, and
Member, Department of Hematology/Oncology,
St Jude Children's Research Hospital, Memphis, Tennessee;
Professor, Department of Pediatrics and Department of Medicine,
University of Tennessee, USA

A. V. Hoffbrand MA DM FRCP FRCPath FRCP(Edin) DSc
Professor of Haematology and Honorary Consultant,
Royal Free Hospital and School of Medicine, London, UK

NUMBER SEVEN

CHURCHILL LIVINGSTONE
EDINBURGH LONDON MADRID MELBOURNE MILAN NEW YORK AND
TOKYO 1993

CHURCHILL LIVINGSTONE
Medical Division of Longman Group UK Limited

Distributed in the United States of America by
Churchill Livingstone Inc., 650 Avenue of the Americas,
New York, N.Y. 10011, and by associated companies,
branches and representatives throughout the world.

First published 1993

ISBN 0-443-04689-1

ISSN 0143-697X

British Library Cataloguing in Publication Data
A catalogue record for this book is available from the British
Library

Library of Congress Cataloging in Publication Data
is available

The
publisher's
policy is to use
**paper manufactured
from sustainable forests**

Produced by Longman Singapore Publishers Pte Ltd
Printed in Singapore

Contents

Preface

The pace of clinical research in haematology has ensured that the 18 months since the publication of *Recent Advances in Haematology 6* has seen a significant number of major changes in the field. Some of these are already having an impact on patient treatment, for example, transplantation for sickle cell disease, while others such as gene therapy, are likely to have their maximum impact over the next decade. Both of these areas are reviewed in the present issue. As in previous volumes, updates are given in other rapidly advancing or important areas of clinical practice and clinical research in haematology. The current book should therefore be considered a companion to No. 6 published in 1992 and continues our intention to try and publish *Recent Advances in Haematology* every eighteen months.

As always, we would like to thank our contributors for their timely and high-quality manuscripts and Yvonne O'Leary at Churchill Livingstone for ensuring the process of compilation of this volume was relatively painless.

Memphis   M. K. Brenner
London   A. V. Hoffbrand
1993

Contributors

F. N. Al-Refaie MB ChB, MRCPath
Clinical Research Fellow, Department of Haematology, Royal Free
Hospital, London, UK

Alain Bernard MD
Professor of Medicine, Hôpital de l'Archet, Nice, France

M. K. Brenner MA MB PhD FRCP MCRPath
Director, Division of Bone Marrow Transplantation, and Member,
Department of Hematology/Oncology, St Jude Children's Research
Hospital, Memphis, Tennessee; Professor, Department of Pediatrics and
Department of Medicine, University of Tennessee, USA

Ernest Briët MD
Professor of Medicine, and Director, Haematology Laboratories, University
Hospital, Leiden, The Netherlands

Dario Campana MD PhD
Assistant Member, Division of Bone Marrow Transplantation, Department
of Hematology/Oncology, St Jude Children's Research Hospital, Memphis,
Tennessee, USA

Dominic J. Culligan BSc MB BS MRCP
Senior Registrar, Department of Haematology, University Hospital of
Wales, Cardiff, UK

S. M. Donohue MRCP MRCPath
Honorary Lecturer, Department of Haematology, Royal Free Hospital and
School of Medicine, London, UK

Geoffrey Dusheiko MB BCh, FCP(SA) FRCP
Reader in Medicine, Royal Free Hospital and School of Medicine,
London, UK

John F. Hancock MA MB PhD MRCP
Honorary Senior Lecturer, Department of Haematology, Royal Free
Hospital and School of Medicine, London, UK; Senior Scientist, Onyx
Pharmaceuticals, Richmond, California, USA

A. V. Hoffbrand MA DM FRCP FRCPath FRCP(Edin) DSc
Professor of Haematology and Honorary Consultant, Royal Free Hospital
and School of Medicine, London, UK

D. C. S. Huang MB BS MRCP
Research Fellow, Department of Haematology, Royal Free Hospital and
School of Medicine, London, UK

A. Jacobs MD FRCPath FRCP
Professorial Fellow, Centre for Applied Public Health Medicine,
University Hospital of Wales, Cardiff, UK

Margaret A. Johnson MD MRCP
Consultant Physician HIV/AIDS, Royal Free Hospital, London, UK

Marc C. I. Lipman MRCP
Clinical Research Fellow, Royal Free Hospital, London UK

Malegapuru W. Makgoba MB ChB(Natal) D Phil(Oxon) FRCP
Reader, and Head, Molecular Endocrinology, and Honorary Consultant,
Department of Chemical Pathology, Royal Postgraduate Medical School,
Hammersmith Hospital, London, UK

Dana C. Matthews MD
Acting Assistant Professor, Division of Hematology/Oncology, Department
of Pediatrics, University of Washington; Assistant Member, Fred
Hutchinson Cancer Research Center, Seattle, Washington, USA

Joseph Mirro, Jr MD
Professor of Pediatrics, University of Pittsburgh, and Children's Hospital of
Pittsburgh, Pittsburgh, Pennsylvania, USA

Robert C. Moen MD PhD
Director of Clinical and Regulatory Affairs, Genetic Therapy Inc.,
Gaithersburg, Maryland, USA

Rose Ann Padua BSc PhD
Reader in Haematology, University of Wales College of Medicine, Cardiff,
UK

F. E. Preston MD FRCP FRCPath
Professor of Haematology, Royal Hallamshire Hospital, Sheffield; Director,
Sheffield Regional Haemophilia Centre, Sheffield, UK

Keith M. Sullivan MD
Professor of Medicine, University of Washington; Member, Fred
Hutchinson Cancer Research Center, Seattle, Washington, USA

Edward G. D. Tuddenham MB BS FRCP FRCPath MD
Director, Haemostasis Research Group, MRC Clinical Research Centre,
Harrow, Middlesex, UK

Mark C. Walters MD
Associate in Clinical Research, Fred Hutchinson Cancer Research Center, Division of Pediatric Oncology, Seattle, Washington, USA

Michael R. Wollman MD
Associate Professor of Pediatrics, University of Pittsburgh, and Children's Hospital of Pittsburgh, Pittsburgh, Pennsylvania, USA

Beatrix Wonke MD FRCPath
Consultant Haematologist, Whittington Hospital, London, UK

Current and prospective gene therapy protocols and their application to hematological disease

R. C. Moen

The first authorized human clinical trial involving gene transfer began in May 1989. Since then many other protocols utilizing gene transfer techniques have begun. The rate of new protocols is accelerating as the number of centers involved and number of target organs increases. Initial protocols were for gene *marking*; the first gene *therapy* protocols began a year later in 1990. Four new protocols opened in 1991, including the first outside the USA. By 1992 over a dozen new protocols are expected to have begun worldwide. The expansion of the field is impressive and the proposed uses of gene therapy have extended from the originally contemplated target of genetic disorders to involve more prevalent maladies such as cancer. Besides the use of gene transfer for its therapeutic aspects, gene marking has proven an extremely useful clinical tool allowing the investigator to answer important questions about various disease processes and treatment. As the trials progress and more information is obtained, more and more uses of gene transfer in clinical situations will be developed.

It is the aim of this chapter to provide the background information and rationale of current and prospective protocols. Given the rapidity with which the field is advancing, this chapter cannot provide an up-to-the-minute report of all protocols. What it can anticipate is the type of protocols which may begin soon and the rationale which will support them. It is in this light that the chapter is written.

DELIVERY SYSTEMS

There are many ways in which genes can be transferred to eukaryotic cells. Brief descriptions of several of them are listed, as are their present and potential future applications.

Physical methods

Initial gene transfer experiments in the laboratory used physical methods to introduce genetic material into cells. Although the most prevalent laboratory method uses calcium phosphate precipitation (Perucho et al 1980, Chen &

Okayama 1988), this method probably will not have wide clinical use. Although calcium phosphate is able to transfer genetic material into a significant proportion of cells, stable gene transfer occurs in only a very small fraction. Moreover, a single oriented copy of genetic material is seldom inserted; more often it is a tandem array of the exogenous DNA that is inserted. Since the physical orientation and gene copy number are difficult to control, problems in appropriate regulation and expression may arise that could be clinically significant. This method will be useful only for clinical protocols in which transient expression of the transferred gene(s) is sufficient; no current protocol or currently proposed protocol utilizes calcium phosphate precipitation as a means of gene transfer.

Electroporation (McNally et al 1988, Kubiniec et al 1990) has many of the same advantages and shortcomings as calcium phosphate transfer. For example, multiple copies of the gene are often transferred and the frequency of stable gene transfer is low. Despite improvements in electroporator machine design and the ability to handle larger number of cells, the approach has not yet found a clinical use.

Liposomes or other forms of lipid-encapsulated genetic material have been increasingly used for gene transfer into tissue culture cells (Hug & Sleight 1991). The physical nature of the introduced DNA is very similar to the above physical techniques, but the overall gentleness and somewhat higher frequency of gene transfer has made it a more appealing system. A gene therapy protocol utilizing this technology has been approved for use (Nabel et al 1992). Interestingly, this protocol is designed to transfer genetic material in vivo, while all previous protocols have used ex vivo methods for gene transfer. This protocol is discussed in more detail later in this chapter.

Microinjection of DNA has been utilized for many years as a method to introduce genetic material into individual cells. The form in which the DNA is introduced and its stability are the same as with all other methods of physical gene transfer. While microinjection can be an effective method, it has the severe limitation that large quantities of cells can not be expeditiously injected. If a stem cell could be obtained, microinjected, and returned to the patient, then it might be possible to consider microinjection techniques for clinical use (Boggs 1990, Gordon 1990). Unfortunately it has not been possible to identify, purify and maintain stem cells for target cells of clinical interest. The problems of returning the stem cells to the patient and finding or making space for these cells also remain unresolved. As cell biology methods improve and purification techniques increase the yield and quality of stem cells, this method may be further explored.

Ballistic techniques, in which 'shotgun' pellets are coated with DNA, have been used both in vitro as well as in vivo. This can be visualized as a microinjection technique which can be applied to large numbers of cells, with the pellets serving the role of the needle. This method is undergoing rapid development and has had substantial success in plant systems. As the technology improves this method may become a preferred method for treating large quantities of cells ex vivo or in vivo.

One final way of microinjecting genetic material into a cell is to allow the cell to inject itself. Various DNA–ligand complexes have been studied with equally variable degrees of success. Most noteworthy are the experiments using DNA–asialoglycoprotein complexes (Wu et al 1991, Wu & Wu 1991), which bind to their corresponding receptors found on many different cell types including hepatocytes. The receptor with the bound DNA complex is taken up by the cell and is then equivalent to the DNA introduced by any other physical method. It can be transiently expressed and will stably integrate into the host cell chromatin at a certain frequency. This system is appealing for its potential for in vivo gene transfer and for the possibility of targeting certain cells by the receptors they express. Protocols using DNA–ligand methods of gene transfer are being developed and will begin the review process shortly.

Viral vectors

Viral vectors represent another large category of gene delivery systems, relying on the ability of viruses to infect host cells and thereby transfer their genetic material. Nature has evolved its own delivery systems which can be modified for use in gene therapy/transfer. Each system has benefits and drawbacks as a vector delivery system which relate to the basic characteristics of each virus type. Several good reviews exist describing retroviral vectors (McLachlin et al 1990, Miller 1990) and only the most developed will be discussed in detail here.

Retroviral vectors

Retroviral-mediated gene transfer (RMGT) was used in all the first clinical gene transfer protocols and continues to be chosen for the vast majority of protocols entering the review process. Perhaps more important than the scientific arguments for using retroviral vectors is the extensive practical experience obtained with Moloney murine leukemia virus (MoMLV) based systems (Fig. 1.1). The most rigorous safety studies in vivo have been performed with this system in mind. Before opening a clinical protocol, a risk–benefit ratio needs to be obtained, and the safety experience in animal models — and now also in human beings — allows some estimation of the risk associated with this method of transfer. RMGT is particularly useful with ex vivo gene transfer — used in almost all clinical protocols approved to date — since the vectors are not then exposed to human complement which inactivates the retrovirus (Cornetta et al 1990). Ex vivo gene transfer was the logical way to begin clinical investigation because it allowed the investigator not only to study and document the status of the vector utilized, but also to study the transduced cells themselves for potential toxicities before returning

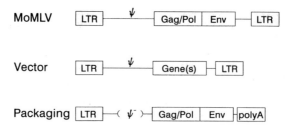

Fig. 1.1   The wild-type Moloney leukemia virus (MoMLV) genome. The LTRs provide important *cis* functions for integration, replication, poly-A signals, as well as promoter/enhancer functions. The Psi (ψ) sequence is needed in *cis* as it supplies the packaging signal. The gag, pol, and env functions can be supplied in *trans* to produce a retroviral particle. A vector can be made by combining the portions needed in *cis* with the gene or genes desired for transfer by the vector. The *trans* functions are provided by a packaging cell which synthesizes the retroviral proteins necessary to produce a retroviral particle. In the packaging cell the gag, pol, and env functions provide the needed proteins but the lack of a 3'-LTR and packaging sequence means the retroviral particles cannot package these *trans* functions and only the vector is packaged. Since the vector genome contains no *trans* functions, no further cycles of infection can be accomplished after integration of the vector genome into the target cells.

them to the patient. More detailed discussion of safety concerns with RMGT is presented in Temin (1990) and Cornetta et al (1990, 1991a, b). Although other vector systems will gain prominence as vector development improves and specific needs arise which are not met by RMGT techniques, the extensive prior experience with RMGT means that this approach will be used for most protocols in the near future.

RMGT takes advantage of the natural life cycle of a retrovirus which involves insertion of its genes into the host cell. The genome of the retrovirus is very simple and can be modified to make an efficient delivery system. The genome contains elements required in *cis*, the long terminal repeats (LTRs) which contain promoter, replication, and integration functions and the Psi region which contains a sequence which designates the piece of RNA for packaging into the viral particle. Other parts of the genome are needed in *trans*, including the coding sequences for the viral proteins gag, pol and env which code for core proteins, polymerase/RNAse/integrase proteins and envelope proteins, respectively. To make a retroviral vector the retroviral proteins gag, pol and env are removed from the genome and replaced by a gene or genes of interest. A packaging cell is prepared which is able to produce empty retroviral particles due to the presence of gag, pol, and env coding sequence. These empty particles therefore package the vector sequence and release infectious particles. When these are delivered to a cell, there is reverse transcription of the RNA strand, and integration of the DNA sequence into the host genome, just as in a wild-type retrovirus infection. However, a productive infection does not result because the vector transferred contains no coding sequences for gag, pol, or env. The integrated vector sequence now becomes a part of the host cell and all its progeny and the genes transferred with the vector code for proteins which will be expressed in the host cell.

Other viral vectors

Other viral vector systems are in various stages of development and can be anticipated to be used in clinical trials after various scientific and safety issues have been addressed. Several of the alternative vector systems will be described briefly with an emphasis on their potential applications.

Adenovirus is a human pathogen which infects a large variety of cell types. Its ability to infect airway cells in vivo has made it an attractive vector system to explore for use in airway disorders. A potential use of this vector system is in the treatment of cystic fibrosis by transferring a functional cystic fibrosis transmembrane conductance regulator (CFTR) gene into affected cells, since the patient's airways are the major area of pathology in this disorder. An adenoviral vector containing the CFTR gene has been constructed and has successfully transferred the human CFTR gene in vivo into the airways of cotton rats (Rosenfeld et al 1992). This particular application of adenoviral vectors will probably be only the first of many. The adenovirus system has two advantages over the retroviral system. It is possible to produce much higher titre vectors and these vectors can be used with non-dividing cells. Its chief disadvantages can be attributed to the relative lack of stable integration in host cell genome and the risks associated with using a vector system which could be subsequently rescued by a common human infection (Cornetta et al 1991a, b). As more experience with this system is obtained and safety/toxicity questions are answered, one can expect to see many uses for this vector system.

The adeno-associated virus (AAV) has also been explored as a gene transfer vehicle with encouraging results (Lebkowski et al 1988, Dixit et al 1991). One of its chief appeals is its potential ability to insert into a specific area of a specific chromosome. This predilection would reduce the risk of insertional mutagenesis and would limit the variable expression associated with random insertion into the host chromatin. The chief drawback of AAV vectors appears to be the limited size of therapeutic genes that can be inserted into the vector backbone. Many of the questions that need to be addressed with adenovirus vectors will have to be addressed with an AAV-based system, but again, as greater understanding of the AAV system develops, clinical uses for this system will follow.

Other vector systems are also being explored which exploit the tissue tropism of the parent virus. Herpes simplex virus is being explored for transferring genes into neural tissue (Fink et al 1992), since this is not amenable to targeting with retroviral vectors. This system would be of obvious use in genetic neurological disorders but might also be appropriate for treating Alzheimer's and Parkinson's disease and other central nervous system related pathology. Other vectors, including the rabies virus, may be even more specifically neurotropic.

Additional virus-based vector delivery systems are also being developed, some of which may have especial relevance for transduction of hemopoietic progenitor cells. One can readily imagine how almost any virus could be exploited to develop an efficient, organ directed, gene delivery vector system. As gene therapy experience increases, understanding of the pathology of human diseases expands, and basic virology progresses, more and more vector systems will be developed to exploit viruses — nature's own gene delivery systems — for therapeutic benefits.

Combinations of delivery systems

As more scientists become involved in gene therapy strategies it is only natural that chimeric delivery systems should also be developed. Eventually the advantages of one system will be combined with the advantages of another, at the same time eliminating any disadvantages as well. One example of a chimeric delivery system will be described to illustrate the benefits of this approach.

Adenovirus–DNA ligands have been developed for delivering genetic material to cells (Curiel et al 1992). In this system a virus particle is used as the ligand to carry the DNA into a cell, much like asialoglycoprotein was used to target DNA to liver cells. The adenovirus particle is inactivated and used to target the desired DNA fragment to cells which can be infected by adenovirus. As the killed particle begins the infection process, it pulls the therapeutic DNA into the cell with a much higher efficiency than can be obtained by other physical means.

CLINICAL PROTOCOLS

(see Table 1.1)

CLINICAL PROTOCOLS USING MARROW-DERIVED CELLS

Marrow cells, by virtue of their ease of harvesting and handling and because of their importance in many different disease processes, were early candidates for inclusion in clinical gene transfer studies.

Lymphocytes

The first gene transfer protocols utilized lymphocytes as the target cells, since these were easy to obtain and expand in vitro (Fig. 1.2). RMGT is most efficient if the target cell is dividing (Springett et al 1989, Miller 1990) and large quantities of transduced lymphocytes could be obtained by expansion with growth factors such as interleukin-2 (IL-2). These transduced

Table 1.1 A listing of gene transfer protocols and their approval status as of 15 July 1992

Location	Principal investigator	Type of protocol
*NCI	Rosenberg	TIL marking
*NCI	Blaese	ADA T-cell therapy
*NCI	Rosenberg	TNF TIL
*Memphis	Brenner	AML ABMT
*Memphis	Brenner	Neuroblastoma ABMT
*Houston	Deisseroth	CML ABMT
*Pittsburgh	Lotze	TIL marking
‡Houston	Ledley/Woo	HCT marking
*Lyon, France	Favrot	TIL marking
*NCI	Rosenberg	TNF tumor therapy/TIL
*NCI	Rosenberg	IL-2 tumor therapy/TIL
*Shanghai, China	Hsueh	Factor IX/fibroblasts
*Ann Arbor	Wilson	LDL receptor for FHC
*Seattle	Greenberg	HIV alloBMT autoCTL clone
*Ann Arbor	Nabel	HLA B7 CA liposome therapy
*Milan, Italy	Bordignon	ADA T & ABMT
†The Netherlands	Vallerio	ADA ABMT
†Rochester	Freeman	hTK ovarian CA
*Indianapolis	Cornetta	ALL/AML AMBT
‡NCI	Blaese	ADA PBSC
‡UCLA/USC	Economou	TIL/PBL marking
*Memphis	Brenner	IL-2/neuroblastoma
¶Viagene	Merchant	HIV gp160 vaccine
*NINDS/NCI	Oldfield/Culver	hTK brain tumor
‡MD Anderson	Deisseroth	CML ABMT dual marker
‡Sloan-Kettering	Gansbacher	IL-2 tumor lines (HLA-A2)
‡CHB/NCI	Dunbar/Nienhuis	ABMT (CML, myeloma, breast)

* Patients enrolled.
† All approvals obtained.
‡ RAC approval, need FDA approval.
¶ FDA approved, RAC approval not sought.

NCI = National Cancer Institute; UCLA = University of California, Los Angeles; USC = University of Southern California; NINDS = National Institute of Neurological Diseases and Stroke; CHB = Clinical Hematology Branch; TIL = Tumor infiltrating lymphocyte; ADA = Adenosine deaminase; TNF = Tumor necrosis factor; AML = Acute myelogenous leukemia; ABMT = Autologous bone marrow transplant; CML = Chronic myelogenous leukemia; HCT = Hepatocellular transplantation; CTL = Cytotoxic T lymphocyte; hTK = Herpes thymidine kinase; ALL = Acute lymphocytic leukemia; PBSC = Peripheral blood stem cell; PBL = Peripheral blood lymphocyte; LDL = ; FHC = Fred Hutchinson Cancer Center

lymphocytes may then be infused into the patient, where they could be therapeutic in their own right by normal lymphocyte actions, or could be used as miniature factories to produce biological factors. All these possible applications are in use or will be tested shortly.

Marking studies with lymphocytes

The first gene transfer trial used RMGT to learn more about a therapeutic modality. It was not designed to give any therapeutic benefit to the patient receiving the transduced lymphocytes, but to provide information about the

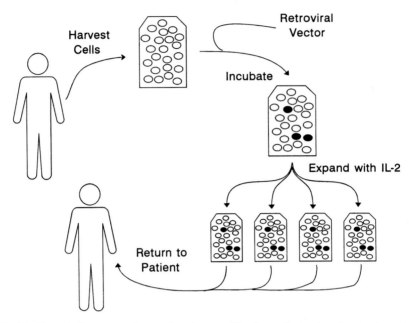

Fig. 1.2 Retroviral gene transfer into lymphocytes. The figure depicts lymphocytes harvested from a patient. These cells are transduced with the retroviral vector ex vivo, expanded, and then returned to the patient. This general protocol is used for TIL cells as well as for ADA replacement therapy.

therapy that might enable improved protocols to be designed for future patients (Rosenberg et al 1990a). The first trial used tumor infiltrating lymphocytes (TIL) as the target cell. These cells are obtained by removing tumor masses from a patient, obtaining a cell suspension, and then expanding in vitro the lymphocytes present within the tumor by using the growth factor IL-2. By this technique it is possible to routinely obtain 10^{11} TIL cells. Previous studies have shown the administration of these large quantities of TIL cells along with IL-2 to patients with renal cell carcinoma or melanoma has resulted in partial and complete responses. Unfortunately, these encouraging results occurred in only a fraction of the patients treated, and analysis of the TIL before infusion provided no clues as to what factors determined outcome. Since the reinfused TIL cells were autologous, there was no way to determine their half-life in the patient, analyze their trafficking, or reisolate them from the patient. By using RMGT in a fraction of the TIL cells it was hoped to use the transferred NEO[R] gene to trace the TIL population by means of sensitive polymerase chain reaction (PCR) techniques.

Gene marking has distinct advantages over other marking systems in that the marker is present in equal concentration in all progeny of the original cell and cannot be transferred to other cells if the marked cells died. This enables the patients to be analyzed for many months after receiving RMGT-marked TIL cells. As the first gene transfer protocol, the proposal was extensively reviewed at local and national levels. The Human Gene Therapy Subcommittee of the Recombinant DNA Advisory Committee as well as the parent committee had to approve the protocol in public meetings. The Director of the National Institutes of Health returned the protocol to both committees for further consideration after their initial approvals. The Food and Drug Administration (FDA) also reviewed the protocol. An FDA advisory committee meeting was also used to obtain expert review of the protocol. Finally, after approvals by the Human Gene Therapy Subcommittee, the Recombinant DNA Advisory Committee, the Director of the National Institutes of Health, and the FDA, the protocol began with its first patient on 22 May 1989.

The results from the first five patients have been published (Rosenberg et al 1990b). The marking enabled the researchers to show that TIL cells persisted for weeks, perhaps months, in the patients. In one patient it was possible to grow and select (with the neomycin analogue G418) transduced TIL cells found in subcutaneous metastasis (Aebersold et al 1990). Although this study did not achieve the aim of determining if TIL cells did indeed specifically home to sites of tumor cells, it established the feasibility of RMGT marking (Fig. 1.3) In none of these patients were any adverse effects seen on

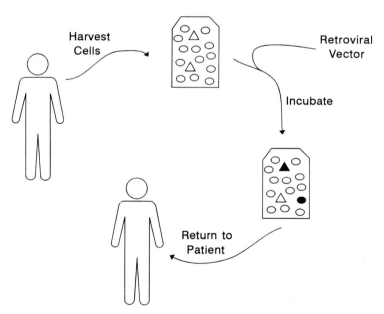

Fig. 1.3 Cell transplant with gene marking. This figure depicts the general protocol for retroviral marking of cells. Cells are removed from the patient, marked with a retroviral vector, and returned to the patient. This approach is also used in the autologous bone marrow transplant protocol. In this case the circles represent normal hematopoietic cells and the triangles contaminating cancer cells. Solid shapes depict retroviral-marked cells returned to the patient. For hepatocellular transplantation, the shapes represent different cell lineages obtained from the liver.

either the transduced cells or the patient that could be attributed to the RMGT.

With the initial usefulness and safety of RMGT established, other clinical centers around the world began to use the marking technology to explore important clinical questions. A similar study of gene marking TIL in patients with malignant melanoma or renal cell carcinoma was begun in Lyon, France, at the end of 1991. Early results confirm the usefulness in studying TIL therapy with RMGT as a marking tool.

Other studies using RMGT to study lymphocyte and TIL trafficking have been approved and began in 1992. Lotze et al (1992) used TIL cells expanded in IL-2 and IL-4 and administered with this combination of growth factors as well. This study uses more sophisticated analyses to more appropriately address the question of TIL trafficking. The number of RMGT-marked cells in tumor biopsies will be compared to their concentration in non-tumor tissues (blood, skin, fat, and muscle). Economou et al (1992) are comparing RMGT-marked TIL populations to a corresponding peripheral blood lymphocyte (PBL) population in patients with melanoma and renal cell carcinoma. The two cell populations will be followed simultaneously and separately by using two different retroviral vectors that can be distinguished by PCR techniques. By comparing the changing ratios of the two populations in tumor biopsies as well as normal tissues, the study should be able both to address trafficking questions and to discover whether TIL cells are significantly different from PBL in their life span, homing, or other characteristics. The study will also explore subpopulation behavior as well determine if any subfraction of TIL may offer certain advantages. As the results of these studies become available a greater understanding of the use of lymphocytes/TIL in cancer therapy may be obtained.

Gene therapy with lymphocytes

After the first successful use of RMGT to mark TIL cells, it was obvious to many observers that RMGT could be used to introduce genes into lymphocytes with therapeutic intent. Severe combined immunodeficiency as a result of adenosine deaminase (ADA) deficiency was the first disease chosen, for reasons that have been summarized elsewhere (Anderson 1984). Although bone marrow transplantation has been curative in ADA-deficient patients, this is a high-risk procedure, particularly in the absence of an HLA-identical sibling. To avoid the dangers associated with ablative treatment, it seemed logical to assume that transduction of autologous hematopoietic stem cells with ADA vectors would allow the patient to be immune reconstituted with similar benefit to that obtained with HLA-matched marrow. Unfortunately, it has proven difficult to demonstrate successful gene transfer into lymphocyte *precursor* cells in primate model studies (Kantoff et al 1987).

Despite the difficulties using marrow stem cells for gene transfer, it has been amply demonstrated that the ADA gene (or other genes) could be successfully transferred into *mature* lymphocytes (see Kasid et al 1990, Culver et al 1991a, and TIL studies mentioned previously). Since ADA-deficient patients have circulating T-cells which could be expanded ex vivo much like TIL, it was reasonable to assume that these lymphocytes might be transduced with ADA vectors and reinfused into the patient with clinical benefit. This was particularly true since experimental models have shown a growth advantage for transduced ADA-deficient T-cells (Culver et al 1991b). If the patient were periodically leukopheresed, the T-cells expanded and transduced in vivo, and returned to the patient, it might be possible to give the patient T-cells with a survival advantage. By obtaining more lymphocytes periodically, it would be expected that a larger and larger immunological repertoire of lymphocytes would be transduced to provide the patient with broader and longer-lived immune function. After extensive review, this first gene therapy protocol (Blaese & Anderson 1990) was approved and the first patient treated on 13 September 1990. Additional patients have subsequently been enrolled and all have had increasing ADA levels in their peripheral blood lymphocyte sample over time. The lymphocytes appear to survive many months and all patients have had a demonstrable improvement in their immune functions and clinical status.

Besides using gene therapy to treat genetic disorders by providing a functional gene to replace a defective or absent gene, the technique can be used to provide functions not normally expected of lymphocytes. For example, by introducing additional genes into TIL cells, it may be possible to increase the antitumor activities seen in the patient. The genes transferred may be able to directly affect the TIL cells so they have enhanced antitumor activities. Alternatively, the TIL may be used to locally deliver biologically active molecules which might recruit additional antitumor responses or change the properties of the tumor cells (MHC expression, etc.) so that they were more readily eliminated. Evidence for the homing of TIL to tumor sites obtained in the initial TIL marking experiments provided further support for the use of TIL as a drug delivery system. Transfer of the tumor necrosis factor (TNF) gene provides one such example. Studies using TNF in animal models have shown significant antitumor effects. Unfortunately, the dosages required in animal experiments could not be achieved in humans with acceptable toxicity. If TNF could be delivered locally at tumor sites then effective concentrations of TNF may be present within the tumor environment without causing systemic toxicities. A protocol using TNF-transduced TIL cells as a delivery system was approved as the second gene therapy experiment (Rosenberg et al 1991) and a phase I dose escalation study has begun at the National Cancer Institute (NCI).

A third protocol approved in 1992 (Greenberg et al 1992) also uses gene transfer into lymphocytes. In this protocol, cloned autologous cytotoxic T-cells are transduced with a vector containing the herpes thymidine kinase (hTK) gene fused to the bacterial hygromycin resistance gene (HyTK). Human immunodeficiency virus (HIV)-positive patients with lymphoma are given bone marrow transplants from HLA-identical siblings while treatment with AZT (zidovudine) continues. The patient will also be given the cytotoxic T-cells in the hopes of eliminating any residual HIV. The goal of the study is to not only cure the patient of their lymphoma but to also to eliminate the HIV. The investigators were concerned that the cytotoxic T-cells may have serious side-effects. The T-cells could attack cells in the central nervous system, bone marrow, or lung and the resulting inflammatory response could have serious consequences. To control these undesired effects the patient could be given ganciclovir which is activated by the transferred TK gene allowing elimination of the transplanted cytotoxic T-cells. Besides this safety factor, the HyTK gene could be used for trafficking and other marking purposes. Although this study is not gene therapy, it is using RMGT for purposes other than just marking; the technique is used to make a cellular-based therapy controllable if unfortunate side-effects are found.

Other gene therapy protocols using lymphocytes are being developed. Applications in lymphocyte genetic disorders or cancer could be broadened to include other disorders such as AIDS, or even to provide insulin for a diabetic. The creativity and ingenuity of the investigator will determine the future uses of gene therapy/transfer with lymphocytes.

Other hematopoietic cells

In genetic disorders in which marrow transplantation had been demonstrated to be useful, scientists assumed gene therapy with autologous marrow would be equally effective. Unfortunately the encouraging results obtained with murine marrow cells have not yet been easily duplicated with larger animal models.

Marking studies with hematopoietic cells

Autologous bone marrow transplantation has gained wide use in the treatment of malignant disease, but the results are limited by a high relapse rate. Since many cancers infiltrate the marrow, a rescuing marrow harvested in remission could still be contaminated with residual malignant cells which may be capable of reintroducing disease to the patient. While there have been many clinical trials which have tried to purge harvested marrow of cancer cells, none have been shown to be effective. Moreover, the purging technique often compromises the hematological recovery of the patient, so that the risk of bleeding or infection is increased. Marking techniques with RMGT could provide a means for determining if purging were necessary or effective, and a number of these studies are underway. The first protocol began in 1991 at St Jude Children's Research Hospital (Brenner et al 1991) and has demonstrated the feasibility of marking hematopoietic progenitor cells. In addition, two gene marked relapses have been seen (Brenner et al 1993).

If further marked relapses are seen, the marking of rescue marrow will be extended to provide information directly comparing one form of purging with another, using the same patient to compare two methods directly. A portion of the marrow would be marked with vector A and purged by Method 1, another portion of the marrow would be marked with vector B and purged by Method 2. The marrows are then returned to the patient and PCR technology used to follow marrow recovery. The relative number of vector A versus vector B marked normal marrow cells would determine the effects of the purging technologies on short- and long-term marrow repopulating cells. If the patient subsequently relapses, the cancer cells could be analyzed for the presence of either vector. In this way, a direct comparison of the two purging techniques could be done without interpatient variability confounding analysis. This approach should be superior to conventional controlled clinical trials comparing one purging technique to another, since a small difference in relapse rates between purging techniques from rescue marrow contamination would be obscured if a majority of relapses occur at least partially from residual cancer cells not eliminated by conditioning from the patient's body. This power of RMGT for marking marrow can thus be used to resolve important clinical issues that could not be expeditiously addressed in any other way.

RMGT marking will also be used to answer other important questions in marrow transplantation. In patients receiving marrow and peripheral blood stem cell transplantation it would be possible to follow, within the same patient, the relative contribution of each source of hematopoietic cells in reconstituting the patient at various time points after transplantation. Many other variations on this theme could also be addressed. Different portions of marrow could be treated ex vivo with various factors or culture conditions and this effect on the time course of marrow reconstitution could be directly compared with other ex vivo treatments. Results from these and related studies would enable the hematologist/transplanter to rapidly take advantage of the rapid development of technology applicable to marrow transplantation.

Gene therapy with hematopoietic cells

The first approved use of marrow stem cells has been to correct the genetic defect, ADA deficiency. Instead of inserting a functioning ADA gene into T-cells as described earlier, this protocol will endeavor to insert the ADA vector into peripheral blood stem cells (Blaese et al 1992), harvested by leucophoresis. After the cells have been returned to the patient, they will be analyzed to see if stem cells were transduced. If so, the patient will now be able to reconstitute his immune system with gene corrected cells. Since the gene transfer would correct cells before T-cell receptor rearrangement, the patient could have his entire repertoire recreated and would not have any 'immunological holes'. This would indeed represent gene therapy as originally envisioned for ADA deficiency — an autologous marrow transplant which mimics the benefits of an allograft, without the potential adverse effects.

Other centers in Italy, The Netherlands, USA and UK have begun similar protocols using bone marrow stem cells transduced with ADA vectors.

If these early studies are successful, gene transfer into marrow or peripheral blood stem cells will be explored for other genetic disorders, since most of the disorders which are successfully treated by allogeneic bone marrow transplantation should respond to gene therapy. Marrow cell function could also be altered for therapeutic purposes, much as lymphocytes can be. The marrow cells could be made resistant to viral infections such as HIV, or to release proteins which the patient is lacking. They could even be altered to release compounds which may be helpful in treating malignancies. Probably the most generically useful alteration — in treatment of malignant disease — would be one in which the marrow cells are made more resistant to standard oncologic therapy by transfer of multidrug resistance (MDR) genes. Since many dose escalation protocols are limited by marrow toxicity, a less sensitive marrow would permit higher doses of chemotherapy than might otherwise be tolerable. Hopefully this dose escalation would eliminate patient tumor cells that were resistant to standard dose therapy. The benefit to the patient would therefore be less morbidity/mortality related to the therapy and perhaps increased efficacy in eliminating the tumor cells related to dose escalation.

Although current proposals are limited by low efficiencies of transfer, transduction with genes (such as the MDR gene) that make the transduced marrow selectable in vivo would permit vectors containing a therapeutic gene along with the selectable gene to be placed into marrow cells, which would be enriched by use of the selectable marker gene (Sorrentino et al 1992). Thus even low transduction efficiencies would be useful in treating many disorders, including hemoglobinopathies. It might even be possible to perform marrow transplantation without first ablating the patient's own marrow, allowing the selective benefit conveyed by the new gene to replace the more dangerous consequences of conditioning with marrow ablative therapy.

CLINICAL PROTOCOLS FOR OTHER HEMATOLOGICAL DISEASES

Hemophilia B

A gene therapy protocol for hemophilia B began in Shanghai, China, at the end of 1991. This protocol is designed to treat hemophilia B patients by using RMGT of the factor IX gene into autologous fibroblast cells. In animal models it has been difficult to obtain prolonged release of proteins from autologous fibroblasts in vivo (Palmer et al 1991). Whether this difficulty can be overcome in humans will be explored by this protocol. A total of four to six patients are expected to be enrolled before the protocol is completed and evaluated.

Other gene therapy protocols

Although few of the remaining protocols described in this chapter have any direct relevance to hematologic disease, they are included because they illustrate basic principles of gene therapy which may be readily adaptable to hematology in the near future.

Gene therapy with hepatocytes

The liver is an attractive target for gene therapy because of its important metabolic role (Grossman et al 1991). Certain gene functions may require they be expressed in the liver where proper enzymatic pathways, cofactors, and anatomical considerations need to be considered.

Gene therapy of patients with the homozygous form of familial hypercholesterolemia has now begun (Wilson et al 1991). This disease has an excellent animal model, the Watanabe rabbit, which enabled preclinical work to demonstrate the possible benefit of RMGT in treating this disorder (Chowdhury et al 1991). In the animal model the cholesterol level of the rabbits could be lowered significantly by transplantation of autologous hepatocytes transduced with a vector containing the low-density lipoprotein receptor gene. The clinical protocol, approved for use in three patients, will use the same procedures in humans. Important questions about the amount of cholesterol-lowering effect, duration of effect, life span of transduced hepatocytes and level of expression in vivo will all be addressed in this protocol.

Gene therapy with tumor cells

Cytokines used systemically may have unacceptable toxicities which could be alleviated if a high concentration were produced locally at the site of the tumor (Asher et at 1991). Cytokine genes transferred into tumor cells may have several effects which could be therapeutic and many studies have now shown that such gene transfer augments the host immune response to the tumor cells. The cytokines being released locally at the tumor site may recruit more immune cells and thus stimulate a stronger immune response which may result in a systemic increase in antitumor immunity. They may also increase MHC antigen expression by the tumor cells and thus make them more antigenic. Finally, the cytokines may have a direct effect on the tumor. This effect would not be systemic, but could result in local destruction of tumor cells followed by systemic immune enhancement. Rosenberg et al at the NCI had two similar protocols that passed the review process at the end of 1991 (Rosenberg et al 1992 a, b). One protocol proposed transferring the TNF gene into patient tumor cells ex vivo, expanding and selecting the transduced cells in vitro, and then giving back the live tumor cells to the patient. The cells would be injected subcutaneously and intradermally in the thigh of the patient. The tumors would not be expected to grow but to survive transiently and release TNF locally. In this protocol the draining lymph node is surgically excised, the lymphocytes therein expanded with IL-2, and returned to the patient as a variation of TIL therapy. This study is in progress in patients with malignant melanoma, colon cancer, and renal cell carcinoma. Preliminary results show local TNF production and the development of strong delayed-type hypersensitivity reaction around the tumor injection site. A second protocol at the NCI uses the same rationale and tumor targets, but transfers instead the gene for IL-2 into the patient tumor lines ex vivo. A similar protocol from St Jude Children's Research Hospital has begun in neuroblastoma (Brenner et al 1992).

Another protocol was approved in early 1992 (Nabel et al 1992). This study proposes to treat cancer cells by transferring the HLA B7 gene into the tumor cells and is novel in several respects. It is based on animal models which show that the exogenous MHC antigen stimulates an immune response to the tumor cell. A second novel feature is that the B7 gene will be transferred with liposomes packaging an expression plasmid for the B7 antigen. This represents the first use of a non-RMGT in an approved gene transfer protocol. Finally, this is the first protocol in which gene transfer into the tumor cells will be performed in vivo. This protocol was approved in 1992.

Another protocol to suggest gene transfer in vivo has recently opened (Oldfield et al 1993). This study uses the in vivo administration of retroviral vector producer cells to transfer the hTK gene into brain tumors. Animal model data imply that direct injection of vector producer cells into tumor mass can result in the transfer of the vector into 50–80% of the tumor cells. In the brain few surrounding cells are transduced, probably because they are not in cell cycle, an event which is important for vector integration. Like the previous hTK protocol, only a fraction of the cells in the tumor mass need to contain the hTK gene to result in the killing of all the tumor cells by administration of ganciclovir. Again the mechanisms which underlie this effect in animals is unknown. Given the dismal outcome of brain tumor patients who have failed conventional therapies, it will be interesting to see if this protocol will show insignificant toxicity with a therapeutic benefit.

The final type of cancer therapy gene transfer protocol considered by the Recombinant DNA Advisory Committee (RAC) and FDA in 1992 uses RMGT of the hTK gene into a ovarian cancer cell line (Freeman et al 1991). Irradiated allogeneic cells will be injected in a phase I study of patients with ovarian cancer. Preclinical studies suggest that the introduction of a relatively small percentage of cells containing the hTK gene can confer sensitivity of cancer cells to the antiviral drug ganciclovir. The exact mechanism of this bystander effect is not clear but it may involve the immune response to the ganciclovir-destroyed cells as well as the uptake of toxic metabolites and/or hTK itself by the surrounding tumor cells. The bystander effect does not appear to have any effect on normal tissues but can result in a substantial killing of tumor cells.

Gene therapy with muscle cells

Another target organ that has been explored for gene therapy includes muscle cells. Multiple gene transfer techniques have been investigated. Cardiac, striated, and vascular smooth muscle cells have all been explored as potential target cells for gene therapy (Salminen et al 1991, Acsadi et al 1991, Barr & Leiden 1991, Dhawan et al 1991, Miller 1992). The cells may be used as targets for gene therapy of inherited disorders of muscle cells (such as muscular dystrophy) or may be used to produce therapeutic proteins (eg. clotting factors) The fusogenic properties of myoblasts and satellite cells make striated muscles an interesting vehicle as a myofiber could begin to make the transferred gene product after a transduced satellite cell fuses with the myofiber.

Gene therapy for cystic fibrosis

Many groups are exploring the use of gene therapy for cystic fibrosis since the CFTR protein has been demonstrated to be responsible for most forms of cystic fibrosis. Adenoviral vectors have been used to transfer the CFTR gene into the cells lining the airways of cotton rats as well as into airway cells brushed from human patients (Rosenfeld et al 1992). Several gene therapy protocols have been submitted and approved, predominantly using adenoviral vectors.

KEY POINTS FOR CLINICAL PRACTICE

- The number of clinical gene marking and gene therapy protocols has increased exponentially since 1989.
- Most clinical protocols to date use retroviral vectors. These are not ideal, and vector systems which are organ specific and can be used in vivo are being developed.
- Lymphocytes and marrow progenitor cells have been the primary target for many of the earliest gene transfer protocols.
- Marker gene expression has been successfully used to trace the source of relapse after autologous bone marrow transplantation and may allow assessment of purging efficacy in a number of malignant diseases.
- Although gene therapy was originally proposed to treat single gene disorders, its most popular current application is in cancer therapy, where it is used to modulate normal or malignant cell function.

REFERENCES

Acsadi G, Dickson G, Love D R et al 1991 Human dystrophin expression in *mdx* mice after intramuscular injection of DNA constructs. Nature 352: 815–818
Aebersold P, Kasid A, Rosenberg S A 1990 Selection of gene-marked tumor infiltrating lymphocytes from post-treatment biopsies: a case study. Hum Gene Ther 1: 373–843
Anderson W F 1984 Prospects for human gene therapy. Science 226: 401–409

Asher A L, Mule J J, Kasid A et al 1991 Murine tumor cells transduced with the gene for tumor necrosis factor-alpha. Evidence for paracrine immune effects of tumor necrosis factor against tumors. J Immunol 146: 3227–3234

Barr E, Leiden J M 1991 Systemic delivery of recombinant proteins by genetically modified myoblasts. Sicence 254: 1507–1509

Blaese R M, Anderson W F 1990 The ADA human gene therapy protocol. Hum Gene Ther 1: 327–329

Blaese, R M et al 1992 RAC Meeting, February 10–11, 1992

Boggs S S 1990 Targeted gene modifiction for gene therapy of stem cells. Int J Cell Cloning 8: 80–96

Brenner M K, Mirro J, Hurwitz C et al 1991 BMT/AML human gene transfer protocol. Hum Gene Ther 2: 137–160

Brenner M K, et al 1992 Immunization with IL-2 transduced neuroblastoma cells. Hum Gene Ther 3: 665–676

Brenner M K, et al 1993 Gene marking to trace origin of relapse after autologous bone marrow transplantation. Lancet 341: 85–86

Chen C A, Okayama H 1988 Calcium phosphate-mediated gene transfer: a highly efficient transfection system for stably transforming cells with plasmid DNA. Biotechniques 6: 632–638

Chowdhury J R, Grossman M, Gupta S et al 1991 Long-term improvement of hypercholesterolemia after ex vivo gene therapy in LDLR-deficient rabbits. Science 254: 1802–1805

Cornetta K, Moen R C, Culver K et al 1990 Amphotropic murine leukemia virus is not an acute pathogen for primates. Hum Gene Ther 1: 15–30

Cornetta K, Morgan R A, Anderson W F 1991a Safety issues related to retroviral-mediated gene transfer in humans. Hum Gene Ther 2: 5–14

Cornetta K, Morgan R A, Gillio A et al 1991b No retroviremia or pathology in long-term follow-up of monkeys exposed to a murine amphotropic retrovirus. Hum Gene Ther 2: 215–220

Culver K, Cornetta K, Morgan R et al 1991a Lymphocytes as cellular vehicles for gene therapy in mouse and man. Proc Natl Acad Sci USA 88: 3155–3159

Culver K W, Osborne W R, Miller A D et al 1991b Correction of ADA deficiency in human T lymphocytes using retroviral-mediated gene transfer. Transplant Proc 23: 170–171

Curiel D T, Wayne E, Cotten M, Birstiel M L, Agarwal S, Li C-M, Loechel S, Hu P-C 1992 High-efficiency gene transfer mediated by adenovirus coupled to DNA–polysine complexes. Hum Gene Ther 3: 147–154

Dhawan J, Pan L C, Pavlath G K et al 1991 Systemic delivery of human growth hormone by injection of genetically engineered myoblasts. Science 254: 1509–1512

Dixit M, Webb M S, Smart W C et al 1991 Construction and expression of a recombinant adeno-associated virus that harbors a human beta-globin-encoding cDNA. Gene 104: 253–257

Economou J et al 1992 The treatment of patients with metastatic expanded and genetically-engineered bulk TIL and/or PBL. Hum Gene Ther 3: 411–430

Fink D J, Sternberg L R, Weber P C et al 1992 In vivo expression β-galactosidase in hippocampal neurons by HSV-mediated gene transfer. Hum Gene Ther 3: 11–20

Freeman S et al 1991 RAC meeting, October 7–8, 1991

Gordon J W 1990 Micromanipulation of embryos and germ cells; an approach to gene therapy? Am J Med Genet 35: 206–214

Greenberg et al 1992 Genetically modified CD8 + HIV-specific T cells for HIV seropositive patients undergoing allogeneic bone marrow transplant. Hum Gene Ther 3: 319–338

Grossman M, Raper S E, Wilson J M 1991 Towards liver-directed gene therapy: retrovirus-mediated gene transfer into human hepatocytes. Somat Cell Mol Genet 17: 601–607

Hug P, Sleight R G 1991 Liposomes for the transformation of eukaryotic cells. Biochim Biophys Acta 1097: 1–17

Kantoff P, Gillio A, McLachlin J R et al 1987 Expression of human adenosine deaminase in nonhuman primates after retroviral mediated gene transfer. J Exp Med 166: 219–234

Kasid A, Morecki S, Aebersold P et al 1990 Human gene transfer: characterization of human tumor-infiltrating lymphocytes as vehicles for retroviral-mediated gene transfer in man. Proc Natl Acad Sci USA 87: 473–477

Kubiniec R T, Liang H, Hui S W 1990 Effects of pulse length and pulse strength on transfection by electroporation. Biotechniques 8: 16–20

Lebkowski J S, McNally M M, Okarma T B et al 1988 Adeno-associated virus: a vector system for efficient introduction and integration of DNA into a variety of mammalian cell types. Mol Cell Biol 8: 3988–3996

Ledley F D, Woo S L C, Ferry G et al 1991 Hepatocellular transplantation in acute hepatic failure and targeting genetic markers to hepatic cells. um Gene Ther 2: 331–359

Lotze et al 1992 The treatment of patients with melanoma using Interleukin-2, Interleukin-4 and tumor-infiltrating lymphocytes. Hum Gene Ther 3: 167–178

McLachlin J R, Cornetta K, Eglitis M A et al 1990 Retroviral-mediated gene transfer. Prog Nucleic Acid Res Mol Biol 38: 91–135

McNally M A, Lebkowski J S, Okarma TB et al 1988 Optimizing electroporation parameters for a variety of human hematopoietic cell lines. Biotechniques 6: 882–886

Miller A D 1990 Retroviral packaging cells. Hum Gene Ther 1: 5–14

Miller A D 1992 Human gene therapy comes of age. Nature 357: 455–460

Miller D G, Adam M A, Miller A D 1990 Gene transfer by retrovirus vectors occurs only in cells that are actively replicating at the time of infection. Mol Cell Biol 10: 4239–4242 (erratum appears in Mol Cell Biol 1992; 12(1): 433)

Moen R C, Horowitz S D, Sondel P M et al 1987 Immunologic reconstitution after haploidentical bone marrow transplantation for immune deficiency disorders: treatment of bone marrow cells with monoclonal antibody CT-2 and complement. Blood 70: 664–669

Nabel G et al 1992 Immunotherapy of malignancy by in vivo gene transfer into tumors. Hum Gene Ther 3: 399–410

Oldfield E H, Ram Z, Culver K W, Blaese R M, DeVroom H L 1993 Gene therapy for the treatment of brain tumors using intra-tumoral transduction with the thymidine kinase gene and intravenous ganciclovir. Hum Gene Ther 4: 36–69

Palmer T D, Rosman G J, Osborne W R et al 1991 Genetically modified skin fibroblasts persist long after transplantation but gradually inactivate introduced genes. Proc Natl Acad Sci USA 88: 1330–1334

Perucho M, Hanahan D, Wigler M 1980 Genetic and physical linkage of exogenous sequences in transformed cells. Cell 22: 309–317

Rosenberg S A, Blaese R M, Anderson W F 1990a The N2-TIL human gene transfer clinical protocol. Hum Gene Ther 1: 73–92

Rosenberg S A, Aebersold P, Cornetta K et al 1990b Gene transfer into humans — immunotherapy of patients with advanced melanoma using tumor-infiltrating lymphocytes modified by retroviral gene transduction. N Engl J Med 323: 570–578

Rosenberg S A, Kasid A, Anderson W F et al 1991 The TNF/TIL human gene therapy clinical protocol. Hum Gene Ther 1: 441–442

Rosenberg S A, Anderson W F, Asher A L et al 1992a Immunization of cancer patients using autologous cancer cells modified by the insertion of the gene for tumor necrosis factor. Hum Gene Ther 3: 57–74

Rosenberg S A, Anderson W F, Blaese R M et al 1992b Immunization of cancer patients using autologous cancer cells modified by the insertion of the gene for interleukin-2. Hum Gene Ther 3: 75–90

Rosenfeld M A, Yoshimura K, Trapnell B C et al 1992 In vivo transfer of the human cystic fibrosis transmembrane conductance regulator gene to the airway epithelium. Cell 68: 143–155

Salminen A, Alson H F, Mickley L A et al 1991 Implantation of recombinant rat myocytes into adult skeletal muscle: a potential gene therapy. Hum Gene Ther 2: 15–26

Sorrentino B P, Brandt S S, Bodine B, Gottesman M et al 1992 Selection of drug-resistant bone marrow cells in vivo after retroviral transfer of human MDRI. Science 257: 99–103

Springett G M, Moen R C, Anderson S et al 1989 Infection efficiency of T lymphocytes with amphotropic retroviral vectors is cell cycle dependent. J Virol 63: 3865–3869

Srivastava C H, Samulski R J, Lu L et al 1989 Construction of a recombinant human parvovirus B19: adeno-associated virus 2 (AAV) DNA inverted terminal repeats are functional in an AAV-B19 hybrid virus. Proc Natl Acad Sci USA 86: 8078–8082

Temin H M 1990 Safety considerations in somatic gene therapy of human disease with retroviral vectors. Hum Gene Ther 1: 111–123

Wilson et al 1991 Ex vivo gene therapy of familial hypercholesterolemia. Hum Gene Ther 3: 179–222

Wu G Y, Wu C H 1991 Delivery systems for gene therapy. Biotherapy 3: 87–95

Wu G Y, Wilson J M, Shalaby F et al 1991 Receptor-mediated gene delivery in vivo. Partial correction of genetic analbuminemia in Nagase rats. J Biol Chem 266: 14338–14342

2

Detection of minimal residual disease in leukemia and lymphoma

D. Campana

Treatment of leukemia and lymphoma is often influenced by the results of peripheral blood (PB), bone marrow (BM) or cerebrospinal fluid (CSF) examination. If neoplastic cells are discovered, more aggressive therapy or the administration of different combinations of anticancer agents may be required.

In acute leukemia, most institutions agree that complete remission is accomplished when BM samples contain <5% morphologically identifiable leukemic blasts. The limitation of this definition is evident: 1–5% of blasts in the BM may correspond to a total of 10^{10}–10^{11} neoplastic cells (Van Bekkum 1984, Ryan & Van Dongen 1988). Although the sensitivity of morphologic studies may be slightly improved by labeling cells with cytochemical stains or by examining smears of a cell fraction enriched with mononucleated cells, a neoplastic infiltration of <1% cannot usually be detected with certainty by morphological examination (Van Dongen et al 1984, Janossy et al 1988).

Because of the clinical importance of an accurate definition of remission in patients with leukemia and lymphoma, considerable ingenuity and resources have been invested in devising techniques able to recognize neoplastic blasts amongst normal cells. In this chapter we will review these techniques and their clinical application.

CLINICAL RELEVANCE OF APPLYING SENSITIVE TECHNIQUES TO DETECT RESIDUAL DISEASE

The application of sensitive methods to estimate the results of treatment on tumor burden is likely to provide important information that could ultimately lead to the improvement of antineoplastic therapy. For example, the degree of tumor cell elimination obtained with different cytotoxic regimens could be evaluated and relapse anticipated. Although the benefits of intensive chemotherapy when the tumor load is relatively low are not well defined, in theory, intensive therapy delivered at such a time could increase the likelihood of eradicating the disease (Goldie et al 1982). Also, patients with persistent low numbers of neoplastic cells are prime candidates to test the value of biological response modifiers and immunotoxins in cancer treatment. Conversely, the initiation of unnecessarily aggressive treatment could be prevented by clarifying the nature of morphologically suspicious cells seen in BM samples after remission induction chemotherapy or cessation of continuation therapy: these cells may represent normal lymphohemopoietic progenitors. Moreover, the presence of residual leukemic cells in the BM harvested for autologous BM transplantation can be evaluated and the efficacy of purging methods assessed (Janossy et al 1988, Negrin et al 1991). Finally, leukemic involvement of the central nervous system can be revealed by unequivocally demonstrating even single leukemic cells in the CSF (Bradstock et al 1980, 1981a, Peiper et al 1980, Hooijkaas et al 1989, Kranz et al 1989).

Methods for detecting residual disease proposed as potential clinical assays require not only sensitivity but also speed and reproducibility. The general limitations of these tests are imposed by the number of cells that can be analyzed and by potentially patchy dissemination of the disease. For example $<5 \times 10^7$ mononuclear cells are available for study from a PB or BM sample taken from a typical patient with acute leukemia in 'remission'; the actual number of cells studied is usually $<5 \times 10^6$. The heterogeneous distribution of leukemia and lymphoma cells is well known to hematologists, and numerous clinical observations supporting this concept have been reported (Mathe et al 1966, Hann et al 1977). This uneven leukemia involvement of marrow has also been documented in animal experiments (Martens et al 1987). Consequently, *minimal* residual disease is not uniformly detectable even with exceptionally sensitive techniques (Table 2.1).

Table 2.1 Comparative sensitivity of methods for detecting residual disease

Technique	Sensitivity*
Morphology	1–5%
Chromosome analysis	
Traditional cytogenetics	?
DNA content	10^{-3}
PCR	10^{-6}
Gene rearrangement studies	
Southern blotting	1–5%
PCR	10^{-6}
Immunophenotyping	10^{-4}
PCR	10^{-6}

* Maximum sensitivity as determined by dilution experiments is listed. In the application of each technique, sensitivity may be lower (see Table 2.2).

A REVIEW OF THE AVAILABLE METHODS

Chromosome analysis

Karyotyping has been used to monitor residual disease, searching for chromosomal abnormalities determined at diagnosis (Arthur et al 1988, Holt et al 1989). The limitations of these studies are related to the number of metaphases examined and to the proliferating activity of malignant cells, which may vary in different cases. These limitations can be overcome by in situ hybridization using chromosome specific probes, which allows the identification of residual cells with karyotypic numerical abnormalities even when these are in interphase (Anastasi et al 1991, Weber-Matthiesen et al 1992). This approach, however, has not yet been systematically applied to residual disease detection.

The sensitivity of conventional cytogenetics techniques in detecting cells with chromosomal abnormalities may be increased by flow cytometry, as follows. Firstly, cells can be labelled with DNA-binding fluorochromes, such as propidium iodide and 7-actinomycin D, to detect aneuploid cells (Krishan 1975, Rabinovitch et al 1986). These techniques can be used in combination with cell marker analysis in double and triple color combinations (Schmid et al 1991): for example, the DNA content of BM CD10$^+$ cells can be selectively examined in patients with aneuploid B lineage acute lymphoblastic leukemia (ALL) (Tsurusawa et al 1989). Secondly, samples can be stained with combinations of dyes which selectively bind to different nucleotide bases, e.g. chromomycin A3 and Hoechst 33258 (Young 1990). In this way, chromosomes can be identified. The former method has the advantage of being simple and requires single-laser flow cytometers. However, only numerical chromosomal abnormalities can be detected. The latter method is technically more complex and requires dual-laser flow cytometry. Although structural chromosomal abnormalities are detectable, reciprocal translocations with no change in DNA content will not be identified.

Gene rearrangement studies

In ALL and in B- and T-cell non-Hodgkin's lymphoma (NHL), either immunoglobulin (Ig) or T-cell receptor (TCR) genes are clonally rearranged in virtually all cases. Because rearrangement is unique for an individual cell and its progeny, analysis of Ig and TCR gene configuration can be used to monitor the presence of residual cells showing clonal rearrangements determined at diagnosis. In B lineage ALL >95%, 54%, 55%, and 33% of cases have rearranged IgH, TCRδ, TCRγ and TCRβ genes, respectively. The same genes are rearranged in 14%, 68%, 91% and 89% of T-ALL cases, respectively (reviewed by Van Dongen & Wolvers-Tettero 1991). Thus, both lineage-associated and inappropriate rearrangements can be used as a target to identify residual disease in ALL (Katz et al 1989). The sensitivity of conventional DNA analysis techniques (e.g. Southern blotting), is, however, limited. After digesting DNA with restriction enzymes, separating DNA fragments with agarose gel electrophoresis, blotting and hybridizing with appropriate probes, no less than 1–5% of cells with clonally rearranged Ig or TCR genes are detectable (Yamada et al 1989). It has been reported that such low sensitivity can be augmented by focusing the DNA analysis on selected subsets of cells, e.g. mononuclear cells isolated with density gradients (Zehnbauer et al 1986), or immunologically defined cells purified by cell sorting with immunomagnetic particles (Bregni et al 1989). While mononuclear cells are used in many laboratories, use of cells purified with immunological techniques has not yet been widely tested.

Polymerase chain reaction

The establishment of methods for enzymatic gene amplification using polymerase chain reaction (PCR) (Saiki et al 1988) has revolutionized many areas of molecular biology, including gene rearrangement analysis for residual disease detection. The sensitivity of PCR is extremely high and 10^{-4}–10^{-6} target cells can be detected. The reaction consists of amplifying selected stretches of DNA using oligonucleotides ('primers') matching DNA regions flanking the target sequence, a mixture of nucleotides and a thermostable DNA polymerase (Taq polymerase). Repeated cycles of DNA denaturation, primer annealing and DNA synthesis are performed. In cases of abnormal gene configurations (e.g. those brought about by chromosomal trans-locations), the simple visualization of the amplified signal may be sufficient to indicate residual disease. However, in the case of t(14;18) caution is necessary since positive signals after PCR have been detected in tissues obtained from individuals free of lymphoma, and it has been speculated that this translocation may be a necessary but not sufficient abnormality for the development of lymphoma (Limpens et al 1990, Price et al 1991, reviewed by Sklar 1991). In the cases where the target sequence is also found in normal cells (e.g. Ig and TCR genes), the leukemia-associated rearrangement must be distinguished from the rest of the amplified DNA by use of specific probes.

A number of chromosomal abnormalities are suitable for use as a target for PCR. In chronic myelocytic leukemia (CML), leukemic cells have a reciprocal translocation between chromosomes 9q34 and 22q11, bearing the c-abl and BCR genes, respectively. Because the breakpoints on chromosome 9 may be scattered along a 150 kb 5' to the second exon of the c-abl, PCR cannot be directly applied to amplify such highly variable DNA sequences. However, the transcribed bcr–abl messenger RNA is consistent, and therefore can be used as a template to synthesize complementary DNA with reverse transcriptase, which can then be amplified using suitable BCR and abl matching primers (Lee et al 1988, 1989, Morgan et al 1989, Hughes et al 1991, Thompson et al 1992, reviewed by Fey et al 1991).

In ALL, identical strategy can be used to study cases with the (9;22) translocation. In addition, the other major translocation in pediatric ALL, the t(1;19)(q23;p13) can also be studied in a similar way, using appropriate primers (Hunger et al 1991, Privitera et al 1992). The possibility of amplifying the breakpoints of the t(9;22) and t(1;19) is of particular interest because patients with such translocations have unfavourable prognosis (Crist et al 1990, Rivera et al 1991). PCR techniques to amplify the *tal*-1 gene, which is altered in approximately 25% of T-ALL cases, have also been described (Jonsson et al 1991).

In most follicular NHLs and in approximately one-quarter of diffuse NHL, the malignant cells bear the t(14;18)(q23;q21) in which the *bcl*-2 gene on chromosome 18 is juxtaposed to the IgH locus on chromosome 14 (Weiss et al 1987). This translocation can be revealed by PCR using a limited set of primers matching any J region of the Ig locus, and the two breakpoint regions on chromosome 18 (reviewed by Sklar 1991 and Fey et al 1991).

It is possible to amplify rearranged Ig and TCR genes with PCR to detect small numbers of residual leukemia and lymphoma cells. IgH (Yamada et al 1990, Deane & Norton 1990), TCRγ (D'Auriol et al 1989) and TCRδ (Hansen-Hagge et al 1989, Campana et al 1990b, Yokota et al 1991, Neale et al 1991) genes have been used as targets for this purpose. In these cases the DNA collected at diagnosis is necessary to construct a leukemia-specific probe suitable to distinguish amplified material derived from leukemic cells from the DNA derived from normal B- or T-lymphocytes.

The most common pitfalls of PCR are related to the possibility of false positive results due to contamination during reagent preparation. Thus, extremely accurate laboratory procedures are mandatory. One limitation of the technology is the difficulty of quantitating the source of a positive signal, i.e. establishing the percentage of target cells present in the cell population assayed. In addition, DNA sequences derived from damaged or dead cells may be sufficient to cause positive signals (Campana et al 1990b, Sklar 1991). Finally, the loci studied may be deleted and/or further rearrangements become predominant during the course of disease (Van Dongen & Wolvers-Tettero 1991, Kiyoi et al 1992).

Immunologic methods

Recognition of leukemia-associated phenotypes with antibodies is a valuable option for monitoring residual disease in a proportion of patients with acute leukemia and T-cell lymphoma. Immunologic methods were amongst the first to be applied to study minimal residual disease: work in this area started soon after the establishment of immunophenotyping for diagnostic purposes (Bradstock et al 1981a,b). Several studies have demonstrated the reliability of this approach. Skepticism about the usefulness of this technology usually originates from insufficient comprehension of fluorescence microscopy and flow cytometry and/or from discouraging experiences with low-quality reagents and equipment. Immunologic methods enable the detection of one leukemic cell amongst $>10^{-4}$ normal hematopoietic cells: this level of sensitivity can only be reached with the best-quality materials and well-standardized methods (Van Dongen et al 1984, Campana et al 1990a).

It is not possible to distinguish neoplastic from normal lympho-hematopoietic cells with a single marker because the same antigens that are found on malignant cells are also present on their normal counterparts (reviewed by Greaves 1986 and Campana et al 1991). An important exception is represented by the protein products of gene fusions such as bcr–abl (Van Denderen et al 1989) or E2A-PBX1 (Kamps et al 1991). Monoclonal antibodies suitable to recognize cells synthesizing these proteins should become available in the near future. The current strategy to detect residual disease with immunologic methods takes advantage of the observation that leukocyte markers may be found on malignant cells in combinations that are normally not seen in PB and BM (Bradstock et al 1981b, 1989, Van Dongen et al 1984, Campana et al 1990a, Terstappen & Loken 1990).

These phenotypes can be identified by double or triple color staining techniques that can be performed using antibodies conjugated to different fluorochromes; cell labeling can be analyzed either with a fluorescence microscope or a flow cytometer (reviewed by Campana et al 1991). Experiments with artificial mixtures of leukemic blasts and normal BM cells have proved that the identification of 10^{-4}–10^{-5} residual leukemic cells is achievable (reviewed by Campana et al 1991).

A potential weakness of the use of immunologic methods to detect residual disease is the possible occurrence of phenotypic switches during treatment (Greaves et al 1980, Stass et al 1984, Bernard et al 1982). However, changes in the expression of the relevant markers are uncommon and failure to detect relapse is not usually attributable to phenotypic changes (Campana et al 1990a).

Tumor-associated phenotypes

Some phenotypic combinations are found in normal tissues but not in BM, PB and/or CSF. For example, the majority of T-ALL cases express nuclear TdT in association with T-cell markers such as CD3, CD5 or CD1 (reviewed by Campana et al 1991). Such phenotypes are also expressed by normal cortical thymocytes, but are not found outside the thymus. Hence, a single CD3/TdT, CD5/TdT or CD1/TdT double-labeled cell in the PB or BM of patients with T-ALL indicates residual disease (Fig. 2.1; reviewed by Campana et al 1991). Identical combinations of reagents can be used to detect residual malignant cells in some cases of NHL. Moreover, TdT$^+$ or CD34$^+$ cells are not found in the CSF but these markers are expressed on the majority of acute leukemias and TdT is found in some T-cell lymphomas. The search for cells expressing phenotypes normally absent in the type of sample studied is the best option for applying immunologic methods for defining remission and has the highest sensitivity.

Phenotype of B-cell progenitors in **normal BM**:

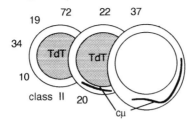

Phenotypic combinations found on **leukemic** lymphoblasts:

B lineage ALL	T-ALL
TdT/cμ (<20% of normal TdT+ cells are cμ+)	TdT/cCD3
TdT/2,13,21,33 and/or w65	
19/2,13,33 and/or w65	

Fig. 2.1 Phenotypic differences between normal and leukemic lymphoblasts. Phenotypic changes which occur during the early stages of normal B-cell differentiation are summarized. In a proportion of ALL cases, leukemic cells express phenotypic features which are rare or absent in normal BM lymphoblasts; these leukemia-associated phenotypes can be used to recognize residual ALL blasts in BM.

In a proportion of B lineage ALL and AML cases, leukemic cells express combinations of normal differentiation antigens which are extremely rare amongst normal hematopoietic cells (reviewed by Campana et al 1991). In B lineage ALL leukemia-associated phenotypes include TdT in combination with cytoplasmic μ, surface Ig, CD13, CD21, CD33, CDw65 and CD2 (Fig. 2.1). In approximately one-third of adult B lineage ALL cases, >80% of blasts have a phenotype absent or extremely rare in normal B-cell precursors (Campana et al 1990a). The relatively high incidence of aberrant immunologic profile is also seen in childhood B lineage ALL (Campana et al 1991).

In acute myeloid leukemia (AML), leukemia-associated features include the expression of 'myeloid-associated' antigens (CD13, CD33, CDw65) with CD2, CD7 and/or nuclear TdT (reviewed by Campana et al 1991). These combinations are found on the majority of blasts in 24% of adult AMLs (Campana et al 1990a) and are also seen in childhood AML (Campana et al 1991). Another interesting combination is CD34/CD4, which is particularly suitable for identifying AMLs with monoblastic differentiation. Recently, we have shown that the combination CD34/CD56, found in approximately 20% of AML, allows the detection of one leukemic myeloblast amongst 10 000 normal BM cells (Coustan-Smith et al 1993).

In T-cell lymphomas in which tumor cells express TdT, strategies identical to those discussed for studying T-ALL can be applied. In B-cell lymphomas that express detectable levels of surface or cytoplasmic Ig, the investigation of light chain expression can be used to detect residual disease. Neoplastic cells would express either kappa or lambda light chains and their presence may alter the normal kappa:lambda ratio of 3:2 (Levy et al 1977). This approach is therefore not useful to detect single lymphoma cells. However, several methods have been proposed to precisely detect alterations in light chain expression (Ault 1979, Wainberg et al 1984). Letwin et al (1990) showed that two-color immunofluorescence analysis by flow cytometry of samples stained with a CD20 monoclonal antibody in combination with either an antikappa or an antilambda reagent allowed the detection of 0.2% monoclonal B-cells admixed with normal lymphocytes. Bagwell et al (1988) and Agrawal et al (1992) suggested that single labelling with anti-light chain reagents followed by Kolmogorov–Smirnov statistics of the resulting histogram could be superior to double color staining to detect abnormal light chain expression.

Detection of leukemia in the CSF

Approximately 5–10% of patients with ALL who achieve remission will have an isolated central nervous system relapse (Rivera et al 1991). The detection of malignant cells in the CSF is frequently the first sign of central nervous disease (Price & Johnson 1973). The discrimination between leukemic lymphoblasts and normal activated lymphocytes by morphology is often difficult. While B- and T-lymphocytes and monocytes are cells normally found in the CSF, cells expressing nuclear TdT (Bradstock et al 1980, Peiper et al 1980, Hooijkaas et al 1989) or membrane CD34 should be absent. Thus, even a single cell with such markers indicates central nervous disease, unless the sample is contaminated by PB, as revealed by the presence of red blood cells. In these cases, TdT^+ or $CD34^+$ cells may represent circulating blasts and the interpretation is problematic.

DETECTION OF RESIDUAL LEUKEMIA AND CLINICAL OUTCOME

The detection of cells expressing leukemia-associated phenotypes in BM samples of patients considered to be in clinical and morphologic remission may forecast the recurrence of leukemia (Bradstock et al 1981b, Campana et al 1990a). In a recent study, residual disease was seen with immunologic methods in approximately 12% of BM samples from patients with leukemia in complete morphologic remission after treatment (Campana et al 1990a). In 19 patients studied, the identification of such cells preceded overt relapse which occurred within 1–6 months after the immunologic analysis (Campana et al 1990a). Another 25 patients were considered to be in morphological *and* immunological remission in repeated testing (Campana et al 1990a); 17 of these patients were in remission after >6 months follow-up whereas eight patients relapsed: two of these relapses were, however, extramedullary (Campana et al 1990a). A high predictive value of immunologic methods was also found by Van Dongen (1990, see also Ryan & Van Dongen 1988).

Detection of residual disease in ALL has been approached with PCR by other investigators. Yokota et al (1991) generated clone-specific probes for

TCRδ sequences in 27 patients with ALL and studied 55 samples obtained during complete clinical remission. Positive signals were seen in all eight patients studied 2–6 months after remission induction, and in six of 11 cases on continuation therapy for 7–19 months from diagnosis. Detection of residual disease was followed by relapse in two T-ALL cases of the latter group. By contrast, 10 of 11 patients, studied 6–41 months after cessation of treatment, were negative with the exception of one patient with residual disease at the 10^{-4}–10^{-5} level after 5.5 years from diagnosis. This patient was still in remission 3 months after the positive PCR analysis at the time of publication. Nizet et al (1991) also obtained positive signals after amplifying Ig heavy chain regions in samples from 16 patients with B lineage ALL. The signal tended to decrease in patients who remained in remission and appeared to persist in patients who eventually relapsed. In a comparative study between immunologic methods and PCR for detection of residual disease in the same samples from patients with ALL, discrepant results were particularly striking in samples obtained after remission induction, where, in some cases, the PCR approach gave strongly positive signals, in contrast to the absence of detectable viable leukemic cells as determined by double color immunofluorescence in the same samples. We speculate that these differences are due to the inability of PCR to distinguish the viability of the DNA source, resulting in amplification of DNA of damaged cells which may be particularly prominent after remission induction chemotherapy. Such damaged cells are easily excluded from the counts when microscopic or cytometric techniques are used (Campana et al 1990b).

Positive PCR in patients with CML in cytogenetic remission has been observed after α-interferon treatment (Lee et al 1989) and after BM transplantation. In the latter situation results are often controversial and difficult to interpret. Morgan et al (1989) found no evidence of PCR signals in patients with CML in long-term remission after BMT transplantation. However, other groups have reported positive data in a similar cohort of patients (Delfau et al 1990, Gabert et al 1989, Bartram et al 1989). The reasons for these discrepancies are difficult to pinpoint but probably include the application of methods with different sensitivity (i.e. one round of PCR versus a 'nested' PCR with two sets of primers) and difficulties in avoiding contamination (Goldman & Hughes 1991).

PCR amplification of the t(14;18) in patients with NHL can detect a positive signal in a tissue sample apparently lacking malignant cells (Lee et al 1987, Crescenzi et al 1988, Negrin et al 1991, Price et al 1991, Lambrechts et al 1992, Gribben et al 1991). In some cases these signals persist after several years of apparent remission. In a study reported by Lambrechts et al (1992), PCR was positive in 15 of 22 samples in remission. On the other hand, in three of 19 patients with clinical evidence of disease, circulating t(14;18) cells were not detectable. Five of 11 patients in remission had circulating t(14;18) cells up to 47 months after discontinuation of treatment. The authors interpret the data as indicating that 300 000 lymphoma cells may circulate for years without evidence of clinical relapse. It should be noted that positive PCR signals have been obtained with similar sets of primers in normal tissues also (Limpens et al 1990). To ensure that the remaining cells after years are the same as those of the original tumor, one may need to sequence the breakpoint regions of the original malignant cells and the follow-up samples, and demonstrate identical sequences, as carried out by Price et al (1991).

The usefulness of immunologic examination of CSF in acute leukemia and NHL using anti-TdT reagents was first demonstrated by Bradstock et al (1980) and Peiper et al (1980). More recently, Hooijkaas et al (1989) have reported the results of a 5-year follow-up study in which the same methods were applied to analyse the CSF of 113 children with TdT$^+$ acute leukemia or T-cell NHL. This study strongly supports the view that immunologic investigations of the CSF are informative.

KEY POINTS FOR CLINICAL PRACTICE

• Several techniques which improve the sensitivity of morphological examination for detecting residual disease in leukemia and lymphoma are available (Table 2.2).

Table 2.2 Sensitive methods for detecting residual leukemia and lymphoma in BM samples

Diagnosis	Method	Percentage of suitable cases	Sensitivity
B lineage ALL	Immunology	50–60	10^{-2}–10^{-4}†
	PCR TCRδ	40–60	10^{-4}–10^{-6}
	PCR IgH	>90	10^{-4}–10^{-6}
	Cytogenetics	5–10	?‡
	PCR on translocations	5–10	10^{-4}–10^{-6}
	Southern blotting for IgH	>90	10^{-2}¶
T-ALL and T-NHL	Immunology	90–95	10^{-4}–10^{-5}
	PCR TCRδ	40–60	10^{-4}–10^{-6}
	PCR tal-1	20–30	10^{-4}–10^{-6}
	Southern blotting for TCRβ	70–90	10^{-2}
B-NHL	Immunology	>90	10^{-2}
	Southern blotting for IgH	>90	10^{-2}
	PCR t(14;18)	70 (follicular)/30 (diffuse)	10^{-4}–10^{-6}
AML	Immunology	50–60	10^{-2}–10^{-4}
	Cytogenetics	70–80★	?

★ 70–80% of AMLs detectable chromosomal translocations.
† Sensitivity changes according to the percentage of cells expressing a given 'leukemia-associated' phenotype in normal BM.
‡ Sensitivity depends on the number of metaphases screened.
¶ Sensitivity may be increased by enriching target cells with immunologic techniques (see Bregni et al 1989).

- It appears that the application of several techniques, each with their specific merits and limitations, will be advantageous because there is no method for residual disease detection that can be universally used.
- The practical question to be answered first is whether positive findings with sensitive methods in patients in morphologic remission predict relapse within individual therapeutic regimes.
- While studies using immunologic methods lacked false-positive results, those using PCR have often yielded positive signals not followed by overt relapse. It remains unclear whether superior sensitivity or technical artefact accounts for these data.
- If detection of residual disease in patients in 'remission' is found to strongly correlate with subsequent relapse, therapeutic strategies could be designed according to the results of these tests. Earlier therapeutic intervention may lead to improved treatment outcome.

ACKNOWLEDGMENTS

This work was supported by a grant from the National Cancer Institute (P30-CA21765) and by American Lebanese Syrian Associated Charities (ALSAC).

REFERENCES

Agrawal Y P, Hamalainen E, Mahlamaki E K et al 1992 Comparison of poly- and monoclonal antibodies for determination of B-cell clonal excess in a routine clinical laboratory. Eur J Haematol 49: 49–55

Anastasi J, Vardiman J W, Rudinsky R et al 1991 Direct correlation of cytogenetic findings with cell morphology using in situ hybridization: an analysis of suspicious cells in bone marrow specimens of two patients completing therapy for acute lymphoblastic leukemia. Blood 77: 2456–2462

Arthur C K, Apperley J F, Guo A P et al 1988 Cytogenetics events after bone marrow transplantation for chronic myeloid leukemia in chronic phase. Blood 71: 1179–1185

Ault K A 1979 Detection of small numbers of monoclonal B lymphocytes in the blood of patients with lymphoma. N Engl J Med 300: 1401–1415

Bagwell C B, Lovett III E J, Ault K A 1988 Localization of monoclonal B-cell populations through the use of Kolmogorov–Smirnov D-value and reduced chi-square contours. Cytometry 9: 469–476

Bartram C R, Janssen J W G, Schmidberger M et al 1989 Minimal residual leukaemia in chronic myeloid leukaemia patients after T-cell depleted bone marrow transplantation. Lancet 1: 1260

Bernard A, Raynal B, Lemerle J et al 1982 Changes in surface antigens on malignant T cells from lymphoblastic lymphomas at relapse: an appraisal with monoclonal antibodies and microfluorimetry. Blood 59: 809–815

Bradstock K F, Papageorgiou E S, Janossy G et al 1980 Detection of leukaemic lymphoblasts in CSF by immunofluorescence for terminal transferase. Lancet 1: 1144

Bradstock K F, Papageorgiou E S, Janossy G 1981a Diagnosis of meningeal involvement in patients with acute lymphoblastic leukemia: immunofluorescence for terminal transferase. Cancer 47: 2478–2481

Bradstock K F, Janossy G, Tidman N et al 1981b Immunological monitoring of residual disease in treated thymic acute lymphoblastic leukaemia. Leuk Res 5: 301–309

Bradstock K F, Kirk J, Grimsley P G et al 1989 Unusual immunophenotypes in acute leukaemias: incidence and clinical correlations. Br J Haematol 72: 512–518

Bregni M, Siena S, Neri A et al 1989 Minimal residual disease in acute lymphoblastic leukemia detected by immune selection and gene rearrangement analysis. J Clin Oncol 7: 338–342

Campana D, Coustan-Smith E, Janossy G 1990a the immunological detection of minimal residual disease in acute leukemia. Blood 76: 163–169

Campana D, Yokota S, Coustan-Smith E et al 1990b The detection of residual acute lymphoblastic leukemia cells with immunologic methods and polymerase chain reaction: a comparative study. Leukemia 9: 609–614

Campana D, Coustan-Smith E, Behm F G 1991 The definition of remission in acute leukemia with immunologic techniques. Bone Marrow Transplant 8: 429–437

Coustan-Smith E, Behm F G, Hurwitz C A, Rivera G K, Campana D 1993 N-CAM (CD56) expression by CD34+ malignant myeloblasts has implications for minimal residual disease detection in acute myeloid leukemia. Leukemia 7 (in press)

Crescenzi M, Seto M, Herzig P G et al 1988 Thermostable DNA polymerase chain amplification of t(14;18) chromosome breakpoints and detection of minimal residual disease. Proc Natl Acad Sci USA 85: 4869–4873

Crist W M, Carroll A J, Shuster J J et al 1990 Poor prognosis of children with pre-B acute lymphoblastic leukemia is associated with the t(1;19) (q23;p13): a Pediatric Oncology Group study. Blood 76: 117–122

D'Auriol L, Macintyre E, Galibert F et al 1989 In vitro amplification of T cell gamma gene rearrangements: a new tool for the assessment of minimal residual disease in acute lymphoblastic leukemias. Leukemia 3: 155–157

Deane M, Norton J D 1990 Detection of immunoglobulin gene rearrangement in B lymphoid malignancies by polymerase chain reaction gene amplification. Br J Haematol 74: 251–256

Delfau M H, Kerckaert J P, Cllyn d'Hooghe M et al 1990 Detection of minimal residual disease in chronic myeloid leukemia patients after bone marrow transplantation by polymerase chain reaction. Leukemia 4: 1–5

Fey M F, Kulozik A E, Hansen-Hagge T E et al 1991 The polymerase chain reaction: a new tool for detection of minimal residual disease in haematological malignancies. Eur J Cancer 27: 89–94

Gabert J, Thuret I, Lafage M et al 1989 Detection of residual bcr–abl translocation by polymerase chain reaction in chronic myeloid leukaemia patients after bone marrow transplantation. Lancet 2: 1125–1128

Goldie J H, Coldman A J, Gudauskas G A 1982 Rationale for the use of alternating non-cross resistant chemotherapy. Cancer Treat Rep 66: 439–449

Goldman J M, Hughes T 1991 Detection and significance of minimal residual disease in patients with leukaemia and lymphoma. Bone Marrow Transplant 7 (Suppl 1): 66–69

Greaves M F 1986 Differentiation-linked leukemogenesis in lymphocytes. Science 1986: 697–704

Greaves M F, Paxton A, Janossy G et al 1980 Acute lymphoblastic leukemia associated antigen. III. Alterations in expression during treatment and in relapse. Leuk Res 4: 1–9

Gribben J G, Freedman A S, Woo S D et al 1991 All advanced stage non-Hodgkin's lymphomas with a polymerase chain reaction amplifiable breakpoint of bcl-2 have residual disease cells containing the bcl-2 rearrangement at evaluation and after treatment. Blood 78: 3275–3280

Hansen-Hagge TE, Yokota S, Bartram C R 1989 Detection of minimal residual disease in acute lymhoblastic leukemia by in vitro amplification of rearranged T-cell receptor delta chain sequences. Blood 74: 1762–1768

Hann I M, Morris-Jones P H, Evans D I K 1977 Discrepancies of bone marrow aspirations in leukaemia. Lancet 1: 1215

Holt C, Arensen E, Carstens B et al 1989 Persistence of pseudodiploidy del (16q) in remission bone marrows of two children with acute lymphoblastic leukemia. Proc Am Soc Clin Oncol 8: 218

Hooijkaas H, Hahlen K, Adriaansen H J et al 1989 Terminal deoxynucleotidyl transferase (TdT)-positive cells in the cerebrospinal fluid and development of overt CNS leukemia: a 5-year follow-up study in 113 children with a TdT-positive leukemia or non-Hodgkin's lymphoma. Blood 74: 416–422

Hughes T P, Ambrosetti A, Barbu V et al 1991 Clinical value of PCR in diagnosis and follow-up of leukaemia and lymphoma: report of the Third Workshop of the Molecular Biology/BMT Study Group. Leukemia 5: 448–451

Hunger S P, Galili N, Carroll A J et al 1991 The t(1;19)(q23;p13) results in consistent fusion of E2A and PBX1 coding sequences in acute lymphoblastic leukemias. Blood 77: 687–693

Janossy G, Campana D, Burnett A K et al 1988 Autologous bone marrow transplantation in acute lymphoblastic leukemia. Preclinical immunologic studies. Leukemia 2: 485–495

Jonsson O G, Kitchens R L, Baer R J et al 1991 Rearrangements of the *tal*-1 locus as clonal markers for T cell acute lymphoblastic leukemia. J Clin Invest 87: 2029–2035

Kamps M P, Look A T, Baltimore D 1991 The human t(1;19) translocation in pre-B ALL produces multiple nuclear E2A–Pbxl fusion proteins with differing transforming potentials. Genes Dev 5: 358–368

Katz F, Ball L, Gibbons B et al 1989 The use of DNA probes to monitor minimal residual disease in childhood acute lymphoblastic leukemia. Br J Haematol 73: 173–180

Kiyoi H, Naoe T, Horibe K et al 1992 Characterization of the immunoglobulin heavy chain complementarity determining region (CDR)-III sequences from human B cell precursor acute lymphoblastic leukemia cells. J Clin Invest 89: 739–746

Kranz B R, Thiel E, Thierfelder S 1989 Immunocytochemical identification of meningeal leukemia and lymphoma: poly-L-lysine-coated slides permit multimarker analysis even with minute cerebrospinal fluid cell specimens. Blood 73: 1942–1950

Krishan A 1975 Rapid cytofluorometric analysis of mammalian cell cycle by propidium iodide staining. J Cell Biol 66: 188–193

Lambrechts A C, de Ruiter P E, Dorssers L C J et al 1992 Detection of residual disease in translocation (14;18) positive non-Hodgkin's lymphoma, using the polymerase chain reaction: a comparison with conventional staging methods. Leukemia 6: 29–34

Lee M S, Chang K S, Cabanillas F et al 1987 Detection of minimal residual cells carrying the t(14;18) by DNA sequence amplification. Science 237: 175–178

Lee M S, Chang K S, Freireich E J et al 1988 Detection of minimal residual bcr/abl transcripts by a modified polymerase chain reaction. Blood 72: 893–897

Lee M S, LeMaistre A, Kantarjian H et al 1989 Detection of two alternative bcr/abl mRNA junctions and minimal residual disease in Philadelphia chromosome positive chronic myelogenous leukemia by polymerase chain reaction. Blood 73: 2165–2170

Letwin B W, Wallace P K, Muirhead K A et al 1990 An improved clonal excess assay using flow cytometry and B-cell gating. Blood 75: 1178–1185

Levy R, Warnke R, Dorfman R F et al 1977 The monoclonality of human B cell lymphomas. J Exp Med 145: 1014–1024

Limpens J, de Jong D, Voetdijk A M H et al 1990 Translocation t(14;18) in benign B lymphocytes. Blood 76 (Suppl 1): 237a

Martens A C M, Schultz, F W, Hagenbeck A 1987 Nonhomogeneous distribution of leukemia in the bone marrow during minimal residual disease. Blood 70: 1073–1078

Mathe G, Schwarzenberg L, Mery A M et al 1966 Extensive histological and cytological survey of patients with acute leukaemia in 'complete remission'. Br Med J 1: 640–642

Morgan G J, Hughes T, Janssen J W G et al 1989 Polymerase chain reaction for detection of residual leukaemia. Lancet 1: 928–929

Neale G A M, Menbarguez J, Kitchingman G R et al 1991 Detection of minimal residual disease in T-cell acute lymphoblastic leukemia using polymerase chain reaction predicts impending relapse. Blood 78: 739–747

Negrin R S, Kiem H-P, Schmidt-Wolf I G H et al 1991 Use of polymerase reaction to monitor the effectiveness of ex vivo tumor cell purging. Blood 77: 654–660

Nizet Y, Martiat P, Vaerman J L et al 1991 Follow-up of residual disease in B lineage acute leukaemias using a simplified PCR strategy: evolution of MRD rather than its detection is correlated with clinical outcome. Br J Haematol 79: 205–210

Peiper S, Stass S A, Bollum F J 1980 Detection of leukaemic lymphoblasts in CSF. Lancet 2: 39

Price R A, Johnson W W 1973 The central nervous system in childhood leukemia: I. The arachnoid. Cancer 31: 520–533

Price C G A, Meerabux J, Murtagh S et al 1991 The significance of circulating cells carrying t(14;18) in long remission from follicular lymphoma. J Clin Oncol 9: 1527–1532

Privitera E, Kamps M P, Hayashi Y et al 1992 Different molecular consequences of the 1;19 chromosomal translocation in childhood B-cell precursor acute lymphoblastic leukemia. Blood 79: 1781–1788

Rabinovitch P S, Torres R M, Engel D 1986 Simultaneous cell cycle analysis and two-color surface immunofluoresnce using 7-amino-actinomycin D and single laser excitation: applications to study cell activation and cell cycle of murine Ly-1 B cells. J Immunol 136: 2769–2775

Rivera G K, Raimondi S C, Hancock M L et al 1991 Improved outcome in childhood acute lymphoblastic leukaemia with reinforced early treatment and rotational combination chemotherapy. Lancet 1: 61–66

Ryan D H, van Dongen J J M 1988 Detection of residual disease in acute leukemia using immunological markers. In: Bennett J M, Foon K A (eds) Immunologic approaches to the classification and management of lymphomas and leukemias. Kluwer, Norwell M A pp 173–207

Saiki R K, Gelfand D H, Stoffel S et al 1988 Primer-directed enzymatic amplification of DNA with thermostable DNA polymerase. Science 239: 487–491

Schmid I, Uittenboggart C H, Giorgi J V 1991 A gentle fixation and permeabilization method for combined cell surface and intracellular staining with improved precision in DNA quantification. Cytometry 12: 279–285

Sklar J 1991 Polymerase chain reaction: the molecular microscope of residual disease. J Clin Oncol 9: 1521–1524

Stass S, Mirro J, Melvin S et al 1984 Lineage switch in acute leukemia. Blood 64: 701–708

Terstappen L W M M, Loken M R 1990 Myeloid cell differentiation in normal bone marrow and acute myeloid leukemia assessed by multidimensional flow cytometry. Anal Cell Pathol 2: 229–236

Thompson J D, Brodsky I, Yunis J J 1992 Molecular quantification of residual disease in chronic myelogenous leukemia after bone marrow transplantation. Blood 79: 1629–1635

Tsurusawa M, Kaneko Y, Katano N et al 1989 Flow cytometric evidence for minimal residual disease and cytological heterogeneities in acute lymphoblastic leukemia with severe hypodiploidy. Am J Hematol 32: 42–49

Van Bekkum D W 1984 Residual reflections on the detection and treatment of leukemia. In: Lowenberg P, Hagenbeck J, (eds) Minimal residual disease in acute leukaemia. Martinus Nijhoff, The Hague, pp 385–389

Van Denderen J, Hermans A, Meeuwsen T et al 1989 Antibody recognition of the tumor-specific bcr–abl joining region in chronic myeloid leukemia. J Exp Med 169: 87–98

Van Dongen J J M 1990 Human T cell differentiation: basic aspects and their clinical applications. PhD Thesis, Department of Immunology, Erasmus University, Rotterdam

Van Dongen J J M, Wolvers-Tettero I L M 1991 Analysis of immunoglobulin and T cell receptor genes. Part II: possibilities and limitations in the diagnosis and management of lymphoproliferative diseases and related disorders. Clin Chim Acta 198: 93–174

Van Dongen J J M, Hooijkaas H, Hahlen K et al 1984 Detection of minimal residual disease in TdT positive T cell malignancies by double immunofluorescence staining. In: Lowenberg P, Hagenbeck J (eds) Minimal residual disease in acute leukaemia. Martinus Nijhoff, The Hague pp 67–81

Wainberg D S, Pinkus G S, Ault K A 1984 Cytofluorometric detection of B cell clonal excess: a new approach to the diagnosis of B cell lymphoma. Blood 63: 1080–1087

Weber-Matthiesen K, Winkemann M, Muller-Hermelink A et al 1992 Simultaneous fluorescence immunophenotyping and interphase cytogenetics: a contribution to the characterization of tumor cells. J Histochem Cytochem 40: 171–175

Weiss L M, Warnke R A, Sklar J et al 1987 Molecular analysis of the t(14;18) chromosomal translocation in malignant lymphomas. N Engl J Med 317: 1185–1987

Yamada M, Hudson S, Tourney O et al 1989 Detection of minimal disease in hematopoietic malignancies of the B lineage by using third-complementarity-determining region specific probes. Proc Natl Acad Sci USA 86: 5123–5127

Yamada M, Wasserman R, Lange B et al 1990 Minimal residual disease in childhood lymphoblastic leukemia. Persistence of leukemic cells during the first 18 months of treatment. N Engl J Med 323: 448–455

Yokota S, Hansen-Hagge T E, Ludwig W-D et al 1991 Use of polymerase chain reactions to monitor minimal residual disease in acute lymphoblastic leukemia patients. Blood 77: 331–339

Young B D 1990 Chromosome analysis and sorting. In: Ormerod M G (ed) Flow cytometry – a practical approach. Oxford University Press, Oxford, pp 145–159

Zehnbauer B A, Pardoll D M, Burke P J et al 1986. Immunoglobulin gene rearrangement in remission bone marrow specimens from patients with acute lymphoblastic leukemia. Blood 67: 835–841

3

The genetic basis of myelodysplasia

D. Culligan   A. Jacobs   R. A. Padua

WHAT IS MYELODYSPLASIA?

The term myelodysplastic syndrome (MDS) is used to describe a group of haematological disorders defined purely in terms of morphological abnormalities (Bennett et al 1982). Further studies show them to be characterized by ineffective production of blood cells (Jacobs & Clark 1986). The common clinical manifestation of peripheral blood cytopenias and a hyper- or normocellular marrow is the result of clonal proliferation of aberrant haemopoietic stem cells whose progeny fail to differentiate or function normally, appear dysplastic and have a high premature death rate (Linman & Bagby 1976). There is variation between the types of MDS in terms of clinical severity, morphology and propensity to evolve into acute leukaemia. Myelodysplasia is an acquired preleukaemic state distinguished from other acquired preleukaemic conditions by its morphologically and functionally dysplastic cells. It represents a transitory, though often prolonged, phase of a multistep leukaemogenic process and in studying its molecular pathogenesis we go some way towards defining the early genetic lesions in this sequence.

Classification and diagnosis of MDS

In 1982 the French–American–British (FAB) group produced a classification system for the myelodysplastic syndromes out of a multitude of haematological abnormalities (Bennett et al 1982). This included the two preleukaemic conditions initially described by Bennett et al (1976) of chronic myelomonocytic leukaemia (CMML) and refractory anaemia with excess of blasts (RAEB), and the three further groups of refractory anaemia (RA), acquired idiopathic sideroblastic anaemia (AISA) and refractory anaemia with excess of blasts in transformation (RAEB-t). This classification of five myelodysplastic syndromes is the mainstay of clinical diagnosis at present; the defining characteristics of each group are shown in Table 3.1.

The practical application of this classification is not always straightforward. Patients have different characteristics at different times, suggesting an evolving process rather than different disease entities. This inherent difficulty in the diagnosis of MDS has been highlighted by a recent multicentre attempt

Table 3.1 The FAB classification of the myelodysplastic syndromes

Category	Blood and marrow characteristics
Refractory anaemia (RA)	Refractory cytopenias, with peripheral monocytes $<1 \times 10^9/l$, peripheral blasts $<1\%$, bone marrow blasts $<5\%$ and ring sideroblasts $<15\%$
Acquired idiopathic sideroblastic anaemia (AISA)	As for RA but with ring sideroblasts $>15\%$
Chronic myelomonocytic leukaemia (CMML)	Monocytes $>1 \times 10^9/l$. Peripheral blasts $<5\%$ and bone marrow blasts $<20\%$
Refractory anaemia with excess blasts (RAEB)	As for RA but with peripheral blasts $<5\%$ and bone marrow blasts 5–20%
Refractory anaemia with excess blasts in transformation (RAEB-t)	As for RA but with peripheral blasts $>20\%$, or marrow blasts 20–30%, or Auer rods present in blasts

to define the minimal diagnostic criteria required for MDS (Hamblin et al 1992). Whilst the various criteria described have much in common, there are also some marked discrepancies. In cases where there is a persistent peripheral blood abnormality and classical dyserythropoiesis, dysgranulopoiesis and dysmegakaryopoiesis (Bennett et al 1982), the diagnosis is clear. However, difficulties occur when dysplasia is minimal, or seems insufficient to account for the abnormalities in the peripheral blood. More sophisticated morphological techniques to define abnormal localization of immature precursors (Mangi et al 1991) or to improve on the subclassification of blast cells depending on their degree of maturation (Goasguen et al 1991), may be of prognostic significance. However, recent attempts to improve the FAB classification (Third MIC Cooperative Study Group 1988) have emphasized the importance of cytogenetic abnormalities and of defining secondary MDS as a distinct entity.

Functional characteristics such as clonal growth patterns in culture are abnormal in up to 80% of cases of MDS (Greenberg 1986, Guyotat et al 1990, Yoshida et al 1989, Tennant et al 1991, Schipperus et al 1990a, Baines et al 1990, Tennant & Jacobs 1988), especially absent growth of peripheral blood erythroid colonies (BFU-E) and peripheral blood myeloid and monocyte colonies. Clonal karyotypic abnormalities and demonstration of X-linked clonality, which is possible in up to 90% of females with MDS, provide useful biological evidence of the preleukaemic state in cases where morphology is inconclusive. The diagnostic groups in Table 3.2 are a useful practical approach to establishing the diagnosis. Equivocal findings may represent early stages of the disease and in these cases careful follow-up with sequential studies will clarify the diagnosis as disease progression occurs.

The FAB classification has proved to have important prognostic significance (Foular et al 1985, Kerkofs et al 1987). The most important prognostic finding is the percentage of blast cells, and therefore patients with RA and

Table 3.2   Diagnostic groups in MDS (in all groups there is a persistent unexplained abnormality in the peripheral blood)

Diagnostic group	Features	Action
1. MDS confirmed	Overt dysplasia or minimal dysplasia with a clonal cytogenetic abnormality or X-linked monoclonality	Treat as clinically indicated
2. Probable MDS	Minimal dysplasia with normal cytogenetics but abnormal progenitors	Careful frequent review with yearly marrow examination
3. Uncertain/possibly very early MDS	Minimal dysplasia, normal cytogenetics, normal progenitor growth	Review every 6 months for evidence of deterioration in the blood

AISA fare better than patients with RAEB or RAEB-t, in terms of both overall survival and incidence of leukaemic transformation. Mean survival for RA and AISA is approximately 35 months, for CMML approximately 12 months, for RAEB 18 months and for RAEB-t 6 months. Similarly, the incidence of leukaemic transformation is between 5% and 30% for RA and AISA, but in the region of 50–70% for RAEB and RAEB-t. Many patients succumb to the effect of cytopenia and bone marrow failure before leukaemic transformation occurs, so the true preleukaemic potential of all these conditions is difficult to assess.

Defining the cellular origin of MDS

Over the past few years strong evidence has emerged that all of these conditions arise from the clonal expansion of aberrant pluripotential stem cells involving myeloid and lymphoid lineages. However, studies have involved only small numbers of patients and very recently the universally pluripotential nature of MDS has been challenged. Given the heterogeneous nature of these disorders it is clearly possible that there may be variations in the level of commitment of the initiating cell. Prchal et al (1978) used the mosaicism of glucose-6-phosphate dehydrogenase isoenzymes to examine a heterozygous female with AISA and demonstrated clonal expression of the same isoenzyme in granulocytes and lymphocytes as well as in red cells and platelets, suggesting that all lineages were part of the neoplastic clone. However, a recent report has emphasized that two subtypes of AISA can be defined on morphological and clinical grounds. One has apparent trilineage dysplasia and the other group has apparent erythroid restricted disease (Gattermann et al 1990). The 5-year cumulative chance of survival is reported as 69% in the 'pure red cell form' and only 19% in the trilineage form of the disease. Lawrence et al (1987) demonstrated the cytogenetic abnormality 13q– to be present in granulocytes and B-cells but not in T-cells in two cases of AISA, and we have recently demonstrated by X-inactivation studies that total peripheral blood lymphocytes are often polyclonal in cases of AISA in the presence of monoclonal granulocytes (Culligan et al 1992). In the other FAB groups there is similar discrepancy between different studies. Kere et al (1987) examined four patients with MDS and monosomy 7. This study demonstrated variable involvement of granulocytes and monocytes but in no case were lymphocytes shown to have the chromosomal abnormality. Janssen et al (1989) and Tefferi et al (1990) used X-inactivation patterns to assess clonality in MDS. These studies, whilst of small numbers, included all FAB types of MDS. The former study showed monoclonality of total bone marrow or blood cell DNA in seven of eight cases and also demonstrated the identical point mutation in the *RAS* oncogene in myeloid and lymphoid fractions from two patients with CMML. Tefferi's study showed monoclonality of granulocytes and T-cells in four of six cases and of monocytes in one of these cases. Abrahamson et al (1991) have used gene dosage studies and X-linked polymorphisms to study cases of refractory anaemia with the 5q− abnormality or monosomy 7. In six out of six cases gene loss was shown in granulocytes but not T-cells, and X-linked monoclonality was proven for granulocytes, but T-cells were polyclonal in all cases and B-cells studied from a single case were also polyclonal. We have recently examined 32 females covering all FAB types who are heterozygous for the X-linked probe M27 beta (Culligan et al 1992) and demonstrated unequivocal lymphoid polyclonality in almost 40% of cases and monoclonality in only 22%. We have found evidence of monoclonal immunoglobulin gene rearrangement by polymerase chain reaction in only 5% of 70 cases. A previous study found no evidence of immunoglobulin or T-cell receptor (TCR) gene rearrangement by Southern blotting (Wainscoat et al 1988). The size of the abnormal clone and therefore its level of detectability along with the persistence of long-lived normal lymphocytes predating the onset of clonal haemopoiesis may account for some of these discrepancies. Furthermore, clonally derived lymphocytes from the aberrant stem cell may be able to undergo normal polyclonal immunoglobulin or TCR rearrangement accounting for the discrepancy between X-linked clonality data and immunoglobulin/TCR rearrangement data. Overall, these diverse studies suggest that not all MDS is pluripotential in origin and the clinical and morphological heterogeneity may reflect heterogeneity of the initiated progenitor.

PATHOGENESIS AND EVOLUTION OF MDS

Human malignancy is now viewed as a multistep process (Land et al 1983, Willecke & Schafer 1984, Shubik 1984, Deuel & Huang 1984, Sporn & Roberts 1985, Jacobs 1987, Weinberg 1989). Initiation produces a somatic mutation in the target cell making it irreversibly altered and giving it a survival advantage. It is susceptible to further insults that lead the cells to evolve through the functional changes resulting from accumulated genetic lesions and clinically from a premalignant to a malignant state. The clinical transition from normality through MDS to acute myeloid leukaemia (AML) is a well-observed example of this sequence. The initiating or subsequent insults causing somatic mutations are usually not known but may involve chemicals, radiation and viruses (Marshall et al 1984, Modan 1987, Farrow et al 1989, Stowers 1987, Brandt et al 1978, Court-Brown & Doll 1965). The incidence of MDS and AML after cytotoxic therapy for other malignancies (Kapadia et al 1980, Rosner & Grunewald 1980, Law & Blom 1980, Kaldor et al 1990a,b, Pedersen-Bjergaad et al 1980, 1984) emphasizes the carcinogenic potential of these mutagenic agents.

The spectrum of lesions acquired by the target cell are now being well documented both at the chromosomal level and within individual genes. Deuel & Huang (1984) suggested that all genes coding for proteins that mediate the cellular response to growth factors are targets for subversion and hence potential oncogenes, as is any gene involved in the control of cell proliferation and differentiation. The sequential acquisition of these lesions over a prolonged period of time appears to give the affected cells a growth advantage. The abnormal clone then expands at the expense of normal haemopoiesis, acquires further genetic change because of its instability and acquires a progressively more malignant phenotype. Clinically, the patient evolves from normality or minimal dysplasia to overt bone marrow failure when the dysfunctional clone has dominated the marrow, to AML when the full malignant phenotype has been acquired. This pattern of evolution of MDS is depicted in Figure 3.1, and a number of chromosomal and genetic lesions are thought to be important in this process.

Cytogenetic abnormalities in MDS

Numerous studies have documented the common finding of clonal chromosomal abnormalities in MDS and emphasized their prognostic significance in terms of survival and incidence of leukaemic transformation. The incidence of these clonal cytogenetic abnormalities in studies using conventional banding techniques varies from 23% to 78% (Second International Workshop on Chromosomes in Leukaemia 1979, Geddes et al 1990, Ayraud et al 1983, Nowell 1982, Knapp et al 1985, Billestrom et al 1986, Pierre et al 1989, Horiike et al 1988, Musilova & Michelova 1988) with some reports, using higher resolution banding, suggesting it to be as high as 85% (Yunis et al 1986, Bendix-Hansen et al 1986).

The common abnormalities found in primary MDS are loss of a whole chromosome 5 or 7 ($-5/-7$) or deletions of the long arm of these chromosomes (del5q/del7q). Trisomy 8 is often described and other abnormalities include deletions of the long arm of chromosomes 11, 13 and 20 (del11q/del13q/del20q), isochromosome 17q, loss of the Y chromosome and balanced translocations especially involving chromosome 3, e.g. t(1;3)(p36;q21)t(3;21)(q26;q22). Specific chromosomal abnormalities found in de novo myeloid leukaemia are rarely found in MDS. These include the

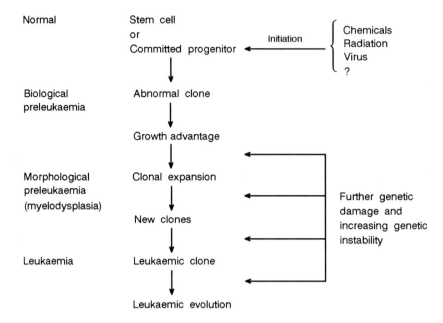

Fig. 3.1   The probable route of evolution from normality, through preleukaemia to leukaemia.

t(8;21) translocation found in AML M4, t(15;17) translocation found in AML M3, and t(9;22) translocation found in CML, suggesting that these disorders do not arise from a pre-existing MDS. However, a minority of patients with AML have a t(6;9) translocation and these are often associated with a preceding preleukaemic phase (Adriaansen et al 1988, Von Lindern et al 1990), although molecular rearrangements of 6;9 are not found in MDS which lacks the chromosomal rearrangement (Soekarman et al 1992).

Except for the so-called 5q– syndrome, specific abnormalities are not associated with specific clinical syndromes or FAB types. Patients with RA and AISA have a lower incidence of karyotypic abnormalities than those with RAEB/RAEB-t, consistent with the observation that chromosomal abnormalities appear to be associated with leukaemic change and a more rapid progression of disease. Similarly, patients with therapy-related MDS (t-MDS) often have complex cytogenetic abnormalities and a high incidence of chromosome 5 and 7 lesions correlating with their poor prognosis (Levine & Bloomfield 1986, Pedersen-Bjergaard et al 1990, Rowley et al 1981). The complexity of the karyotypic abnormalities — i.e. multiple versus single abnormalities — the emergence of new clones, especially in a patient with a normal karyotype at diagnosis, and the presence of residual normal cells provide important prognostic information (Geddes et al 1990). The fact that specific cytogenetic abnormalities are found in primary MDS and that clinical evolution is often marked by the appearance of new karyotypic abnormalities, suggest the existence of target genes at these loci which are involved in the pathogenesis of preleukaemia.

5q− abnormality and the FMS proto-oncogene

A distinct clinical syndrome was first described by Van den Berghe et al (1974, 1985). It affects elderly females predominantly who present with a macrocytic anaemia associated with marked dyserythopoiesis, thrombocytosis or normal platelet counts, but with micromegakaryocytes, and megakaryocytes with hypolobulation of the nuclei. The cytogenetic abnormality is often found in cases of MDS that do not fit the clinical syndrome. Two-thirds of these patients have less than 5% blast counts and hence fall into the FAB group of RA or AISA. However, the 5q− abnormality is also found in patients with RAEB and RAEB-t. In patients with 5q− as the sole abnormality the prognosis is good, with a chronic stable course and a low rate of transformation to acute leukaemia. However, in association with other cytogenetic abnormalities, leukaemic transformation is common (Hoelzer et al 1984).

Careful analysis of the breakpoint on the long arm of chromosome 5 has resulted in the identification of a critical region at band q31 which is always deleted (Hoelzer et al 1984, Le Beau et al 1986a) despite variations in the overall size of the interstitial deletion. A host of genes important to haemopoiesis have been allocated to this critical region and are summarized in Table 3.3. It is possible that loss of one or more genes by this deletion (Le Beau et al 1986b, 1989) exposes a mutant gene on the other allele or renders the remaining allele susceptible to mutations. Work has especially concentrated on FMS and granulocyte-macrophage colony-stimulating factor (GM-CSF) as these may be involved in autocrine regulation of leukaemic cell growth. Homozygous loss of the FMS proto-oncogene has been described in a patient with 5q− (Boultwood et al 1990a). However, major structural rearrangements of the GM-CSF gene on the normal allele have not been found in MDS (Boultwood et al 1990b) though it has been seen in AML (Cheng et al 1988). Obviously, a tumour suppressor gene would be a good candidate for the target gene within the critical deletion region of 5q.

Table 3.3 Genes located within or adjacent to the critical region 5q31

GM-CSF	EGR-1
IL-3	ADRB2R
IL-4	GRL
IL-5	FGFA
IL-9	CSF-1R/FMS
CD14	PDGFRB

The *FMS* gene encodes the functional receptor for the growth factor colony-stimulating factor-1 (CSF-1 or M-CSF) (Sherr et al 1985, Sherr 1990). Interestingly, until recently the M-CSF gene was also thought to be on 5q but has been relocated to chromosome 1 (Morris et al 1991). M-CSF is required for normal proliferation and survival of monocytes and M-CSF/ FMS ligand receptor binding leads to receptor autophosphorylation on tyrosine and phosphorylation of other downstream proteins (Van den Geer & Hunter 1990, Tapley et al 1990, Downing et al 1988, Sengupta et al 1988). Mutations at codon 301 of *FMS* mimic the ligand-induced conformational change produced by M-CSF binding, which in turn produces constitutional protein tyrosine kinase activity and transforming ability in NIH3T3 cells (Roussel et al 1988, 1990, Woolford et al 1988). Further mutations at codon 969 which enhance this transforming effect are not transforming on their own (Roussel et al 1987). However, a recent study of site-directed mutagenesis of the extracellular domain has suggested that mutations in several sites have transforming ability, but whether or not they occur in vivo is not known (van Daalen Wetters et al 1992). Mutations at both codons 301 and 969 have been demonstrated in up to 18% of cases of MDS and 25% of AML using polymerase chain reaction and oligonucleotide hybridization (Ridge et al 1990, Tobal et al 1990). The majority of the mutations have been predominantly at codon 969, the putative negative regulatory domain and the region which is lost upon viral transduction of v-*fms* (Coussens et al 1986, Roussel et al 1987, Hampe et al 1984). However, subsequent confirmation of the presence of these mutations by sequencing has been difficult as a result of the variably small size of the abnormal clone and hence of the mutant gene copy number. More sensitive techniques such as single-stranded conformational polymorphism (SSCP) (Orita et al 1989) and single nucleotide primer extension (Kuppuswamy et al 1991) should overcome these problems. As might be predicted from the normal function of CSF-1, diseases with a predominant monocytic component have a higher incidence of *FMS* mutations, i.e. CMML and AML M4 and M5. Recently, increased levels of CSF-1 have been demonstrated in the serum of all types of MDS (Janowska-Wieczorek et al 1991), suggesting that dysfunctional factor dependent growth or abnormal autocrine growth loops may exist in cases of MDS.

Another candidate tumour suppressor gene on 5q and the only gene in the critical region to possess transcription-regulating activity in the mould of classical tumour suppressor genes such as p53 and the Wilms' tumour gene is the early growth response gene (EGR-1) at 5q23–31 (Sukhatme et al 1988). This possesses a zinc finger DNA-binding motif as do the genes *FOS* and *JUN* which are also early response genes and as such probably have important roles in initiating the gene transcription required for the protracted response of cells to various growth stimuli. We still await evidence for homozygous loss or mutations of this gene in MDS.

Chromosome 7 abnormalities

Monosomy 7 or deletion 7q is a common finding in adults and children with MDS (Dezza et al 1983, Wegelius 1986) and in de novo AML (Rowley 1990). MDS with monosomy 7 is associated with a hypoproliferative marrow with pancytopenia, defective neutrophil chemotaxis and recurrent infection. Progression to a resistant AML is common, and de novo AML with monosomy 7 is similarly difficult to treat and of poor prognosis. Genes localized to chromosome 7 include the proto-oncogenes *ERB*-B, and *MET*, the multidrug-resistant gene *MDR*-1 and growth factors interleukin-6 (IL-6) and erythropoietin (EPO).

Serum levels of EPO have been shown to be generally related to the degree of anaemia in MDS (Jacobs et al 1989, 1991) although there is a wide range of values between patients with similar haemoglobin concentrations, and some patients show relatively low levels for the particular degree of anaemia. In general, erythroid colony growth is usually decreased or absent in marrow and peripheral blood from patients with MDS (Baines et al 1990, Ruutu et al 1984, Amato & Khan 1983, Chui & Clarke 1982) and does not respond to supernormal levels of added EPO. The EPO receptor gene is found on chromosome 19 and to date no gross structural rearrangements of the EPO receptor gene have been demonstrated in MDS (Bowen 1992). However, mutations in the EPO receptor gene have been described in cell lines (Yoshimura et al 1990) and recently transfection of an EPO receptor mutation has been demonstrated to produce an erythroleukaemia (Longmore & Lodish 1991). Several studies have shown beneficial effects of intravenous or subcutaneous EPO in approximately 20% of patients with MDS (Bowen et al 1991, Hirashima et al 1989, Schouten et al 1991, Van Kamp et al 1991, Cazzola et al 1992). All FAB types can respond, although it is unusual for patients with AISA to respond, and modest rather than severe anaemia, detectable BFU-E prior to treatment and relatively low basal EPO levels are potential indicators of those patients who will respond. It is possible, therefore, that point mutations in the EPO receptor gene or subnormal production of EPO from chromosome 7 either in the renal producing cell or locally in the marrow in some autocrine manner may contribute to the dysfunctional anaemia in some cases of MDS.

There have been studies on the MDR-1 gene on chromosome 7, and increased levels of MDR-1 expression have been shown in AML and MDS (Holmes et al 1989) which may contribute to the difficulty in treating MDS and secondary AML. As with chromosome 5, the search for a potential tumour suppressor gene on chromosome 7 accounting for the effects of monosomy 7 or deletion 7q continues.

The RAS genes

The *RAS* family of proto-oncogenes consists of H-*RAS*, K-*RAS* and N-*RAS* found on chromosomes 11p15.1–15.5, 12p12.1–ter, and 1p22–32, respectively. They all code for a 21 kDa inner membrane protein (p21), which binds GTP and probably has a pivotal role in signal transduction from cell surface stimulated receptors to internal second messengers, such as non-receptor tyrosine kinases and protein kinase C (Downward et al 1990, Ellis et al 1990, Molloy et al 1989, Moran et al 1991). These genes can be activated by point mutations at codons 12, 13 and 61 which correspond to the GTP-binding sites, and in these active states can transform NIH3T3 fibroblasts which are in turn tumorigenic in immunodeficient nude mice. Such mutations in the *RAS* family have been found in several haematological malignancies including AML (Bos et al 1987, Farr et al 1988), acute lymphoblastic leukaemia (ALL) (Neri et al 1988, Ahuja et al 1990) and myeloma (Neri et al 1989). However, the highest incidence of *RAS* mutations in haematological disease is found in MDS (Padua et al 1988, Lyons et al 1988, Yunis et al 1989, Bar-Eli et al 1989, Melani et al 1990, Hirai et al 1987, Liu et al 1987, Van Kamp et al 1992), reported in the order of 3–50%, with the highest incidence being found in CMML.

The role of the mutated *RAS* genes in the preleukaemic process seems to be variable. The fact that mutated *RAS* genes are found in a higher number of MDS cases than AML cases, and that there are reports of *RAS* genes being lost in progression of MDS to AML or on relapse of AML with a more aggressive clone (Farr et al 1988), suggest that in some cases *RAS* mutations are early lesions involved in the early stage of the malignant process, but are then lost and not required for subsequent clonal evolution. However, contrary to this, some patients are described in whom *RAS* mutations appear late in the disease and may represent acquisition during clonal evolution (Van Kamp et al 1992). In general the presence of detectable *RAS* mutations in MDS is associated with poor prognosis in terms of survival and progression to AML (Padua et al 1988, Yunis et al 1989, Carter et al 1991).

The p53 gene

The p53 gene which is localized on chromosome 17p codes for a nuclear binding protein. Normal p53 appears to function as a tumour suppressor gene (Baker et al 1990, Eliyaha et al 1989, Finlay et al 1989) in that the malignant phenotype is associated with loss of one chromosome 17 and simultaneous mutation of the remaining gene. Loss of chromosome 17p is a common finding in colon cancer (Baker et al 1989) and p53 is thought to play a vital role in the oncogenic process (Fearon & Vogelstein 1990). p53 mutations have also been found in cases of small cell lung cancer, breast cancer, liver cancer and mesenchymal tumours (Nigro et al 1989, Prokocimer et al 1989). It is also described in AML blasts especially from transformed CML (Ahuja et al 1989, Marshal et al 1990, Slingerland et al 1991) and HL60 (Wolf & Rotter 1985) and T-cell leukaemia cell lines (Cheng & Haas 1990) and recently in a high percentage of adult T-cell leukaemia/lymphoma patients (Sakashita et al 1992). A large study by Jonveaux et al (1991) has examined over 150 cases of MDS for point mutations in p53 using the SSCP technique and found mutations in only five cases covering all of the conserved exons (5–8). In keeping with the tumour suppressor role of p53, three of the five cases also had a cytogenetic abnormality involving 17p. Furthermore, Fenaux et al (1991) have shown only eight mutations in 112 cases of AML and several of these had complex cytogenetic abnormalities including abnormality of chromosomes 5 and 7, suggesting that overall p53 may not have an important role in myeloid malignancy.

THERAPY-RELATED MDS (t-MDS)

Of all the human malignancies related to previous cancer therapy, AML is the most common and a preceding MDS phase is usual (Court-Brown & Doll 1965, Kapadia et al 1980, Law & Blom 1980, Rosner & Grunewald 1980, Kaldor et al 1990a,b, Pedersen-Bjergaard et al 1980, 1984, Rosner et al 1978). The median interval between the initial treatment and the occurrence of secondary clonal disease is 3–5 years. The incidence depends on the type of drug regimen, dosage and combination with radiotherapy. Alkylating agents and etoposide are particularly implicated.

Secondary AML is most commonly described after treatment for Hodgkin's disease (Kaldor et al 1990a), ovarian cancer (Pedersen-Bjergaard et al 1980, 1990, Kaldor et al 1990b), myeloma (Law & Blom 1980) and childhood ALL (Neglia et al 1991). The preceding MDS phase is often of the type RAEB or RAEB-t with severe pancytopenia and complex karyotypic abnormalities. Of 216 cases of secondary MDS, Bloomfield (1986) found that 66% had a cytogenetic abnormality and the most common single abnormalities were monosomy 7 in 35%, 5q– in 18% and monosomy 5 in 14%. Other studies have emphasized the high proportion of cases of t-MDS with loss of part or the whole of chromosomes 5 and/or 7. These abnormalities also occur in de novo AML following occupational exposure to myelotoxic chemicals (Van den Berghe et al 1979, Mitelman et al 1978, Mitelman 1980). A study by Fenaux et al (1990) of young people with MDS confirms the high incidence of complex karyotypic abnormalities involving chromosome 7 and their poor prognosis. In this respect, in this young group of de novo MDS patients, MDS mimics t-MDS, suggesting it is the result of exposure to some occupational mutagen.

It is likely that damaged cells or a reduced stem cell pool in heavily treated patients are less able to deal with subsequent toxic damage or have proceeded part way along the path of malignant transformation. As such these patients are an ideal group of people to study in order to assess the very early genetic lesions of the leukaemic process during careful follow-up. Evidence of this early genetic damage is beginning to emerge and mutations in the *RAS* and *FMS* gene have been found in patients treated for lymphoma between 1 and 13 years previously. These patients had no residual disease, haematological or karyotypic abnormality at the time of analysis (Carter et al 1990, 1991, Jacobs et al 1990, Cachia et al 1993c). Amongst these patients, we have identified one young woman with normal haematology 4 years after treatment for Hodgkin's disease who on sequential studies has developed a small cytogenetic clone of 7q– cells, followed by an activated N-*RAS* gene which was found to transform NIH3T3 cells in a nude mouse tumorigenicity assay. She also developed abnormal peripheral blood colony growth, despite the persistence of normal blood counts and normal peripheral blood and bone marrow morphology (Cachia et al 1993b). We suspect this represents the early stages in the transformation process and is preleukaemia without myelodysplasia.

Further evidence of the extensive damage to the stem cell population in heavily treated patients can be found in clonality studies. We have found clonal haemopoiesis by X-inactivation analysis in women post chemotherapy to be statistically higher than age-matched normals (Cachia et al 1993a). However, a recent similar study (Gale et al 1991) failed to find a significant difference between treated and normal women owing to the high incidence of skewed X-inactivation in their normal population. It is emerging, therefore, that the presence of preleukaemia can be demonstrated before the morphological manifestations of myelodysplasia in some of these patients. Functional and genetic markers may allow comparative follow-up studies and define those patients most at risk of secondary MDS or leukaemia.

CONCLUSION

Over the past 10 years the myelodysplastic syndromes have emerged as variations in clonal haemopoiesis which represent the morphological manifestations of a preleukaemic state. These variations may represent progressive stages in the leukaemic process from early biological abnormalities in the presence of normal morphology or minimal dysplasia to domination of the marrow by the abnormal clone resulting in bone marrow failure and the eventual emergence of frankly leukaemic cells. Some of these cases represent disease originating in a pluripotential stem cell and others may represent disease originating in a myeloid or erythroid committed progenitor cell. In some cases evidence of preleukaemia may exist with no dyplastic changes. The acquired genetic lesions associated with the progression of preleukaemia to leukaemia and their effect on cell growth and differentiation mechanisms are slowly being defined and hopefully will provide a fuller understanding of leukaemogenesis and provide new targets for more effective therapy.

KEY POINTS OF CLINICAL PRACTICE

- Patients with peripheral blood findings suggesting myelodysplasia must have a bone marrow sample taken for morphological and cytogenetic analysis.
- When the diagnosis remains uncertain an annual follow-up is required.

- Measurement of clonal growth patterns in culture, karyotyping and analysis of X-linked clonality if technically available can provide evidence of preleukaemia if the morphological diagnosis is in doubt.
- Patients with bone marrow cytogenetic abnormalities have a higher incidence of leukaemic transformation and a relatively poor prognosis.
- RAEB patients with cytogenetic abnormalities respond poorly to cytotoxic therapy.

REFERENCES

Abrahamson G, Boultwood J, Madden J et al 1991 Clonality of cell populations in refractory anaemia using combined approach of gene loss and X-linked restriction length polymorphism-methylation analyses. Br J Haematol 79: 550–555

Adriaansen H J, van Dongen J J M, Hooijkaas H 1988 Translocation (6;9) may be associated with a specific Tdt-positive immunological phenotype in ANLL. Leukaemia 2: 136–140

Ahuja H, Bar-Eli M, Advani S et al 1989 Alterations in the p53 gene and the clonal evolution of the blast crisis of chronic myelocytic leukaemia. Proc Natl Acad Sci USA 86: 6783–6787

Ahuja H G, Foti A, Bar-Eli M et al 1990 The pattern of mutational involvement of RAS genes in human haematologic malignancies determined by DNA amplification and direct sequencing. Blood 75: 1684–1690

Amato D, Khan N R 1983 Erythroid burst formation in cultures of bone marrow and peripheral blood from patients with refractory anaemia. Acta Haematol 70: 1–10

Ayraud N, Donzeau M, Raynaud S et al 1983 Cytogenetic study of 88 cases of refractory anaemia. Cancer Genet Cytogenet 8: 243–248

Baines P, Bowen D, Jacobs A 1990 Clonal growth of haemopoietic progenitor cells from myelodysplastic marrow in response to recombinant haemopoietins. Br J Haematol 14: 247–252

Baker S J, Fearon E R, Nigro J M et al 1989 Chromosome 17 deletions and p53 gene mutations in colorectal carcinomas. Science 244: 217–220

Baker S J, Markowitz S, Fearon E R et al 1990 Suppression of human colorectal carcinoma cell growth by wild type p53. Science 249: 912–915

Bar-Eli M, Ahuja H, Gonzalez-Cadavid N et al 1989 Analysis of NRAS exon 1 mutations in myelodysplastic syndromes by polymerase chain reaction and direct sequencing. Blood 73: 281–283

Bendix-Hansen K, Kerndrup G, Pedersen B 1986 Myeloperoxidase-deficient polymorphonuclear leucocytes (VI): relation to cytogenetic abnormalities in primary myelodysplastic syndromes. Scand J Haematol 36: 3–7

Bennett J M, Catovsky D, Daniel M T et al 1976 Proposals for the classification of the acute leukaemias. Br J Haematol 33: 451–458

Bennett J M, Catovsky D, Daniel M T 1982 Proposals for the classification of the myelodysplastic syndromes. Br J Haematol 51: 189–199

Beran M, Hast R 1978 Studies on human preleukaemia II. In vitro colony forming capacity in a regenerative anaemia with hypercellular bone marrow. Scand J Haematol 21: 139–149

Billestrom R, Nilsson P G, Mitelman F et al 1986 Cytogenetic analysis in 941 consecutive patients with haematologic disorders. Scand J Haematol 37: 29–40

Bloomfield C D 1986 Chromosome abnormalities in secondary myelodysplastic syndromes. Scand J Haematol 45 (Suppl 82)

Bos J L, Verlaan de Vries M, van der Eb A et al 1987 Mutations in N-ras predominate in acute myeloid leukaemia. Blood 69: 1237–1241

Boultwood J, Rack K, Buchck V J et al 1990a Homozygote deletion of fms in a patient with the 5q– syndrome. Br J Haematol 55: 217–227

Boultwood J, Abrahamson G, Buckle V et al 1990b Structure of the granulocyte macrophage colony-stimulating factor gene in patients with the myelodysplastic syndromes. Am J Hematol 34: 157–158

Bowen D 1992 Personal communication

Bowen D T, Culligan D, Jacobs A 1991 The treatment of anaemia in the myelodysplastic syndromes with recombinant human erythropoietin. Br J Haematol 77: 419–423

Brandt L, Nilsson P G, Mitleman F 1978 Occupational exposure to petroleum products in men with acute non-lymphocytic leukaemia. Br Med J 1: 553

Cachia P G, Culligan D J, Clarke R et al 1993a Clonal haemopoiesis following cytotoxic therapy for lymphoma. Leukaemia 7 (in press)

Cachia P G, Taylor C, Thompson P W et al 1993b Non dysplastic myelodysplasia (submitted)

Cachia P G, Ridge S A, Baker A et al 1993c FMS mutations in patients following cytotoxic therapy for lymphoma (in preparation)

Carter G, Hughes D C, Clark R E et al 1990 RAS mutations in patients following cytotoxic therapy for lymphoma. Oncogene 5: 411–416

Carter G, Hughes N, Warren N et al 1991 RAS mutations in pre-leukaemia, in patients following cytotoxic therapy and in normal subjects. In: Spandidos D A (ed) The superfamily of ras-related genes. Plenum Press, New York, pp 89–94

Cazzola M, Ponchio L, Beguin Y et al 1992 Subcutaneous erythropoietin for treatment of refractory anaemia in haematologic disorders. Results of phase I/II clinical trial. Blood 79: 29–37

Cheng J, Haas M 1990 Frequent mutations in the p53 tumour suppressor gene in human leukaemia T cell lines. Mol Cell Biol 10: 5502–5509

Cheng G, Kelleher C A, Miyauchi J et al 1988 Structure and expression of genes of GM-CSF and G-CSF in blast cells from patients with acute myelodysplastic leukaemia. Blood 71: 204–208

Chui D H K, Clarke B J 1982 Abnormal erythroid progenitor cells in human preleukaemia. Blood 60: 362–367

Court-Brown W H, Doll R 1965 Mortality from cancer and other causes after radiotherapy for ankylosing spondylitis. Br Med J 2: 1327–1332

Coussens L, Van Beveren C, Smith D et al 1986 Structural alteration of viral homologue of receptor proto-oncogene fms at the carboxyl terminus. Nature 320: 277–280

Culligan D J, Cachia P, Whittaker J A et al 1992 Clonal lymphocytes are detected in only some cases of MDS. Br J Haematol 81: 346–352

Deuel T A, Huang J S 1984 Roles of growth factor activities in oncogenesis. Blood 64: 951–958

Dezza L, Cazzola M, Bergamaschi G et al 1983 Myelodysplastic syndrome with monosomy 7 in adulthood: a distinct preleukaemic disorder. Haematologica 68: 723–725

Downing J R, Rettenmier C W, Sherr C J 1988 Ligand-induced tyrosine kinase activity of the colony stimulating factor-1 receptor in a murine macrophage cell line. Mol Cell Biol 8: 1795–1799

Downward J, Graves J D, Warne P H et al 1990 Stimulation of p21 ras upon T cell activation. Nature 346: 719–723

Eliyaha D, Michalovitz D, Eliyahu S et al 1989 Wild type p53 can inhibit oncogene mediated focus formation. Proc Natl Acad Sci USA 86: 8763–8767

Ellis C, Moran M, McCormick F et al 1990 Phosphorylation of GAP and GAP associated proteins by transforming and mitogenic tyrosine kinases. Nature 343: 377–381

Farr C J, Saiki R K, Erlich H A et al 1988 Analysis of RAS gene mutations in acute myeloid leukaemia by polymerase chain reaction and oligonucleotide probes. Proc Nat Acad Sci USA 85: 1629–1633

Farrow A, Jacobs A, West R R 1989 Myelodysplasia, chemical exposure and other environmental factors. Leukaemia 3: 33–35

Fearon E R, Vogelstein B 1990 A genetic model for colorectal tumorigenesis. Cell 61: 759–767

Fenaux P, Preudhomme C, Estienne MH 1990 De novo myelodysplastic syndromes in adults aged 50 or less. A report on 37 cases. Leuk Res 14: 1053–1059

Fenaux P, Jonveaux P, Quiquandon I et al 1991 p53 gene mutations in acute myeloid leukaemia with 17P monosomy. Blood 78: 1652–1657

Finlay C A, Hinds P W, Levine A et al 1989 The p53 protooncogene can act as a suppressor of transformation. Cell 57: 1083–1093

Foular K, Langdon R M, Armitage J O et al 1985 Myelodysplastic syndromes. A clinical and pathological analysis of 109 cases. Cancer 56: 553–561

Gale R E, Wheadon H Linch D C 1991 X-chromosome inactivation patterns using HPRT and PGK polymorphisms in haematologically normal and post chemotherapy females. Br J Haematol 79: 193–197

Gattermann N, Aul C, Schneider W 1990 Two types of acquired idiopathic sideroblastic anaemia (AISA). Br J Haematol 74: 45–52

Geddes A D, Bowen D T, Jacobs A 1990 Clonal karyotype abnormalities and clinical progress in the myelodysplastic syndromes. Br J Haematol 76: 194–202

Goasguen J-E, Bennett J M, Cox C et al 1991 Prognostic implication and characterisation of the blast cell population in the myelodysplastic syndrome. Leuk Res 15: 1159–1165

Greenberg P L 1986 In vitro culture techniques defining biological abnormalities in the myelodysplastic and myeloproliferative disorders. Clin Haematol 15: 973–993

Guyotat D, Campos L, Thomas X et al 1990 Myelodysplastic syndromes. A study of surface markers and in vitro growth patterns. Am J Hematol 34: 26–31

Hamblin T, Culligan D J, Jacobs A et al 1992 Minimal diagnostic criteria for the myelodysplastic syndrome in clinical practice. Leuk Res 16: 3–11

Hampe A, Gobet M, Scherr C J et al 1984 Nucleotide sequence of the feline retroviral oncogene V-*fms* shows unexpected homology with oncogenes encoding tyrosine-specific protein kinases. Proc Natl Acad Sci USA 81: 85–89

Hirai H, Kobayashi Y, Mano H et al 1987 A point mutation at codon 13 of the N*ras* oncogene in myelodysplasia. Nature 327: 430–432

Hirashima K, Besho M, Susaki L et al 1989 Improvement of anaemia by IV injection of recombinant erythropoietin in patients with MDS and aplastic anaemia. Exp Hematol 17: 385

Hoelzer D E, Ganser A, Heimpel H 1984 'Atypical' leukaemias: preleukaemia, smouldering leukaemia and hypoplastic leukaemia. Recent Results Cancer Res 93: 69–101

Holmes J, Jacobs A, Carter G et al 1989 Multidrug resistance in haemopoietic cell lines, myelodysplastic syndromes and acute myeloblastic leukaemia. Br J Haematol 72: 40–44

Horiike S, Taniwaki M, Misawa S et al 1988 Chromosome abnormalities and karyotypic evolution in 83 patients with myelodysplastic syndrome and predictive value for prognosis. Cancer 62: 1129–1138

Jacobs A 1987 Human leukaemia, do we have a model? Br J Cancer 55: 1–5

Jacobs A, Clark R 1986 Pathogenesis and clinical variations in the myelodysplastic syndrome. Clin Haematol 15: 925–951

Jacobs A, Janowska-Wieczorek A, Caro J et al 1989 Circulating erythropoietin in patients with myelodysplastic syndromes. Br J Haematol 73: 36–39

Jacobs A, Ridge S A, Carter G et al 1990 *FMS* and *RAS* mutations following cytotoxic therapy for lymphoma. Exp Hematol 18: 648

Jacobs A, Culligan D, Bowen D T 1991 Erythropoietin and the myelodysplastic syndrome. Contrib Nephrol 88: 266–270

Janowska-Wieczorek A, Belch A R, Jacobs A et al 1991 Increased circulating colony stimulating factor 1 in patients with preleukaemia, leukemia and lymphoid malignancies. Blood 77: 1796–1803

Janssen J W G, Buschle M, Layton M et al 1989 Clonal analysis of myelodysplastic syndromes: evidence of multipotent stem cell origin. Blood 73: 248–254

Jonveaux P H, Fenaux P, Quiquandon I et al 1991 Mutations in the p53 gene in myelodysplastic syndromes. Oncogene 6: 2243–2247

Kaldor J M, Day N E, Clarke A et al 1990a Leukaemia following Hodgkin's disease. N Engl J Med 322: 7–13

Kaldor J M, Day N E, Pettersson F et al 1990b Leukaemia following chemotherapy for ovarian cancer. N Engl J Med 322: 1–6

Kapadia S B, Krawse J R, Ellis L D et al 1980 Induced acute non-lymphocytic leukaemia following long-term chemotherapy. A study of 20 cases. Cancer 45: 1315–1321

Kuppuswamy M N, Hoffmann J W, Kasper C K et al 1991 Single nucleotide primer extension to detect genetic diseases. Experimental application to haemophilia B (factor IX) and cystic fibrosis genes. Proc Natl Acad Sci USA 88: 1143–1147

Kere J, Ruutu T, De La Chapelle A 1987 Monosomy 7 in granulocytes and monocytes in myelodysplastic syndrome. N Engl J Med 316: 499–503

Kerkofs H, Hermans J, Haak H L et al 1987 Utility of the FAB classification for myelodysplastic syndromes; investigation of prognostic factors in 237 cases. Br J Haematol 65: 73–81

Knapp R H, Dewald G W, Pierre R V et al 1985 Cytogenetic studies on 174 consecutive patients with preleukaemic or myelodysplastic syndromes. Mayo Clinic Proc 60: 507

Land H, Parada L F, Weinberg R A 1983 Cellular oncogenes and multistep carcinogenesis. Science 222: 771–778

Law I P, Blom J 1980 Second malignancies in patients with multiple myeloma. Oncology 34: 20–24

Lawrence H J, Broudy V C, Magenis R E et al 1987 Cytogenetic evidence for involvement of B lymphocytes in acquired idiopathic sideroblastic anaemia. Blood 70: 1003–1005

Le Beau M M, Albain K S, Larson R A et al 1986a Clinical and cytogenetic correlation in 63 patients with therapy related myelodysplastic syndromes and acute nonlymphocytic leukaemia: further evidence for characteristic abnormalities of chromosome 5 and 7. J Clin Oncol 4: 325–345

Le Beau M, Westbrook C A, Diaz M O et al 1986b Evidence of the involvement of GM-CSF and FMS in the deletion 5q in myeloid disorders. Science 231: 984–987

Le Beau M, Lemons R S, Espinosal R 1989 IL-4 and IL-5 map to human chromosome 5 in a region encoding growth factors and receptors and are related to myeloid leukaemia with a del 5q. Blood 73: 647–650

Levine E, Bloomfield C 1986 Secondary MDS and leukaemia. Clin Haematol 15: 1037–1080

Linman J W, Bagby G C 1976 The preleukaemic syndrome: clinical and laboratory features, natural course, and management. Blood Cells 2: 11–31

Liu E, Hjelle B, Morgan R et al 1987 Mutations of the kirsten *ras* proto-oncogene in human preleukaemia. Nature 330: 186–188

Longmore G D, Lodish H F 1991 An activating mutation in the murine erythropoietin receptor induces erythroleukaemia in mice: a cytokine receptor superfamily oncogene. Cell 67: 1089–1102

Lyons J, Janssen J W G, Bartam C et al 1988 Mutation of Ki *ras* and N *ras* oncogenes in myelodysplastic syndromes. Blood 71: 1707–1712

Mangi M H, Salisbury J R, Mufti G J 1991 Abnormal localisation of immature precursors (ALIP) in the bone marrow of myelodysplastic syndromes: current state of knowledge and future direction. Leuk Res 15: 627–639

Marshal R, Shtalrid M, Talpaz M et al 1990 Rearrangement and expression of p53 in the chronic phase and blast crisis of chronic myelogenous leukaemia. Blood 75: 180–189

Marshall C J, Rigby P W J 1984 Viral and cellular genes involved in oncogenesis. Cancer Surv 3: 183–214

Melani C, Haliassos A, Chomel J C et al 1990 *Ras* activation in myelodysplastic syndromes: clinical and molecular study of the chronic phase of the disease. Br J Haematol 74: 408–413

Mitelman F 1980 Cytogenetics of experimental neoplasms and non-random chromosome correlations in man. Clin Haematol 9: 195–219

Mitelman F, Brandt L, Nilsson P G 1978 Relation among occupational exposure to potential mutagenic/carcinogenic agents, clinical findings and bone marrow chromosomes in acute non-lymphocytic leukaemia. Blood 52: 1229–1237

Modan M 1987 Cancer and leukaemia risks after low level radiation. Med Oncol Tumour Pharmacother 4: 151–161

Molloy C J, Bottaro D P, Flemming T P et al 1989 PDGF induction of tyrosine phosphorylation of GTPase activating protein. Nature 342: 711–714

Moran M F, Polakis P, McCormick F et al 1991 Protein tyrosine kinases regulate the phosphorylation, protein interactions, subcellular distribution and activity of p21^{ras}GTPase activating protein. Mol Cell Biol 11: 1804–1812

Morris S W, Valentine M B, Shapiro D N et al 1991 Reassignment of the human CSF1 gene to chromosome 1p13–p21. Blood 78: 2013–2020

Musilova J, Michelova K 1988 Chromosome study of 85 patients with myelodysplastic syndrome. Cancer Genet Cytogenet 33: 39–50

Neglia J P, Meadows A T, Robinson L L et al 1991 Second neoplasms after acute lymphoblastic leukaemia in childhood. N Engl J Med 325: 1330–1336

Neri A, Knowles D M, Greco A et al 1988 Analysis of *RAS* oncogene mutations in human lymphoid malignancies. Proc Nat Acad Sci USA 85: 9268–9272

Neri A, Murphy J P, Cro L et al 1989 *Ras* oncogene mutations in multiple myeloma. J Exp Med 170: 1715–1725

Nigro J M, Baker S J, Preisinger A C et al 1989 Mutations in the p53 gene occur in diverse human tumour types. Nature 342: 705–708

Nowell P C 1982 Cytogenetics of preleukaemia. Cancer Genet Cytogenet 5: 265–278

Orita M, Suzuki Y, Sekiya T et al 1989 Rapid and sensitive detection of point mutations and DNA polymorphisms using the polymerase chain reaction. Genomics 5: 874–879

Padua R A, Carter G, Hughes D et al 1988 *RAS* mutations in myelodysplasia detected by oligonucleotide hybridisation and transformation. Leukemia 2: 503–510

Pedersen-Bjergaard J, Nissen N I, Sorensen H M et al 1980 Acute non-lymphocytic leukaemia in patients with ovarian carcinoma following long-term treatment with Treosulfan (= dihydroxybusulphan). Cancer 45: 19–29

Pedersen-Bjergaard J, Philip P, Pedersen N T et al 1984 Acute non-lymphocytic leukaemia, preleukaemia and acute myeloproliferative syndrome secondary to treatment of other malignant diseases. Cancer 52: 452–462

Pedersen-Bjergaard J, Philip P, Larsen S D et al 1990 Chromosome aberrations and prognostic factors in therapy related MDS and acute non-lymphocytic leukaemia. Blood 76: 1087–1091

Pierre R V, Catovsky D, Mufti G J et al 1989 Clinical–cytogenetic correlations in myelodysplasia (preleukaemia). Cancer Genet Cytogenet 40: 149–161

Prchal J T, Throckmorton D W, Carol A J et al 1978 A common progenitor for human myeloid and lymphoid cells. Nature 274: 590–591

Prokocimer M, Shaklai M, Benbassat H et al 1989 p53: a frequent target for genetic abnormalities in lung cancer. Science 246: 491–494

Ridge S A, Worwood M, Oscier D et al 1990 *FMS* mutations in myelodysplastic leukaemic and normal subjects. Proc Natl Acad Sci USA 87: 1377–1380

Rosner F, Grunewald H W 1980 Cytotoxic drugs and leukaemogenesis. Clin Haematol 9: 663–681

Rosner F, Carey R A W, Zarrabi M H 1978 Breast cancer and acute leukaemia: report of 24 cases and review of the literature. Am J Hematol 4: 151–172

Roussel M F, Dull T J, Rettenmier C W et al 1987 Transforming potential of the c-*fms* proto-oncogene (CSF-1 receptor). Nature 325: 549–552

Roussel M F, Downing J R, Rettenmier C W et al 1988 A point mutation in the extracellular domain of the human CSF-1 receptor (c-*fms* proto-oncogene product) activates its transforming potential. Cell 55: 979–988

Roussel M F, Downing J R, Sherr C J 1990 Transforming activities at codon 301 in their extracellular domain. Oncogene 5: 25–30

Rowley J D 1990 Recurring chromosome abnormalities in leukaemia and lymphoma. Semin Hematol 27: 122–136

Rowley J D, Golomb H M, Vardiman J W 1981 Non-random chromosome abnormalities in acute leukaemia and dysmyelopoietic syndromes in patients with previously treated malignant disease. Blood 58: 759–767

Ruutu T, Partanen S, Lintula R et al 1984 Erythroid and granulocyte-macrophage colony formation in myelodysplastic syndromes. Scand J Haematol 32: 395–402

Sakashita A, Hattori T, Miller C W et al 1992 Mutations of the p53 gene in adult T-cell leukaemia. Blood 79: 477–480

Schipperus M, Sonneveld P, Lindermans J et al 1990a The effects of interleukin-3, GM-CSF on the growth kinetics of colony forming cells in myelodysplastic syndromes. Leukemia 4: 267–272

Schipperus M, Sonneveld P, Lindermans J 1990b The combined effects of IL-3, GM-CSF and G-CSF on the in vitro growth of myelodysplastic myeloid progenitor cells. Leuk Res 14: 1019–1025

Schouten H C, Vellenga E, Van Rhenen D J et al 1991 Recombinant human erythropoietin in patients with myelodysplastic syndromes. Leukemia 5: 432

Second International Workshop on Chromosomes in Leukaemia 1979 Chromosomes in preleukaemia. Cancer Genet Cytogenet 2: 108–113

Sengupta A, Liu W K, Yeung Y G et al 1988 Identification and subcellular localisation of proteins that are rapidly phosphorylated in tyrosine in response to CSF-1. Proc Natl Acad Sci USA 85: 8062–8066

Sherr C J 1990 Colony stimulating factor-1 receptor. Blood 75: 1–12

Sherr C J, Rettenmier C W, Sacca R et al 1985 The c-*fms* proto-oncogene product is related to the receptor for the mononuclear phagocyte growth factor, CSF-1. Cell 41: 665–676

Shubik P 1984 Progression and promotion. Natl Cancer Inst 73: 1005–1011

Slingerland J M, Minden M D, Benchimaol S et al 1991 Mutation of the p53 gene in human acute leukaemia. Blood 77: 1500–1507

Soekarman D, Von Lindern M, Van der Plas L et al 1992 Dek–can rearrangement in translocation (6;9)(p23:q34). Leukemia 6(6): 489–494

Sporn M B, Roberts A B 1985 Autocrine growth factors and cancer. Nature 313: 745–747

Stowers S J 1987 The role of oncogenes in chemical carcinogenesis. Environ Health Perspect 75: 81–86

Sukhatme V P, Cao X, Chang L C et al 1988 A zinc finger encoding gene coregulated with c-*fos* during growth and differentiation and after cellular depolarisation. Cell 53: 37–43

Tapley P, Kazlauskas A, Cooper A et al 1990 Macrophage colony stimulating factor induced tyrosine phosphorylation of c-*fms* proteins expressed in FDC-P1 and Balb/c3T3 cells. Mol Cell Biol 10: 2528–2538

Tefferi A, Thibodeau S N, Soldberg L A 1990 Clonal studies in the myelodysplastic syndrome using X-linked restriction fragment length polymorphisms. Blood 75: 1770–1773

Tennant G B, Jacobs A 1988 Undetectable peripheral blood CFU-GM as a prognostic indicator in myelodysplastic syndromes. Leuk Res 13: 385–389

Tennant G B, Bowen D T, Jacobs A 1991 Colony–cluster ratio and cluster number in cultures of circulating myeloid progenitors as indicators of high-risk myelodysplasia. Br J Haematol 77: 296–300

Third M I C Cooperative Study Group 1988 Recommendation for morphologic, immunologic and cytogenetic (MIC) working classification of the primary and therapy related myelodysplastic disorders. Cancer Genet Cytogenet 32: 1–10

Tobal K, Pagliuca A, Bhatt B et al 1990 Mutation of the human *FMS* gene (M-CSF receptor) in myelodysplastic syndromes and acute myeloid leukaemia. Leukemia 4: 486–489

Van Daalen Wetters T, Hawkins S A, Roussel M F et al 1992 Random mutagenesis of CSF-1 receptor (*FMS*) reveals multiple sites for activating mutations within the extracellular domain. EMBO J 11:2 551–557

Van den Berghe H, Cassiman J, David G 1974 Distinct haematological disorder with deletion of long arm of no. 5 chromosome. Nature 251: 437–438

Van den Berghe H, Louwagie A, Broeckaert-Van Orshoven A et al 1979 Chromosome analysis in two unusual malignant blood disorders presumably induced by benzene. Blood 53: 558–566

Van den Berghe H, Vermaden K, Mecucci C et al 1985 The 5q– anomaly. Cancer Genet Cytogenet 17: 189–255

Van den Geer P, Hunter T 1990 Identification of tyrosine 706 in the kinase insert as the major colony stimulating factor 1 (CSF-1) stimulated autophosphorylation site in the CSF-1 receptor in a murine macrophage cell line. Mol Cell Biol 10: 2991–3002

Van Kamp H, Prinsze-Postema T C, Kluin P M et al 1991 Effect of subcutaneously administered human recombinant erythropoietin on erythropoiesis in patients with myelodysplasia. Br J Haematol 78: 488–493

Van Kamp H, de Piper C, Verlaan-de Vries M 1992 Longitudinal analysis of point mutations of the N-*RAS* proto-oncogene in patients with myelodysplasia using archived blood smears. Blood 795: 1266–1270

Verma D S, Spitzer G, Dicke K A et al 1979 In vitro agar culture patterns in preleukaemia and their clinical significance. Leuk Res 3: 41–49

Von Lindern M, Poustka A, Lerach H et al 1990 The (6;9) translocation associated with a specific subtype of acute non-lymphocytic leukaemia leads to aberrant transcription of a target gene on 9q34. Mol Cell Biol 10: 4016–4026

Wainscoat J S, Fey M F, Pilkington S et al 1988 Absence of immunoglobulin and T-cell receptor gene rearrangements in myelodysplastic syndromes and acute non-lymphocytic leukaemias. Am J Hematol 25: 95–97

Wegelius R 1986 Preleukaemia states in children. Scand J Haematol 36: 133–139

Weinberg R A 1989 Oncogenesis, anti-oncogenes and the molecular bases of multistep carcinogenesis. Cancer Res 49: 3713–3721

Willecke K, Schafer R 1984 Human oncogenes. Hum Genet 66: 132–142

Wolf D, Rotter V 1985 Major deletions in the gene encoding the p53 tumour antigen cause lack of p53 expression in HL-60 cells. Proc Natl Acad Sci USA 82: 790–794

Woolford J, McAuliffe A, Rohrschneider L R 1988 Activation of the feline c-*fms* proto-oncogene: multiple alterations are required to generate a fully transformed phenotype. Cell 55: 965–977

Yoshida Y, Yoshida C, Tohyamma K et al 1989 Prognostic implication of sequential bone marrow cultures in the myelodysplastic syndromes. Leuk Res 13: 967–972

Yoshimura A, Longmore G, Lodish H F 1990 Point mutation in the exoplasmic domain of the erythropoietin receptor resulting in hormone-independent activation and tumorigenicity. Nature 348: 647–649

Yunis J J, Rydell R E, Oken M M et al 1986 Refined chromosome analysis as an independent prognostic indicator in de novo myelodysplastic syndromes. Blood 67: 1721–1730

Yunis J J, Boot A J M, Mayer M G et al 1989 Mechanisms of *ras* mutation in myelodysplastic syndrome. Oncogene 4: 609–614

4

New drug treatment for acute myeloblastic leukemia

M. R. Wollman   J. Mirro Jr

Acute myelogenous leukemia (AML) is the name applied to a heterogeneous group of leukemias which have a poor prognosis (Dutcher 1990, Krischer et al 1989). AML can be divided into distinct clinical subgroups described by morphologic characteristics (French–American–British, or FAB, classification), surface antigen expression (immunophenotyping) and, most importantly, cytogenetic abnormalities (Creutzig et al 1990, Cuneo et al 1992, Kalwinsky et al 1990, Raimondi et al 1989, Schiffer et al 1989). Because of their poor response to treatment these disease entities were initially grouped together and called nonlymphocytic leukemia. To the oncologist, the treatment of AML has been extremely frustrating with only a very slight improvement in long-term outcome over the past 10 years (Buckley et al 1989, Creutzig et al 1985, Steuber et al 1991). Unlike the therapy of lymphoblastic leukemia, the therapy of AML requires intensive treatment with extremely toxic agents. The severe hematopoietic and gastrointestinal toxicity of therapy has limited attempts to increase treatment because of increased mortality, but attempts at limiting toxicity by decreasing therapy have resulted in decreased survival except in elderly patients.

AML therapy has generally been divided into two phases. The first phase, induction therapy, is designed to eliminate large numbers of leukemic cells and permit return of hematopoiesis. This phase is followed by some type of postremission therapy administered after the patient has recovered from toxicity. The induction phase, in most studies, results in a complete remission rate between 65% and 85% (Amadori et al 1991, Berman et al 1989a,b, 1991, Carella et al 1989, Creutzig et al 1985, Dahl et al 1987, Hicsonmez et al 1989, Kalwinsky et al 1990). Generally, the patients failing to achieve a complete remission are nearly equally divided between those with resistant disease and those who die of toxicity. Despite successful induction therapy in most patients, the long-term disease-free survival in most large series is a disappointing 30–40% (Dutcher 1990, Krischer et al 1989). The consistently high relapse rate in clinical trials strongly supports the hypothesis that the residual malignant precursors remaining after induction therapy are relatively resistant to standard chemotherapy agents. Therefore, in an effort to improve long-term outcome, oncologists have been intensifying the postremission therapy (Büchner et al 1992, Cassileth et al 1988, Dillman et al 1991, Mayer et al 1992), and bone marrow transplantation (BMT) is being used more often in an attempt to eliminate residual leukemic cells (Gale et al 1989, 1991, Lowenberg et al 1990).

Recent clinical trial results provide some optimism for physicians treating AML. The induction success rate has been significantly improved by using a new anthracycline (idarubicin), and improved supportive care with growth factors may also further improve the induction rate. New drugs, including fludarabine, 2-chlorodeoxyadenosine, and carboplatinum, have been shown to be effective. However, their exact role in AML therapy still needs to be defined. In addition to a higher complete remission rate, long-term survival also appears to be improving as a result of increased postremission therapy, particularly the use of BMT. Immune augmentation post-BMT to eliminate residual leukemia may provide an additional 'new drug' that improves disease-free survival. This review will discuss the use of new drugs in the two phases of treatment, induction therapy and postremission treatment.

INDUCTION THERAPY

In young adults and children with AML, complete remission rates have ranged from 70% to 85%, while the remission rates have been lower in the very young (< 2 years of age) because of refractory disease and in the very old (> 65 years of age) because of mortality from the complications of therapy. For the past two decades, induction therapy has combined cytosine arabinoside (ara-C) with an anthracycline drug. The 'standard' schedule has been to combine ara-C at $100–200$ mg/m^2 per day as a continuous intravenous infusion for 7 days with daunorubicin 45 mg/m^2 per dose $\times 3$ (commonly referred to as 'Standard $7 + 3$'). Attempts to improve the complete remission (CR) rate by varying the ara-C dose (between 100 and 500 mg/m^2 per day) or duration (between 5 and 10 days) have been unsuccessful. The therapeutic effect of ara-C requires intracellular transport and phosphorylation of the drug to its active form (ara-CTP) and therefore the response to this drug is not directly correlated with dose. The therapeutic efficacy of ara-C and the intracellular concentration of the active agent (ara-CTP) are more closely correlated with membrane transport and metabolism of the agent in leukemic blasts than with the plasma concentration (Heinemann et al 1990).

A promising new agent, fludarabine, may be particularly helpful during remission induction because of its biochemical interaction with ara-C. Investigators at M. D. Anderson have shown that fludarabine administered prior to ara-C results in good therapeutic effects (Estey et al 1992). Although the fludarabine, or FAMP, is cytotoxic in itself, when it is administered before ara-C, it blocks ara-C metabolism resulting in a marked increase in the intracellular concentration of ara-CTP (Gandhi & Plunkett 1988, Gandhi et al 1989). Since the intracellular concentration of ara-CTP correlates directly with cytotoxicity, the combination of fludarabine and ara-C should decrease the percentage of patients failing to achieve remission because of refractory disease. Preliminary trials using fludarabine with ara-C have been reported. From phase I studies, it would appear that fludarabine given as a 10.5 mg/m^2 bolus followed by 30 mg/m^2 per day as a continuous infusion for 2 days followed by ara-C at approximately 100 mg/m^2 for 72 hours are the maximally tolerated doses in combination. Clinical trials using the combination of fludarabine, ara-C, and idarubicin for induction therapy are now beginning.

One recent advance in AML induction therapy has been determining the best anthracycline to use in combination with ara-C. Although idarubicin is not a new drug, recent randomized adult AML trials have demonstrated that idarubicin is superior to daunorubicin when combined with ara-C for remission induction in patients under the age of 50 years (Wiernik et al 1992). More patients treated with the combination of idarubicin and ara-C achieved remission after one course, a greater proportion achieved remission if two courses were required, and the duration of remission was found to be better for those patients receiving idarubicin (Berman et al 1989b, 1991, Carella et al 1989, Mandelli et al 1991). Additional benefits of idarubicin include better central nervous system (CNS) penetration (Reid et al 1990), the lack of modulation by p-glycoprotein (Berman & McBride 1992, Marie et al 1991), and the major metabolite of idarubicin having a long half-life and being cytotoxic (Speth et al 1986, Tan et al 1987). Unfortunately, idarubicin has slightly greater myelosuppression and hepatotoxicity and possibly produces a higher incidence of infectious complications, thereby making it more difficult to use in elderly patients (Berman et al 1989b, 1991). The pharmacokinetics of idarubicin appear to be the same in children and adults, and replacing the standard daunorubicin dose of 45 mg/m^2 with idarubicin at 12.5 mg/m^2 should result in similar toxicity but with better therapeutic efficacy in patients younger than 50 years. Based on multiple studies, idarubicin should now be considered the anthracycline of choice for induction therapy (Wiernik et al 1992).

Combinations of ara-C with amsacrine or ara-C with mitoxantrone have also been shown to be effective remission induction therapy (Amadori et al 1991, Berman et al 1989a, Kalwinsky et al 1988, Latagliata et al 1990, Rowe et al 1992). Whether or not these are equivalent to idarubicin plus ara-C for induction has yet to be tested. The effect of adding additional drugs like 6-thioguanine (6-TG) or VP-16 has not been shown to improve the remission induction rate except in a few small trials (Amadori et al 1991, Kalwinsky et al 1988).

High-dose ara-C alone at a dose of 3.0 g/m^2 every 12 hours for 4–6 days has been evaluated an alternative to 'standard' remission induction therapy. Uncontrolled trials have reported high remission rates but as yet there are no data comparing the outcome with high-dose ara-C alone to that of standard-dose ara-C in combination with idarubicin. The latter combination should now be considered the best therapy for patients under the age of 60 years.

In an attempt to decrease the number of patients dying of toxicity during remission therapy, a number of investigators have been using hematopoietic growth factors (e.g. G-CSF or GM-CSF) following induction therapy (Büchner et al 1991). Many oncologists are reluctant to administer growth factors to patients with AML because of the fear that such therapy would increase leukemic cell growth (Ikeda et al 1991, Park et al 1989). Initially growth factors were given to patients over 60 years of age since these patients have an increased death rate from infection or bleeding and would be the most likely to benefit from such therapy. Patients over the age of 60 years also have a higher incidence of antecedent hematologic disorders and therefore have a poorer prognosis. To date, no study has demonstrated a therapeutic benefit of G-CSF in patients receiving therapy for AML, but the ongoing German Cooperative Trial (BFM) should answer this question (Büchner et al 1991).

A completely alternative approach to improve induction therapy has been to use hematopoietic growth factors to recruit leukemic cells into cycle, thereby increasing their sensitivity to cell cycle active agents. When G-CSF or GM-CSF is given to patients with AML, there is an increase in DNA synthesis and the number of circulating leukemic blasts. Theoretically, when leukemic blasts are in cell cycle, they should be more sensitive to agents such as ara-C or VP-16. Laboratory evidence has demonstrated increased leukemic cell killing by cytotoxic agents when the drugs are administered with growth factors (Reuter et al 1992, Zühlsdorf et al 1992). However, there is no clinical evidence yet that remission rate or duration will be increased by these drugs in clinical trials.

Induction therapy for patients with acute promyelocytic leukemia

Among patients with AML, some unique groups have specific remission induction requirements. Patients with acute promyelocytic leukemia (APML) almost uniformly have been found to contain the 15;17 translocation (Larson et al 1984). This t(15;17) results in the fusion of the α-retinoic acid receptor with the PML gene which interferes with normal myeloid differentiation (Chomienne et al 1990). All-*trans*-retinoic acid (TRA) administered to patients with APML results in a high remission rate (Castaigne et al 1990, Chen et al 1991). However, patients treated only with TRA relapsed; so this drug does not eliminate the leukemic clone, but only results in cell differentiation. Complications of TRA during induction therapy include an increase in leukocyte count with leukostasis, a clinical picture similar to septic shock and adult respiratory distress syndrome. This syndrome can be controlled by the use of steroids and leukophoresis; nonetheless, whether TRA will result in a higher complete remission rate than standard 7 + 3 therapy and a longer duration of event-free survival than standard maintenance therapy is unknown. Therefore, a large multinational trial for all patients with APML is currently underway. Patients are first randomized between the standard 7 + 3 and TRA for induction. After achieving complete remission, all patients receive consolidation with high-dose ara-C; patients are then randomized a second time to maintenance with TRA for 1 year or no further therapy. This study should clarify the best way to use TRA in patients with APML.

Induction therapy for patients with secondary AML

Patients who develop AML following preleukemia, myelodysplasia, or after previous exposure to cytotoxic drugs, require special attention during induction therapy. Such patients generally have a poorer prognosis because they have more resistant disease which is often associated with cytogenetic abnormalities of chromosome 5 or 7 (Narod & Dube 1989, Rubin et al 1991).

Patients who develop secondary leukemia after treatment with cytotoxic drugs for previous malignancy are a particularly difficult problem. The first cases of secondary AML reported occurred most often in patients treated for Hodgkin's disease. These patients had chromosome 5 or 7 abnormalities and a poor complete remission rate. Such cases continue to have very poor induction rates, and BMT, when possible, appears to be a reasonable alternative to induction chemotherapy as initial treatment.

More recently, patients with secondary AML following therapy with epipodophyllins have been identified. These patients usually have FAB-M4 or FAB-M5 AML and have cytogenetic abnormalities of chromosome 11 at band q23 (Pui et al 1989). Patients with secondary AML and abnormalities of 11q23 generally have a short preleukemic phase. It is important for clinicians to be aware that these patients generally respond well to induction therapy and they should be treated as soon as the diagnosis is made. In our experience, the complete remission rate for such patients is approximately 70%. Despite the high CR rate, these patients have a poor disease-free survival and the best clinical management would appear to be allogeneic BMT in first remission.

Pharmacokinetics may also be an important consideration in planning induction therapy. Many drugs have a three- to four-fold variability in plasma concentrations. Therefore the plasma concentration achieved in some patients may be inadequate while in others it may result in significant toxicity (Avramis et al 1989, Heinemann & Jehn 1990, Ratain et al 1991).

POSTREMISSION CHEMOTHERAPY

Initially, in a small study, some patients who received only induction therapy (timed sequential pulses) had long-term leukemic-free survival (Vaughan et al 1984). However, in a recent large randomized study, patients achieving remission were randomized to no further therapy versus high-dose or low-dose postremission chemotherapy. The median duration of remission in the no maintenance therapy arm was only 4 months and the study proved that some form of postremission therapy prolongs remission duration (Cassileth et al 1988). The ideal number of maintenance courses (or duration) remains controversial. The German childhood studies have reported excellent results where children receive protracted treatment for 2 years (Creutzig et al 1985). Alternatively, extremely exciting results were obtained in one nonrandomized study when young patients where given high-dose ara-C (Wolff et al 1989). Although this study was nonrandomized and had some preselection of patients, it and other studies emphasize that intensive therapy with ara-C should be included in maintenance therapy (Dillman et al 1991, Phillips et al 1991, Ravindranath et al 1991).

The intensity of maintenance therapy has been analyzed in a very recently completed randomized trial by the Cancer Chemotherapy Group B in which patients were assigned to receive standard ara-C, increased ara-C, or intensive ara-C. The remission duration was significantly longer in those patients who received intensive therapy. Those receiving increased therapy also fared better than those receiving standard ara-C, suggesting that the intensity of maintenance therapy with ara-C clearly contributes to long-term disease-free survival (Mayer et al 1992). The old oncology belief that more is better may after all be true for the use of ara-C in postremission therapy.

It is unknown whether noncross-resistant drugs are important in postremission treatment. A number of chemotherapy trials have included AMSA, 5-azacytidine, VP-16, high-dose ara-C, and 6-TG. To date, no studies have shown an advantage of alternating noncross-resistant drugs over the same drugs used repeatedly for postremission therapy.

Because of the low incidence of CNS involvement in patients with AML, CNS prophylactic therapy has not been a major component of most trials, particularly in adult patients. However, patients with elevated leukocyte counts, monocytic or myelomonocytic leukemia, or those with abnormalities of chromosome 16 may have an increased risk of CNS disease. In pediatric series of AML, where FAB-M4 or -M5 morphology is more common, CNS prophylactic therapy has generally been administered without undue complications. Recently, the German (BFM) investigators have analyzed their results in a clinical trial which eliminated cranial irradiation. The children who did not receive CNS prophylactic radiation had a higher incidence of systemic relapse (Creutzig et al 1993). The relationship between the lack of CNS irradiation and the higher systemic relapse rate led these investigators to reinstitute CNS irradiation. Nonetheless, the role of CNS irradiation in AML therapy remains unclear. Randomized studies are required to determine if CNS irradiation can improve systemic disease control. Until such evidence is available, most physicians will not use CNS irradiation since CNS disease is rarely an isolated site of initial relapse.

Effective new drugs

New drugs which have demonstrated some efficacy and may prove to be important in AML therapy include 2-chlorodeoxyadenosine (Petzer et al

1991, Santana et al 1992). This agent is exciting since its mechanism of cytotoxicity does not require cell division, and therefore it may be effective for noncycling cells. In the phase I and II trials in children with relapsed AML (Santana et al 1992) the drug has demonstrated marked efficacy, with only hematopoietic toxicity. A study using the drug as initial induction therapy in children is under way and relapse studies in adults have also been started. The drug should be commercially available in the near future because of its excellent therapeutic effects in hairy cell leukemia.

Additionally, carboplatinum has been proven effective without undue extramedullary toxicity in relapsed patients (Martinez et al 1991, Meyers et al 1989). Whether this drug has a role in maintenance or remission induction is still unknown. Carboplatinum's predominant toxicity is hematopoietic and therefore it may be difficult to use the drug for induction therapy, but it might be used in postremission therapy.

Bone marrow transplantation as postremission therapy

A number of studies have compared intensive maintenance chemotherapy with either allogeneic or autologous BMT for disease control (Büchner et al 1992, Dahl et al 1987, Gale et al 1989, Mayer 1988, Schiller et al 1992). Marrow transplantation has generally been used for two reasons. First, it allows further intensification of effective chemotherapy. Second, in allogeneic BMT, the graft itself has been shown to have significant antileukemic effects (graft versus leukemia) (Horowitz et al 1990, Sullivan et al 1989). These benefits are partially offset by the problems associated with allogeneic BMT, which include a higher mortality risk at the time of transplant and the risk of graft versus host disease (GVHD). An additional problem with allogeneic BMT is that it is only suitable for patients less than 45–50 years of age with an acceptable donor (Berman et al 1992).

Allogeneic BMT in first remission results in about 50% 5-year leukemia-free survival. The actual relapse rate is approximately 20%. Outcome is related to age, with 50–60% event-free survival in persons under the age of 20 years versus 40% in those between the age of 20 and 50 years. In a recent study no difference was detected in transplant recipients between the age of 30 and 55 years (Gale et al 1989, 1991). Patients older than 55 years can rarely undergo allogeneic BMT, and unfortunately most AML cases are in patients over the age of 55 years, severely limiting the use of this treatment.

The standard ablative or pretransplant therapy for allogeneic BMT has been cyclophosphamide and total body irradiation (Brochstein et al 1987). Other regimens include busulfan and cyclophosphamide which has been found to be very effective (Blaise et al 1992, Copelan et al 1991). Busulfan, however, is poorly absorbed in young children, which may limit its usefulness, and busulfan pharmacokinetics may be helpful in this clinical situation. High-dose ara-C or etoposide has been incorporated into the pretransplant therapy with promising preliminary results (Forman et al 1991).

As yet, however, the use of additional drugs preallogeneic BMT have not demonstrated improved leukemia-free survival (Aurer & Gale 1991, Gale et al 1991).

There remains considerable controversy as to whether patients with AML in first remission having an HLA-identical sibling should receive a bone marrow transplant immediately, or when they develop early relapse, or in second complete remission. A number of ongoing trials in the cooperative pediatric groups are addressing this question. Although the overall survival with BMT appears superior to chemotherapy, almost 25–30% of patients will be cured with chemotherapy alone and therefore they can avoid transplantation. In addition, a number of patients who relapse can be salvaged with bone marrow transplant. When clinical trials comparing transplant with postremission chemotherapy are summarized, the vast majority demonstrate that sibling transplant recipients have a higher disease-free survival and overall survival. Thus, until results from randomized trials are available, BMT from sibling donors appears to be the treatment of choice for young patients (< 20 years of age) not being treated on protocols. Long-term follow-up of patients undergoing transplant in early relapse or in second complete remission is needed to help select the best therapy for such patients. For patients with disease refractory to induction therapy, bone marrow transplant may be the treatment of choice and the only treatment with curative potential (Forman et al 1991).

The use of alternative matched unrelated donor (MUD) bone marrow transplant is being explored for patients without a suitable sibling donor. Results demonstrate that successful transplants are possible but the risk of graft rejection and GVHD is considerably greater (McGlave et al 1990, 1993). With further development of molecular typing and specific subtyping in the DR region, it may be possible to better select matched unrelated donors in the future and overcome these problems. Nonetheless, until further reports of MUD transplants are available, most clinicians feel they should be reserved for patients who relapse or are at extremely high risk for relapse.

Autologous bone marrow transplants

Autologous bone marrow transplant has been evaluated in patients with AML. Typically, bone marrow or blood cells are collected and cryopreserved when the patient is in remission. The patient later receives high-dose chemotherapy followed by reinfusion of the cryopreserved marrow. Autologous BMT is safely performed in patients with AML under the age of 55 years. Thus, like allogeneic BMT, a large percentage of older patients with AML cannot be treated with autologous BMT. The significant limitation of this type of therapy is the fact that the cryopreserved marrow is likely to be contaminated with leukemic cells.

Attempts to decrease the number of residual leukemic cells have led most investigators to purge the autologous marrow before cryopreservation.

Methods for purging autologous marrow of leukemic cells have included the use of drugs, monoclonal antibody and complement lysis (Ball et al 1990, Stiff et al 1991), lecithin separation, monoclonal antibody positive selection (Lebkowski et al 1992), or long-term in vitro bone marrow culture (Dexter 1992). More recently, interleukin (IL-2) or lymphokine activated killer cells have been proposed as a method to purge bone marrow (Charak et al 1990). There is a large amount of laboratory evidence that purging can eliminate leukemic cells from the bone marrow (Rowley et al 1989). A number of studies have reported good results with purged marrows (Ball et al 1990, Stewart et al 1985); however, other studies have demonstrated similar outcomes when purging was not used (Gorin et al 1990). In one study, patients in second complete remission were transplanted without purging and some patients achieved long-term survival (Chopra et al 1991). No trials randomizing between purging or no purging have been undertaken since the number of patients required to answer this question is quite large.

Recently, using retroviral vectors to mark leukemic cells, evidence that relapse can occur from morphologically and cytogenetically normal marrow has been obtained. This work demonstrates that at least some relapses following autologous BMT have been from the infused marrow (Brenner et al 1993, Rill et al 1992). These studies have not yet answered the question as to whether purging is capable of eliminating these clonogenic leukemic cells or whether those patients surviving after purging survive because the marrows were leukemia free or contained a lower number of viable leukemic cells. Purging may only be effective in a small group of patients with leukemic cells that are eliminated by the purging agent.

As described previously, one advantage of allogeneic BMT over autologous BMT is that GVL provides a significant improvement in leukemic control. Relapse occurs in only 20% of patients undergoing allogeneic BMT compared with about 60% in patients receiving chemotherapy. The beneficial effect of GVL has resulted in a number of investigators attempting to induce GVL in the autologous transplant setting. Most investigators are using IL-2 to activate T-cells and hopefully these will eliminate any residual leukemia (Foa et al 1991). Many studies have demonstrated a period of T-cell disregulation following autologous BMT, and IL-2 during this period increases in vitro leukemic cell killing (Heslop et al 1991, Higuchi et al 1991). Alternatively, cyclosporine has been used to disregulate T-cells following autologous transplant, thereby inducing some effects of GVL and hopefully improving outcome (Yeager et al 1992). Immune augmentation post transplant is becoming a very exciting area of research and may provide additional therapeutic tool in the therapy of AML.

We are at a turning point in the therapy of AML. We are now beginning to improve the remission/induction rate through the addition of idarubicin. A number of new agents have become available which might be very helpful, especially fludarabine and 2-chlorodeoxyadenosine. The role of growth factors in AML therapy is unknown but these drugs may be very useful in decreasing mortality or increasing cell killing. Finally, we are developing the ability to manipulate the immune system post transplant in an attempt to improve outcome through GVL effect. Therefore, for oncologists involved in the therapy of AML, the next 5 years may prove to be very rewarding.

KEY POINTS FOR CLINICAL PRACTICE

- Fludarabine is an active new drug which shows great promise for improving the efficacy of ara-C because of its biochemical modulation of ara-C.
- Idarubicin is the anthracycline of choice for induction therapy in younger patients.
- Growth factor use during induction has not yet been shown to change the induction success rates except possibly in older patients.
- 2-Chlorodeoxyadenosine is effective in AML but its specific role in therapy of AML is unknown.
- Carboplatinum appears to be effective in AML.
- When used in postremission therapy, the higher the dose of ara-C the better the disease-free survival.
- All-*trans*-retinoic acid is useful in acute progranulocytic leukemia.
- Allogeneic bone marrow transplant in first complete remission results in the best disease control but survival is only slightly improved over the use of maintenance chemotherapy.
- In autologous bone marrow transplants, relapse may arise from the cryopreserved marrow, but the efficacy of purging autologous marrow remains unproven.

REFERENCES

Amadori S, Arcese W, Isacchi G et al 1991 Mitoxantrone, etoposide, and intermediate-dose cytarabine: an effective and tolerable regimen for the treatment of refractory acute myeloid leukemia. J Clin Oncol 9(7): 1210–1214

Aurer I, Gale R P 1991 Are new conditioning regimens for transplants in acute myelogenous leukemia better? Bone Marrow Transplant 7: 255–261

Avramis V I, Weinberg K I, Sato J K et al 1989 Pharmacology studies of 1-β-D-arabinofuranosylcytosine in pediatric patients with leukemia and lymphoma after a biochemically optimal regimen of loading bolus plus continuous infusion of the drug. Cancer Res 49: 241–247

Ball E D, Mills L E, Cornwell G G et al 1990 Autologous bone marrow transplantation for acute myeloid leukemia using monoclonal antibody-purged bone marrow. Blood 75(5): 1199–1206

Berman E, Arlin Z A, Gaynor J et al 1989a Comparative trial of cytarabine and thioguanine in combination with amsacrine or daunorubicin in patients with untreated acute nonlymphocytic leukemia: results of the L-16M protocol. Leukemia 3(2): 115–121

Berman E, Raymond V, Gee T S et al 1989b Idarubicin in acute leukemia: results of US trials. Bone Marrow Transplant 4 (Suppl 1): 49

Berman E, Heller G, Santorsa J et al 1991 Results of a randomized trial comparing idarubicin and cytosine arabinoside with daunorubicin and cytosine arabinoside in adult patients with newly diagnosed acute myelogenous leukemia. Blood 77(8): 1666–1674

Berman E, McBride M 1992 Comparative cellular pharmacology of daunorubicin and idarubicin in human multidrug-resistant leukemia cells. Blood 79(12): 3267–3273

Berman E, Little C, Gee T et al 1992 Reasons that patients with acute myelogenous leukemia do not undergo allogeneic bone marrow transplantation. N Engl J Med 326(3): 156–160

Blaise D, Maraninchi D, Archimbaud E et al 1992 Allogeneic bone marrow transplantation for acute myeloid leukemia in first remission: a randomized trial of a busulfan–cytoxan versus cytoxan–total body irradiation as preparative regimen: a report from the Groupe d'Etudes de la Greffe de Moelle Osseuse. Blood 79(10): 2578–2582

Brenner M K, Rill D R, Moen R C et al 1993 Gene marking to trace origin of relapse after autologous bone marrow transplantation. Lancet 341: 85–86

Brochstein J A, Kernan N A, Groshen S et al 1987 Allogeneic bone marrow transplantation after hyperfractionated total-body irradiation and cyclophosphamide in children with acute leukemia. N Engl J Med 317(26): 1618–1624

Büchner Th, Hiddemann W, Koenigsmann M et al 1991 Recombinant human granulocyte-macrophage colony-stimulating factor after chemotherapy in patients with acute myeloid leukemia at higher age or after relapse. Blood 78(5): 1190–1197

Büchner Th, Hiddemann W, Wörmann B et al 1992 Long-term results in adult AML: conventional induction with maintenance versus double induction with maintenance versus allogeneic or autologous BMT. Data from AMLCG. Ann Hematol 64 (Suppl): A113

Buckley J D, Chard R L, Baehner R L et al 1989 Improvement in outcome for children with acute nonlymphocytic leukemia: a report from the Childrens Cancer Study Group. Cancer 63: 1457–1475

Carella A M, Pungolino E, Piatti G et al 1989 Idarubicin in combination with etoposide and cytarabine in adult acute nonlymphoblastic leukaemia (ANLL). Bone Marrow Transplant 4 (Suppl 1): 50–51

Cassileth P A, Harrington D P, Hines J D et al 1988 Maintenance chemotherapy prolongs remission duration in adult acute nonlymphocytic leukemia. J Clin Oncol 6: 583–587

Castaigne S, Chomienne C, Daniel M T et al 1990 All-trans retinoic acid as a differentiating therapy for acute promyelocytic leukemia. I. Clinical results. Blood 76(9): 1704–1709

Charak B S, Malloy B, Agah R, Mazumder A 1990 A novel approach to purging of leukemia by activation of bone marrow with interleukin 2. Bone Marrow Transplant 6: 193–198

Chen Z X, Xue Y Q, Zhang R et al 1991 A clinical and experimental study on all-trans retinoic acid-treated acute promyelocytic leukemia in patients. Blood 78(6): 1413–1419

Chomienne C, Ballerini P, Balitrand N et al 1990 The retinoic acid receptor alpha gene is rearranged in retinoic acid-sensitive promyelocytic leukemias. Leukemia 4: 802

Chopra R, Goldstone A H, McMillan A K et al 1991 Successful treatment of acute myeloid leukemia beyond first remission with autologous bone marrow transplantation using busulfan/cyclophosphamide and unpurged marrow: the British Autograft Group experience. J Clin Oncol 9(10): 1840–1847

Copelan E A, Biggs J C, Thompson J M et al 1991 Treatment for acute myelocytic leukemia with allogeneic bone marrow transplantation following preparation with BuCy2. Blood 78(3): 838–843

Creutzig U, Ritter J, Riehm H et al 1985 Improved treatment results in childhood acute myelogenous leukemia: a report of the German cooperative study AML-BFM-78. Blood 65: 298–304

Creutzig U, Ritter J, Schellong G 1990 Identification of two risk groups in childhood acute myelogenous leukemia fter therapy intensification in study AML-BFM-83 as compared with study AML-BFM-78. Blood 75(10): 1932–1940

Creutzig U, Ritter J, Zimmermann M, Schellong G 1993 Does cranial irradiation reduce the risk for bone marrow relapse in acute myelogenous leukemia? Unexpected results of the childhood acute myelogenous leukemia study BFM-87. J Clin Oncol 11(2): 279–286

Cuneo A, Michaux J L, Ferrant A et al 1992 Correlation of cytogenetic patterns and clinicobiological features in adult acute myeloid leukemia expressing lymphoid markers. Blood 79(3): 720–727

Dahl G V, Kalwinsky D K, Mirro J, Look A T 1987 A comparison of cytokinetically based versus intensive chemotherapy for childhood acute myelogenous leukemia. Haematol Blood Trans 30: 83–87

Dexter T M 1992 Autologous marrow transplantation using cultured cells. Ann Hematol 64 (Suppl): A77

Dillman R O, Davis R B, Green M R et al 1991 A comparative study of two different doses of cytarabine for acute myeloid leukemia: a phase III trial of Cancer and Leukemia Group B. Blood 78(10): 2520–2526

Dutcher J P 1990 Therapy for acute leukemia in adults. Curr Opin Oncol 2(1): 41–48

Estey E, Kantarjian H, Plunkett W et al 1992 Treatment of refractory acute myelogenous leukemia with fludarabine + cytosine arabinoside. Am Soc Clin Oncol (ASCO) 11: 268 (Abstract)

Foa R, Meloni G, Tosti S et al 1991 Treatment of acute myeloid leukaemia patients with recombinant interleukin 2: a pilot study. Br J Haematol 77: 491–496

Forman S J, Schmidt G M, Nademanee A P et al 1991 Allogeneic bone marrow transplantation as therapy for primary induction failure for patients with acute leukemia. J Clin Oncol 9(9): 1570–1574

Gale R P, Horowitz M M, Biggs J C et al 1989 Transplant or chemotherapy in acute myelogenous leukaemia. Lancet 1: 1119–1122

Gale R P, Butturini A, Horowitz M M 1991 Does more intensive therapy increase cures in acute leukemia? Semin Hematol 28(3): 93–94

Gandhi V, Plunkett W 1988 Modulation of arabinosylnucleoside metabolism by arabinosylnucleotides in human leukemia cells. Cancer Res 48: 329–334

Gandhi V, Nowak B, Keating M J, Plunkett W 1989 Modulation of arabinosylcytosine metabolism by arabinosyl-2-fluoroadenine in lymphocytes from patients with chronic lymphocytic leukemia: implications for combination therapy. Blood 74(6): 2070–2075

Gorin N C, Aegerter P, Auvert B et al 1990 Autologous bone marrow transplantation for acute myelocytic leukemia in first remission: a European survey of the role of marrow purging. Blood 75: 1606–1614

Heinemann V, Jehn U 1990 Rationales for a pharmacologically optimized treatment of acute nonlymphocytic leukemia with cytosine arabinoside. Leukemia 4(11): 790–796

Heslop H E, Duncombe A S, Reittie J E et al 1991 Interleukin 2 infusion induces haemopoietic growth factors and modifies marrow regeneration after chemotherapy or autologous marrow transplantation. Br J Haematol 77: 237–244

Hicsonmez G, Ozsoylu S, Gurgey A et al 1989 High-dose methylprednisolone for remission induction in children with acute nonlymphoblastic leukemia. Eur J Haematol 42(5): 498–500

Higuchi C M, Thompson J A, Petersen F B et al 1991 Toxicity and immunomodulatory effects of interleukin-2 after autologous bone marrow transplantation for hematologic malignancies. Blood 77(12): 2561–2568

Horowitz M M, Gale R P, Sondel P M et al 1990 Graft-versus-leukemia reaction after bone marrow transplantation. Blood 75: 555–562

Ikeda H, Kanakura Y, Tamaki T et al 1991 Expression of functional role of the proto-oncogene c-*kit* in acute myeloblastic leukemia cells. Blood 78(11): 2962–2968

Kalwinsky D, Mirro J, Schell M et al 1988 Early intensification of chemotherapy for childhood acute nonlymphoblastic leukemia: improved remission induction with a five-drug regimen including etoposide. J Clin Oncol 6: 1134–1143

Kalwinsky D K, Raimondi S, Schell M J et al 1990 Prognostic importance of cytogenetic subgroups in de novo pediatric acute nonlymphocytic leukemia. J Clin Oncol 8: 75–83

Krischer J P, Steuber C P, Vietti T J 1989 Long-term results in the treatment of acute non-lymphocytic leukemia: a Pediatric Oncology Group Study. Med Pediatr Oncol 17(5): 401–408

Larson R A, Kondo K, Vardiman J W 1984 Evidence for a 15;17 translocation in every patient with acute promyelocytic leukemia. Am J Med 76: 827

Latagliata R, Petti M C, Spiriti M A et al 1990 High doses of ara-C and m-AMSA in the treatment of refractory acute nonlymphocytic leukemia. Haematologica 75(3): 249–251

Lebkowski J S, Schain L R, Okrongly D et al 1992 Rapid isolation of human CD34 hematopoietic stem cells — purging of human tumor cells. Transplantation 53: 1011–1019

Lowenberg B, Verdonck L J, Dekker A W et al 1990 Autologous bone marrow transplantation in acute myeloid leukemia in first remission: results of a Dutch prospective study. J Clin Oncol 8(2): 287–294

McGlave P B, Beatty P, Ash R et al 1990 Therapy for chronic myelogenous leukemia with unrelated donor bone marrow transplantation: results in 102 cases. Blood 75: 1728–1732

McGlave P, Bartsch G, Andselti C et al 1993 Unrelated donor marrow transplantation therapy for chronic myelogenous leukemia: initial experience of the national marrow donor program. Blood 81(2): 543–550

Mandelli F, Petti M C, Ardia A et al 1991 A randomized clinical trial comparing idarubicin and cytarabine to daunorubicin and cytarabine in the treatment of acute nonlymphoid leukaemia: a multicentric study from the Italian Cooperative Group GIMEMA. Eur J Cancer 27(6): 750–755

Marie J P, Zittoun R, Sikic B I 1991 Mkultidrug resistance (mdr1) gene expression in adult acute leukemias: correlations with treatment outcome and in vitro drug sensitivity. Blood 78(3): 586–592

Martinez J A, Martin G, Sanz G F 1991 A phase II clinical trial of carboplatin infusion in high-risk acute nonlymphoblastic leukemia. J Clin Oncol 9(1): 39–43

Mayer R J 1988 Allogeneic transplantation versus intensive chemotherapy in first remission acute leukemia: Is there a 'best choice'? J Clin Oncol 6(10): 1532–1536

Mayer R J, Davis R B, Schiffer C A et al 1992 Comparative evaluation of intensive post remission therapy with different dose schedules of ara-C in adults with acute myeloid leukemia (AML): initial results of a CALGB phase III study. Ann Hematol 64 (Suppl): A113

Meyers F J, Welborn J, Lewis J P et al 1989 Infusion carboplatin treatment of relapsed and refractory acute leukemia: evidence of efficacy with minimal extramedullary toxicity at intermediate doses. J Clin Oncol 7(2): 173–178

Narod S A, Dube I D 1989 Occupational history and involvement of chromosomes 5 and 7 in acute nonlymphocytic leukemia. Cancer Genet Cytogenet 38(2): 261–269

Park L S, Waldron P E, Friend D et al 1989 Interleukin-3, GM-CSF, and G-CSF receptor expression on cell lines and primary leukemia cells: receptor heterogeneity and relationship to growth factor responsiveness. Blood 74(1): 56–65

Petzer A L, Bilgeri R, Zilian U et al 1991 Inhibitory effect of 2-chlorodeoxyadenosine on granulocytic, erythroid, and T-lymphocytic colony growth. Blood 78(10): 2583–2587

Phillips G L, Reece D E, Shepard J D et al 1991 High dose cytarabine and daunorubicin induction and post-remission chemotherapy for the treatment of acute myelogenous leukemia in adults. Blood 77: 1429–1435

Pui C-H, Behm F G, Raimondi S C et al 1989 Secondary acute myeloid leukemia in children treated for acute lymphoid leukemia. N Engl J Med 321: 136–142

Raimondi S C, Kalwinsky D K, Hayashi Y et al 1989 The cytogenetics of childhood acute nonlymphocytic leukemia. Cancer Genet Cytogenet 40(1): 13–27

Ratain M J, Mick R, Schilsky R L et al 1991 Pharmacologically based dosing of etoposide: a means of safely increasing dose intensity. J Clin Oncol 9(8): 1480–1486

Ravindranath Y, Steuber C P, Krischer J et al 1991 High dose cytarabine for intensification of early therapy of childhood acute myeloid leukemia: a Pediatric Oncology Group study. J Clin Oncol 9: 572–580

Reid J M, Pendergrass T W, Krailo M D et al 1990 Plasma pharmacokinetics and cerebrospinal fluid concentrations of idarubicin and idarubicinol in pediatric leukemia patients: a Childrens Cancer Study Group report. Cancer Res 50: 6525–6528

Reuter C, Landwehr U, Kiehl M et al 1992 Modulation of intracellular ara-C metabolism in AML blasts by GM-CSF pretreatment in vitro. Ann Hematol 64 (Suppl): A98

Rill D R, Moen R C, Buschle M et al 1992 An approach for the analysis of relapse and marrow reconstitution after autologous marrow transplantation using retrovirus-mediated gene transfer. Blood 79: 2694–2700

Rowe J M, Andersen J W, Mazza J J 1992 Mitoxantrone in the treatment of acute myelogenous and lymphoblastic leukemia: the ECOG and University of Rochester experience. Ann Hematol 64 (Suppl): A75

Rowley S D, Jones R J, Piantadosi S et al 1989 Efficacy of ex vivo purging for autologous bone marrow transplantation in the treatment of acute nonlymphoblastic leukemia. Blood 74(1): 501–506

Rubin C M, Arthur D C, Woods W G et al 1991 Therapy-related myelodysplastic syndrome and acute myeloid leukemia in children: correlation between chromosomal abnormalities and prior therapy. Blood 78(11): 2982–2988

Santana V M, Mirro J, Kearns C et al 1992 2-Chlorodeoxyadenosine produces a high rate of complete hematologic remission in relapsed acute myeloid leukemia. J Clin Oncol 10: 364–370

Schiffer C A, Lee E J, Tomiyasu T et al 1989 Prognostic impact of cytogenetic abnormalities in patients with de novo acute nonlymphocytic leukemia. Blood 73(1): 263–270

Schiller G J, Nimer S D, Territo M C et al 1992 Bone marrow transplantation versus high-dose cytarabine-based consolidation chemotherapy for acute myelogenous leukemia in first remission. J Clin Oncol 10: 41–46

Speth P A J, van de Loo F A J, Linssen P C M et al 1986 Plasma and human leukemic cell pharmacokinetics of oral and intravenous 4-demethoxydaunomycin. Clin Pharmacol Ther 40(6): 643–649

Steuber C P, Civin C, Krischer J et al 1991 A comparison of induction and maintenance therapy for acute nonlymphocytic leukemia in childhood: results of a Pediatric Oncology Group study. J Clin Oncol 9(2): 247–258

Stewart P, Buckner C D, Bensinger W et al 1985 Autologous marrow transplantation in patients with acute nonlymphocytic leukemia in first remission. Exp Hematol 13: 267–272

Stiff P J, Schulz W C, Bishop M, Marks L 1991 Anti-CD33 monoclonal antibody and etoposide/cytosine arabinoside combinations for the ex vivo purification of bone marrow in acute nonlymphocytic leukemia. Blood 77(2): 355–362

Sullivan K M, Weiden P L, Storb R et al 1989 Influence of acute and chronic graft-versus-host disease on relapse and survival after bone marrow transplantation from HLA-identical siblings as treatment of acute and chronic leukemia. Blood 73(6): 1720–1728

Tan C T C, Hancock C, Steinherz P et al 1987 Phase I and clinical pharmacological study of 4-demethoxydaunorubicin (idarubicin) in children with advanced cancer. Cancer Res 47: 2990–2995

Vaughan W P, Karp J E, Burke P J 1984 Two-cycle timed-sequential chemotherapy for adult acute nonlymphocytic leukemia. Blood 64: 975–980

Wiernik P H, Banks P L C, Case D C Jr et al 1992 Cytarabine plus idarubicin or daunorubicin as induction and consolidation therapy for previously untreated adult patients with acute myeloid leukemia. Blood 79(2): 313–319

Wolff S N, Herzig R H, Fay J W et al 1989 High dose cytarabine and daunorubicin as consolidation therapy for acute myeloid leukemia in first remission: long-term follow up and results. J Clin Oncol 7: 1260–1267

Yeager A M, Vogelsang G B, Jones R J et al 1992 Induction of cutaneous graft-versus-host disease by administration of cyclosporine to patients undergoing autologous bone marrow transplantation for acute myeloid leukemia. Blood 79: 3031–3035

Zühlsdorf M, Busemann C, Ameling C et al 1992 Effects on ara-C cytotoxicity for AML-colony forming cells by priming with rh GM-CSF and rhIL-3 in vitro and in vivo. Ann Hematol 64 (Suppl): A73

5

Ras and GAP

D. C. S. Huang   J. F. Hancock

Our understanding of the genetic basis of human cancer has been enhanced by the identification of an ever increasing number of oncogenes. In recent years, there has been intensive research into the function of proteins encoded by these genes since it is clear that they play key roles in the regulation of cell growth and differentiation.

One of the first oncogenes to be identified was *ras*. The *ras* genes are frequently mutated in a wide range of human malignancies including the acute leukaemias and the myelodysplastic syndromes. The normal function of Ras proteins and the signal transduction pathways in which they operate continue to be the focus of extensive investigation. Our aim here is to highlight recent results on Ras and the proteins it interacts with (such as GAP) rather than to provide a comprehensive review (for which see Barbacid 1987, Bourne et al 1990, 1991, Hall 1990, Lacal & McCormick 1993). In particular, we will consider how Ras and GAP interact with each other and with other cellular proteins in a putative signal transduction pathway from the cell surface to the nucleus. In discussing this area, we will also address the putative function of certain other Ras-related proteins and their own GAP molecules. Only with this background, for example, can all the possible biological consequences of the Bcr–Abl translocation in chronic myeloid leukaemia be fully appreciated.

Given that *ras* mutation is one of the commonest defects in human tumours, chemotherapeutic agents which interfere with Ras function might in future have a significant role to play in the management of these malignancies. Recent work on one aspect of Ras biology, namely how the Ras protein is translocated from its site of synthesis in the cytosol to its site of action on the plasma membrane, has identified an approach for designing such drugs. This will be discussed at the end of the chapter.

RAS STRUCTURE AND BIOCHEMISTRY

The three *ras* genes (H-*ras*, K-*ras* and N-*ras*) encode small 21 kDa guanine nucleotide binding proteins which are highly conserved in evolution and are ubiquitously expressed in mammalian tissues. Studies in vivo and in vitro indicate that the Ras proteins play an important role in signalling for cell growth and differentiation and the biochemical pathways in which they operate are only now starting to be unravelled.

Ras proteins bind GTP (guanosine triphosphate) and GDP (guanosine diphosphate) and are localized to the inner surface of the plasma membrane. They function as molecular switches, being active when bound to GTP and inactive when bound to GDP (Fig. 5.1A). In a signal transduction pathway, it is envisaged that upstream events activate Ras by promoting the formation of the active GTP-bound form. The Ras proteins possess an intrinsic GTPase activity which hydrolyses GTP to GDP and thus returns Ras to the inactive GDP-bound ground state. Specific conformational changes are associated

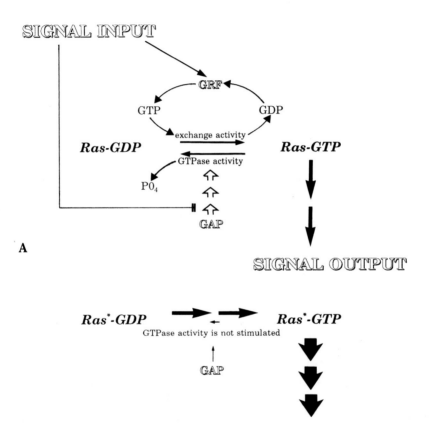

Fig. 5.1 A The GTPase cycle of Ras. Signal input leads to the activation of Ras either by stimulating the activity of the exchange factor (e.g. *ras*GRF) or by inhibiting the activity of GAP. The net result is increased levels of GTP-bound Ras which signals downstream for cell growth and differentiation. **B** Oncogenic mutant Ras escapes control by GAP. The intrinsic GTPase activity of oncogenic mutant Ras* is not stimulated by GAP even though GAP binds normally to the GTP-bound form of oncogenic Ras*. As the GTPase activity is not stimulated, oncogenic mutant Ras* remains locked in the GTP-bound form and continues to signal in an uncontrolled manner.

with the active and inactive states which allow Ras to interact with specific proteins.

Two classes of proteins which interact directly with Ras have been identified. These are the guanine nucleotide releasing factors (GRFs) and the GTPase activating proteins (GAPs), which will be discussed in the next section. GRFs are exchange proteins which stimulate dissociation of GDP from Ras. The effect is to switch Ras into the activated GTP-bound form since GTP is in a 10–20 molar excess over GDP in the cell. A mammalian GRF (*ras*GRF) which has recently been cloned is homologous to a yeast exchange protein CDC25 (Shou et al 1992) (Fig. 5.2C). Overexpression of yeast CDC25 transforms fibroblasts by switching Ras into the active GTP-bound state.

*ras*GAP AND NEUROFIBROMIN

The Ras proteins have intrinsic GTPase (guanosine triphosphatase) activity which slowly hydrolyses bound GTP to GDP. This activity is greatly enhanced by *ras*GAP, a 120 kDa cytoplasmic protein, which binds to GTP-bound Ras and stimulates GTP hydrolysis 1000-fold (Trahey & McCormick 1987). One function of *ras*GAP is therefore to switch Ras from the active GTP-bound form to the inactive GDP-bound form. Although *ras*GAP clearly functions as a downregulator of Ras, a number of experiments suggest that it may have other roles. For example, amino acids 32–40 of Ras constitute a domain which is known to interact with downstream 'effector' proteins. *ras*GAP also binds to this domain (Adari et al 1988, Cales et al 1988) implying that *ras*GAP itself may be an effector protein for Ras, and it has been suggested that *ras*GAP may function both as a signal transducer and as a signal terminator for Ras (McCormick 1989).

A number of functional domains of *ras*GAP have been defined by analysis of *ras*GAP deletion mutants. The C-terminal third of the protein alone is sufficient to stimulate the GTPase activity of Ras and is called the catalytic domain (Marshall et al 1989). At the N-terminus of *ras*GAP are found two SH2 domains (SH:Src homology) and a single SH3 domain. SH2 and SH3 domains are being found in an increasing number of proteins (Fig. 5.2A) involved in signal transduction, including tyrosine kinases such as Abl, and cytoskeletal proteins (reviewed by Koch et al 1991 and by Pawson & Gish 1992). SH2 and SH3 domains mediate protein–protein interactions and may provide a mechanism by which signalling proteins talk to each other. Specific SH2 domains bind with high affinity to phosphotyrosine residues within a specified amino acid sequence. The SH3 domains binds proline/serine-rich domains of cytoskeletal and other proteins. There is therefore intense interest in the role *ras*GAP may play in signal transduction not only via Ras but also by its interaction with other signalling proteins, which will be discussed in the next section.

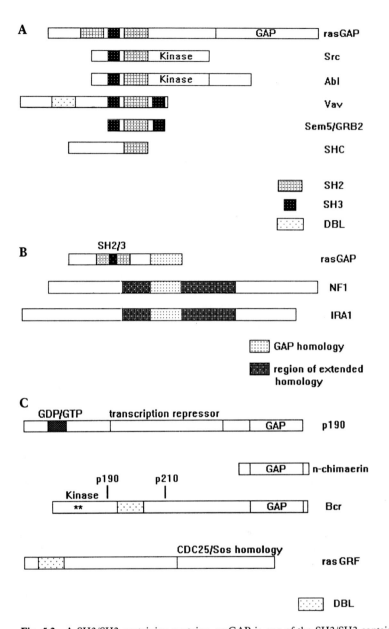

Fig. 5.2 A SH2/SH3-containing proteins. *ras*GAP is one of the SH2/SH3-containing proteins which also contains a domain with enzymatic activity. Src and Abl have tyrosine kinase activity. However, other SH2/SH3-containing proteins, such as Sem5/GRB2, do not contain separate enzymatic activity and these proteins have been termed 'adaptors'. **B** Sequence homology between *ras*GAP and NF1. (neurofibromin) NF1 contains a domain that has sequence (and functional homology) to *ras*GAP; however, it does not have SH2/SH3 domains. Instead it has extended sequence homology with the downregulators of RAS in yeast, IRA1 and IRA2. **C** Proteins with GAP activity on the Ras-related proteins. p190 and Bcr are both multidomain proteins. p190 can function as a GAP for Rho, Rac and CDC42; Bcr and n-chimaerin can function as a GAP for Rac. Bcr also has a serine/threonine kinase domain at the N-terminus as well as a domain with homology to the *dbl* oncogene. The p210 Bcr–Abl fusion protein formed as the result of the 9;22 translocation in CML retains the Dbl homology domain whereas in the p190 fusion protein characteristic of Ph + ve ALL does not. Another Dbl-containing protein is the exchange factor for Ras, *ras*GRF. The domain of *ras*GRF with exchange activity is homologous to two other known exchange factors, CDC25 (in yeast) and Sos (in *Drosophila*).

A second GAP for Ras was accidentally discovered in 1990 by two separate groups who were searching for the gene involved in Type 1 (von Recklinghausen's) neurofibromatosis (Ballester et al 1990, Xu et al 1990). A large gene encoding for a 280 kDa protein, neurofibromin (also known as NF1), was identified. Sequence analysis revealed a domain within the gene that is significantly homologous to the C-terminal catalytic domain of *ras*GAP. It was then demonstrated that full-length neurofibromin or the GAP-related domain (NF1GRD) alone can function as a GAP for Ras, although the kinetics of the interaction between neurofibromin and Ras are different from that of *ras*GAP and Ras. Neurofibromin also interacts with the effector binding domain (between amino acids 32–40) of Ras (Martin et al 1990). However, neurofibromin, unlike *ras*GAP, has no SH2 or SH3 domains and neurofibromin shows more extensive homologies with the yeast proteins IRA1 and IRA2 which function as GAPs for yeast RAS (Fig. 5.2B).

Why Ras should require two GAPs is as yet unclear. An attractive hypothesis is that the interaction of *ras*GAP or neurofibromin with Ras results in different signal outputs although there is little evidence for this at the present time. Interestingly, there is accumulating evidence that neurofibromin is a tumour suppressor gene and that loss of this gene by translocations, missense mutations or inactivating mutations predisposes to tumorigenesis (Basu et al 1992, DeClue et al 1992, Li et al 1992).

HOW DOES Ras FUNCTION?

In fibroblasts, Ras is required for signalling from membrane associated tyrosine kinases, such as the PDGF (platelet derived growth factor) receptor, Fms and Src (Smith et al 1986). Also, following cross linking of the T-cell receptor, Ras accumulates in the active GTP-bound form, suggesting a role for Ras in T-cell activation (Downward et al 1990). The key questions are: how does activation of membrane-associated tyrosine kinases regulate the nucleotide bound to Ras? And what proteins lie immediately downstream of activated Ras in a signal transduction pathway which ultimately results in altered transcription from Ras responsive genes?

In activated T-cells, some 50% of Ras is switched to the GTP-bound form following T-cell receptor activation. However, the rate of exchange of nucleotide on and off Ras is unchanged and activation correlates instead with a protein kinase C-dependent inhibition of total GAP activity within the T-cell. These data indicate that inhibiting the activity of a negative regulator of Ras rather than stimulating the activity of its exchange factor may be a mechanism of accumulating Ras–GTP (Downward et al 1990). A related observation has been made in Schwann tumour cell lines derived from patients with neurofibromatosis. These cells lack functional neurofibromin and, in the absence of this potent downregulator, 50% of Ras is in the GTP-bound state. It is as yet unclear why the *ras*GAP in these cells, which is functional, is insufficient to maintain Ras in the GDP-bound state (Basu et al 1992, DeClue et al 1992). Recently proteins with guanine nucleotide exchange activity have been cloned and are being characterized (Kaibuchi et al 1991, Martegani et al 1992, Shou et al 1992). These studies should rapidly throw light on whether the activity of any of these exchange factors is directly regulated by activated tyrosine kinases as this may be an alternative mechanism for activating Ras.

That Ras plays a key role in signal transduction from the cell surface to the nucleus has been highlighted by recent studies on MAP (mitogen-activated protein) kinases. These proteins are activated in response to mitogens such as PDGF and participate in a phosphorylation cascade resulting in the induction of gene expression. It has now been shown that Ras function is required for activation of MAP kinase (De Vries-Smits et al 1992, Leevers & Marshall 1992, Thomas et al 1992, Wood et al 1992). The oncogene *raf* has also been slotted into this cascade (Howe et al 1992, Kyriakis et al 1992). Ras is upstream of Raf, a serine/threonine kinase, which can activate a MAP kinase kinase which in turn phosphorylates and activates MAP kinase (Fig. 5.3). Amongst the known substrates of activated MAP kinase are the nuclear oncoproteins such as Jun and Myc as well as the S6 kinases.

What other proteins are potentially involved in Ras signalling? In cells transformed by v-*src* or mitogenically stimulated with growth factors such as PDGF, *ras*GAP associates with two phosphoproteins known by their molecular weights as p62 and p190 (Ellis et al 1990, Kaplan et al 1990, Molloy et al 1989). p190 is phosphorylated on tyrosine and serine residues and forms a stoichiometric complex with *ras*GAP in the cytosol following tyrosine kinase activation. Some 50% of cellular *ras*GAP is complexed with p190 and this p190–*ras*GAP complex has reduced GAP activity on Ras compared with non-complexed *ras*GAP (Moran et al 1991). p62 is highly phosphorylated in cells transformed by tyrosine kinases but is less abundant in *ras*GAP complexes than is p190. Both of these proteins have recently been cloned and the predicted amino acid sequences contain some remarkable surprises.

Sequence analysis of p62 reveals that it has an RNA binding domain and indeed p62 binds to RNA and to DNA in vitro (Wong et al 1992). Thus it may be a direct link between signalling from tyrosine kinases and regulation of mRNA processing.

p190 turns out to be a multidomain protein (Settleman et al 1992) (Fig. 5.2C). At the N-terminus is a domain which binds guanine nucleotides (like the Ras proteins) and at the C-terminus is a domain with homology to n-chimaerin (a protein related to Bcr). n-Chimaerin homology is cropping up in an increasing number of proteins. One of the first was Bcr. Hall and coworkers (Diekmann et al 1991) whilst sequencing the GAP for a Ras-related protein Rho identified a peptide which was identical to part of the C-terminus of Bcr and which was highly homologous to n-chimaerin. They therefore tested whether the C-terminal domain of Bcr and n-chimaerin had GAP activity on Rho. They did not. However, they had GAP activity on a related protein, Rac, which is expressed at high levels in myeloid cells. It is therefore

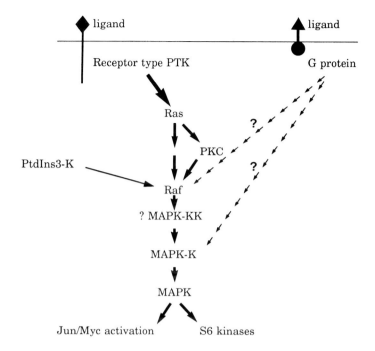

Fig. 5.3 Model of receptor stimulated protein phosphorylation cascade. A number of different stimuli can set off a phosphorylation cascade resulting in the induction of gene expression. Raf is a key protein in this cascade. It is unclear whether Raf is a MAP kinase kinase kinase or whether it is upstream of an as yet unidentified MAP kinase kinase kinase. Abbreviations: MAPK-KK, MAP kinase kinase kinase; MAPK-K, MAP kinase kinase; MAPK, mitogen activated protein kinase; PKC, protein kinase C; PtdIns-3K, phosphatidylinositol 3-kinase; PTK, protein tyrosine kinase.

not surprising that the C-terminal domain of p190 which is homologous to n-chimaerin indeed turns out to have GAP activity on Rac as well as Rho and yet another Ras-related protein, CDC42. In the middle of the p190 protein is a domain which is highly homologous to, and which probably is, a protein cloned previously as the glucocorticoid suppressor, that is a transcription factor. Thus the p190 protein may function as a Ras-related protein (binding guanine nucleotides), a GAP (for Rho, Rac and CDC42) and a transcription factor; indeed it is conceivable that the C-terminus of p190 may function as a GAP for the N-terminus!

What is to be made of the transcription factor domain? The molecule clearly provides a direct link between tyrosine kinase activation and nuclear events. One can envisage, for example, that tyrosine kinase activation reduces the amount of p190 in the nucleus by sequestering it in the cytosol as a p190–*ras*GAP complex thus derepressing genes normally suppressed by this transcription factor. Alternatively, p190 and *ras*GAP form complexes in the nucleus where the complex may lose novel activity possessed by the p190 monomer in terms of regulating gene expression.

Like p190, Bcr is also a multidomain protein (Fig. 5.2C). Bcr has C-terminal GAP activity on Rac (as already discussed); in addition it has serine/threonine kinase activity and a domain homologous to the *dbl* oncogene. The *dbl* oncogene encodes for a protein which stimulates nucleotide exchange on CDC42, a Ras-related protein homologous to Rho and Rac. In the p210 Bcr–Abl fusion protein generated as the result of the 9;22 Philadelphia translocation of chronic myeloid leukaemia, the *rac*GAP homology domain of Bcr is lost from the fusion protein. The implications this has for regulation of Rac are as yet unclear since it is not known whether the *rac*GAP activity in CML cells is lost or enhanced. Interestingly, the Dbl as well as the *rac*GAP homology domain is lost in the p190 Bcr–Abl fusion protein characteristic of Philadelphia–positive acute lymphoblastic leukaemia (Ph + ve ALL) (Fig. 5.2C). And, if this is not complicated enough, recent work in CML cells has shown that the p210 Bcr–Abl fusion protein (like Src in v-Src transformed cells) also forms complexes with *ras*GAP and its associated phosphoproteins, p62 and p190 (Druker et al 1992). The significance of this is unknown.

Ras SIGNALLING IN INVERTEBRATES

Given the enormous complexity of these signalling pathways, what alternative systems are there available to dissect them? Intriguing insights into the possible mechanisms of Ras function have come recently from studying eye development in the fruitfly, *Drosophila*, and vulval development in the nematode worm, *Caenorhabditis elegans*. The advantages of studying such invertebrates are that morphogenetic abnormalities are relatively easy to identify and the organisms can be genetically manipulated.

The *Drosophila* compound eye comprises a series of repeating units called ommatidia each consisting of eight photoreceptor cells, numbered R1 to R8, and accessory cells. Some years ago, Rubin and others described a *Drosophila* mutant called *sevenless* in which the majority of ommatidia in the eye lacked an R7 cell. The *sevenless* gene turns out to encode a tyrosine kinase receptor (Sev) expressed on the R7 precursor cell and certain other cell types (Hafen et al 1987). A mutation in another gene called *bride of sevenless* (*Boss*) which encodes the ligand for the Sev protein also blocks R7 development. Boss is a protein expressed only on the R8 cell surface. The model is therefore that the ligand Boss on R8 is presented to the receptor Sev on the R7 cell, activating the tyrosine kinase activity of Sev which triggers expression of the genes required for R7 differentiation.

Elegant genetic screens have revealed other genes involved in signalling via this Sev pathway. The first turns out to be *Drosophila Ras 1* (D-*Ras1*) and the second, *Sos* (*son of sevenless*), which on the basis of significant homology to the *Saccharomyces cerevisiae* CDC25 gene, encodes a guanine nucleotide exchange factor for D-Ras 1 (Bonfini et al 1992, Simon et al 1991). Moreover, the expression of a constitutively activated D-*Ras1* (Gly → Val12) gene (homologous to oncogenic mutant *ras*) in *sevenless* flies or in flies which lack *Boss*, restores R7 differentiation and indeed leads to the formation of supernumery R7 cells in many ommatidia. Thus D-Ras1 fixed in the GTP-bound form activates Sev-dependent pathways in the absence of an activated Sev receptor (Fortini et al 1992). Moreover, inactivation of *Gap1* (*Drosophila rasGAP*) also leads to the formation of supernumerary R7 cells, which is consistent with Gap1 being purely a downregulator of D-Ras1 (Gaul et al 1992).

A Ras-related protein, Rap1 can antagonize Ras function in NIH3T3 fibroblasts, and a mutation (*roughened*) which suppresses R7 development in the presence of a normal Sev protein has recently been identified as a gain of function mutation in the *Drosophila* homologue of *Rap1* (Hariharan et al 1991). The scene is therefore set for Rubin and colleagues to solve Ras function by characterizing other proteins involved in the Sev pathway and as a starting point they have five further genes to investigate. It seems certain that the mammalian homologues of these proteins will be key players in mammalian Ras-dependent signalling pathways and that the fruitfly eye may therefore yield the elusive immediate Ras effector (Fig. 5.4A).

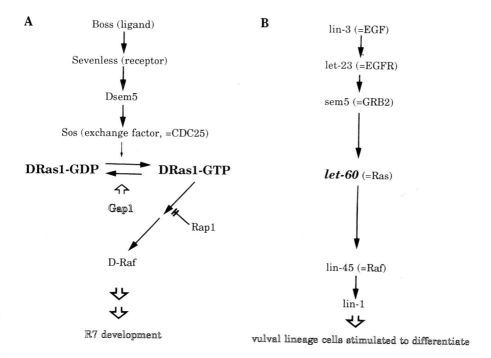

Fig. 5.4 A Ras signalling in *Drosophila* eye development. See text for discussion. **B** Ras signalling for vulval induction in *C. elegans*. See text for discussion

Vulval development in *C. elegans* operates through an analogous system with a tyrosine kinase receptor (let23) on a vulval precursor cell receiving an inductive signal from neighbouring cells. let23 requires a Ras protein (let60) for its signal transduction (Han & Sternberg 1990, Beitel et al 1990). An interesting additional player here, however, is a protein (Sem5) which comprises two SH3 domains separated by a SH2 domain (Clark et al 1992) (Fig. 5.2A). It seems probable that the Sem5 protein binds directly to tyrosine phosphorylated let23 via its SH2 domain and assembles a protein complex using its SH3 domains which results in nucleotide exchange on Ras (let60) (Fig. 5.4B). The mammalian homologue of Sem5, GRB2, has just been identified (Lowenstein et al 1992) and potentially provides the link between activated tyrosine kinases, possibly another SH2 adaptor protein (SHC) (Pelicci et al 1992) and Ras. Such SH2/3 domains may allow the assembly of multiprotein complexes in signal transduction pathways.

Ras IN ONCOGENESIS

ras mutation is one of the commonest genetic lesions in human malignancy. Activating point mutations of *ras* occur at one of three different codons: 12, 13 or 61. The effect of these mutations is to render Ras insensitive to GAP activity since the intrinsic GTPase activity of the mutant protein is not stimulated when GAP binds to the oncogenic Ras protein. Oncogenic mutant Ras protein is therefore locked in the active GTP-bound state and interacts constitutively with the Ras effector protein(s) to produce an unregulated signal output (Fig. 5.1B).

The incidence of *ras* mutations varies enormously between different malignancies (Bos 1989). For instance, *ras* mutation is very rare in patients with carcinoma of the breast whilst over 90% of pancreatic carcinomas, 50% of colorectal carcinomas and 20–30% of all cases of acute myeloblastic leukaemia, acute lymphoblastic leukaemia and myelodysplastia studied have *ras* mutations. This difference in incidence may reflect the differences in Ras function between different cell types or differential exposure of these tissues to carcinogenic agents. An intriguing and related question is why the predominantly activated *ras* gene varies between different tumours. For example, why do K-*ras* mutations predominate in pancreatic and colonic tumours whereas N-*ras* mutations predominate in haematological malignancies? The Ras proteins are highly homologous over most of their sequence and to date no functional differences between them have been identified.

Recently, it has become evident that GTP-bound Ras may be elevated in the absence of *ras* mutation. An example of this is the demonstration that Ras–GTP levels are elevated in neurofibrosarcoma cell lines derived from patients with neurofibromatosis compared with control cell lines. Thus although *ras* mutations are rare in neurofibromatosis, loss of functional neurofibromin has a similar consequence to oncogenic mutation of *ras* (Basu et al 1992, DeClue et al 1992). It has also been shown that loss of functional neurofibromin (due to inactivating point mutations) in colonic carcinoma tissue from non-neurofibromatosis patients leads to elevation of Ras–GTP levels even though the *ras* genes were not mutated (Li et al 1992).

Activating *ras* mutations cooperate with the activation of other cellular oncogenes (e.g. *myc*) or loss of tumour suppressor genes (e.g. p53) to lead to tumour formation. Vogelstein and others have shown for colorectal carcinoma that a series of up to 4–6 different genetic events are required to convert a normal colonic epithelial cell to a highly malignant and metastatic cell (Fearon & Vogelstein 1990). This multistep process probably holds true for the majority of human malignancies including leukaemias. In colonic neoplasms, activating *ras* mutations are a relatively early genetic event whereas *ras* mutation may be a later event in leukaemogenesis.

PLASMA MEMBRANE TARGETING OF Ras AND PROSPECTS FOR ANTI-Ras CHEMOTHERAPY

Given that the Ras signalling pathway is complicated and incompletely understood, is there any prospect, in the immediate future, of drugs to selectively inhibit Ras function? The answer is probably yes, but comes from a completely different area of Ras biology.

The Ras proteins require translocation to the inner surface of the plasma membrane in order to be biologically active. All Ras and many Ras-related proteins terminate at their C-terminus with a tetrapeptide CAAX motif, where C is cysteine, A an aliphatic amino acid and X any amino acid. This motif undergoes a series of post-translational modifications (Fig. 5.5). First, a prenoid group is attached to the cysteine residue. Prenoids are branched chain, unsaturated fatty acids which are precursors in the cholesterol bio-synthetic pathway. Ras is prenylated with a C_{15} prenoid group called farnesyl (Hancock et al 1989, Schafer et al 1990) whereas all other Ras-related proteins are prenylated on the cysteine of their CAAX motifs with a C_{20} geranylgeranyl group (reviewed in Hancock & Marshall 1993). The prenoid group used (C_{15} or C_{20}) to modify a CAAX motif is determined by the X amino acid and by different enzymes, farnesyl transferase (FTase) or geranylgeranyl transferase (GGTaseI) which catalyse the prenylation. These share a common alpha-subunit (Seabra et al 1991) which binds the prenoid group but have different beta-subunits which bind the different CAAX motifs (Reiss et al 1990, 1991, Schaber et al 1990). Following farnesylation, the -AAX amino acids are removed from the CAAX motif by an endopeptidase and the free α-carboxyl group exposed on the now C-terminal cysteine residue is methylated (Gutierrez et al 1989). This triplet of C-terminal modifications is essential for membrane association of the Ras protein (Hancock et al 1989, 1991a). The targeting of Ras proteins specifically to the plasma membrane is more complicated since this requires a second signal in addition to the -CAAX modifications (Fig. 5.5; Hancock et al 1990, 1991b).

PLASMA MEMBRANE

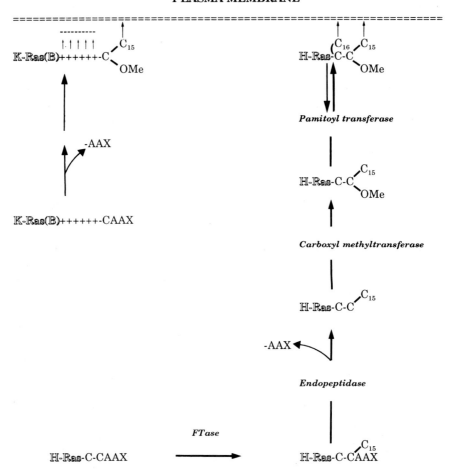

CYTOPLASM

Fig. 5.5 Post-translational processing of Ras. In order for Ras to be biologically active, it must undergo post-translational modifications and localization to the inner surface of the plasma membrane. The processing consists of three modifications to the -CAAX motif which is common to all the Ras proteins (see text for discussion). This signal is read in conjunction with a second signal which is required for efficient plasma membrane localization. The second signal is palmitoylation (addition of a C_{16} group) of upstream cysteine residues in all the Ras proteins except for K-Ras(B) in which a polybasic domain (consisting of six positively charged lysine residues) instead acts as the second signal. The enzymes responsible for the post-translational modifications are indicated in italics.

However, if prenylation is blocked then none of the other CAAX modifications can take place and the Ras protein remains cytosolic and biologically inactive. This was first demonstrated by replacing the cysteine residue in the CAAX motif with a serine residue that cannot be prenylated; this mutation renders an oncogenic mutant Ras protein non-transforming by preventing its attachment to the plasma membrane (Willumsen et al 1984). Ras proteins can also be confined to the cytosol by blocking the biosynthesis of all cellular prenoids with lovastatin or related compounds (Hancock et al 1989, Kim et al 1990). These drugs inhibit HMG-CoA (3-hydroxy-3-methylglutaryl coenzyme A) reductase, the rate-limiting enzyme for prenoid synthesis (reviewed in Goldstein & Brown 1990). However, whilst an inhibition of Ras processing can be demonstrated in vitro with these compounds, this can only achieved in vivo at concentrations some 50 times greater than that required to completely inhibit cholesterol synthesis (Sinensky et al 1990). Moreover the clinical effect of an efficient inhibitor of prenoid synthesis is uncertain since all prenylated proteins would be affected.

Much interest, however, is focused on developing inhibitors of FTase, since apart from Ras proteins there only a few other proteins that are farnesylated. These agents would therefore be expected to have a much narrower range of toxicity since geranylgeranylated proteins (proteins prenylated by a C_{20} prenoid) would not be affected. If FTase inhibitors can be developed is there any reason to suppose that they may have selective toxicity for cells expressing oncogenic mutant *ras*? As discussed by Gibbs (1991), there are at least two reasons why this might be the case. First, in certain biological systems non-farnesylated oncogenic mutant Ras has a dominant negative phenotype (inhibiting Ras function) whereas non-farnesylated wild-type Ras does not have such a phenotype (Gibbs et al 1989, Stacey et al 1991). Second, since Rap1, a Ras-related protein which has Ras suppressor activity, is geranylgeranylated the relative balance of active Rap1 to active Ras in a cell might be shifted in favour of Rap1 following FTase inhibition (Gibbs 1991). Whatever the theoretical arguments the appearance of FTase inhibitors is anxiously awaited.

SUMMARY

A discussion of Ras biology is now incomplete without considering mammalian cells, yeasts, fruitflies and worms. A massive amount of data is being generated in each of these systems which will allow us to answer the question of what exactly Ras does. This is not possible as yet although, as we have highlighted in this review, the answer may not be that distant. Given that *ras* mutation is such a frequent event in human malignancies, including some of the leukaemias, it is to be hoped that a detailed knowledge of how Ras functions may lead eventually to development of novel therapeutic approaches to human malignancy.

KEY POINTS FOR CLINICAL PRACTICE

- The epidemiological data that *ras* mutations play an important part in the genetic events leading towards malignancy have been complemented by studies on Ras biology.
- The biological function of Ras and the proteins (such as *ras*GAP and neurofibromin) which regulate its activity are being progressively unravelled.
- The complex signalling pathways for cell growth and differentiation are slowly becoming clearer; it is clear that oncogenes are in one way or another linked with each other in putative signalling pathways.
- Understanding the biology of oncogenes such as *ras* may allow the development of specific inhibitors (such as those of Ras function) to treat malignancies.

ACKNOWLEDGEMENTS

The authors are supported by the Cancer Research Campaign, UK.

REFERENCES

Adari H, Lowy D R, Willumsen B M et al 1988 Guanosine triphosphatase activating protein (GAP) interacts with the p21*ras* effector binding domain. Science 240: 518–521

Ballester R, Marchuk D, Boguski M et al 1990 The NF1 locus encodes a protein functionally related to mammalian GAP and yeast *IRA* proteins. Cell 63: 851–859

Barbacid M 1987 *ras* genes. Annu Rev Biochem 56: 779–827 (Review)

Basu T H, Gutmann D H, Fletcher J A et al 1992 Aberrant regulation of Ras proteins in malignant tumour cells from type 1 neurofibromatosis patients. Nature 356: 713–715

Beitel G J, Clark S G, Horvitz H R 1990 *Caenorhabditis elegans ras* gene *let-60* acts as a switch in the pathway of vulval induction. Nature 348: 503–509

Bonfini L, Karlovich C A, Dasgupta C et al 1992 The *Son of sevenless* gene product: a putative activator of Ras. Science 255: 603–606

Bos J (1989) *ras* oncogenes in human cancer: a review. Cancer Res 49: 4682–4689

Bourne H R, Sanders D A, McCormick F 1990 The GTPase superfamily: a conserved switch for diverse cell functions. Nature 348: 125–132 (Review)

Bourne H R, Sanders D A, McCormick F 1991 The GTPase superfamily: conserved structure and molecular mechanism. Nature 349: 117–127 (Review)

Cales C, Hancock J F, Marshall C J et al 1988 The cytoplasmic protein GAP is implicated as the target for regulation by the *ras* gene product. Nature 332: 548–551

Clark S G, Stern M J, Horvitz H R 1992 *C. elegans* cell-signalling gene *sem-5* encodes a protein with SH2 and SH3 domains. Nature 356: 340–344

DeClue J E, Papageorge A G, Fletcher J A et al 1992 Abnormal regulation of mammalian p21*ras* contributes to malignant tumor growth in von Recklinghausen (type 1) neurofibromatosis. Cell 69: 265–273

De Vries-Smits A M M, Burgering B M Th, Leevers S et al 1992 Involvement of p21*ras* in activation of extracellular signal-regulated kinase 2. Nature 357: 602–604

Diekmann D, Brill S, Garrett M D et al 1991 Bcr encodes a GTPase-activating protein for p21*rac*. Nature 351: 400–402

Downward J, Graves J D, Warne P H et al 1990 Stimulation of p21*ras* upon T-cell activation. Nature 346: 719–723

Druker B, Okuda K, Matulonis U et al 1992 Tyrosine phosphorylation of *ras*GAP and associated proteins in chronic myelogenous leukaemia cell lines. Blood 79: 2215–2220

Ellis C, Moran M, McCormick F et al 1990 Phosphorylation of GAP and GAP-associated proteins by transforming and mitogenic tyrosine kinases. Nature 343: 377–381

Fearon E R, Vogelstein B 1990 A genetic model for colorectal tumorigenesis. Cell 61: 759–767 (Review)

Fortini M E, Simon M A, Rubin G M 1992 Signalling by the *sevenless* protein kinase is mimicked by Ras 1 activation. Nature 355: 559–561

Gaul U, Mardon G, Rubin G 1992 A putative *Ras* GTPase activating protein acts as a negative regulator of signalling by the *Sevenless* receptor tyrosine kinase. Cell 68: 1001–1019

Gibbs J 1991 Ras C-terminal processing enzymes-new drug targets? Cell 65: 1–4 (Minireview)

Gibbs J B, Schaber M D, Schofield T L et al 1989 *Xenopus* oocyte germinal-vescicle breakdown induced by (Val12) Ras is inhibited by a cytosol-localized Ras mutant. Proc Natl Acad Sci USA 86: 6630–6634

Goldstein J L, Brown M S 1990 Regulation of the mevalonate pathway. Nature 343: 425–430 (Review)

Gutierrez L, Magee A I, Marshall C J et al 1989 Post-translational processing of p21^{ras} is two-step and involves carboxyl-methylation and carboxyl-terminal proteolysis. EMBO J 8: 1093–1098

Hafen E, Basler K, Edstroem J-E et al 1987 *Sevenless*, a cell-specific homeotic gene of Drosophila, encodes a putative transmembrane receptor with a tyrosine kinase domain. Science 236: 55–63

Hall A 1990 The cellular functions of small GTP-binding proteins. Science 249: 635–640 (Review)

Han M, Sternberg P W 1990 *let-60*, a gene that specifies cell fates during *C. elegans* vulval induction, encodes a Ras protein. Cell 63: 921–931

Hancock J F, Marshall C J 1993 Post-translational processing of Ras and Ras-related proteins. In: Lacal J C, McCormick F (eds) The Ras superfamily of GTPases. CRC Press, Florida (in press)

Hancock J F, Magee A I, Childs J et al 1989 All Ras proteins are polyisoprenylated but only some are palmitoylated. Cell 57: 1167–1177

Hancock J F, Paterson H, Marshall C J 1990 A polybasic domain or palmitoylation is required in addition to the CAAX motif to localize p21^{ras} to the plasma membrane. Cell 63: 133–139

Hancock J F, Cadwallader K, Marshall C J 1991a Methylation and proteolysis are essential for efficient membrane binding of prenylated p21$^{K-ras(B)}$. EMBO J 10: 641–646

Hancock J F, Cadwallader K, Paterson H et al 1991b A CAAX or a CAAL motif and a second signal are sufficient for plasma membrane targeting of Ras proteins. EMBO J 10: 4033–4039

Hariharan I K, Carthew R W, Rubin G M 1991 The Drosophila *roughened* mutation: activation of a *rap* homolog disrupts eye development and interferes with cell determination. Cell 67: 717–722

Howe L R, Leevers S J, Gomez N et al 1992 Activation of MAP kinase pathway by the protein kinase Raf. Cell 71: 335–342

Kaibuchi K, Mizuno T, Fujioka H et al 1991 Molecular cloning of the cDNA for stimulatory GDP/GTP exchange protein for *smg* p21s (*ras* p 21-like small GTP-binding proteins) and characterization of stimulatory GDP/GTP exchange protein. Mol Cell Biol 11: 2873–2880

Kaplan D R, Morrison D K, Wong G et al 1990 PDGF beta-receptor stimulates tyrosine phosphorylation of GAP and association of GAP with a signalling complex. Cell 61: 125–133

Kim R, Rine J, Kim S-H 1990 Prenylation of mammalian Ras proteins in *Xenopus* oocytes. Mol Cell Biol 10: 5945–5949

Koch C A, Anderson D, Moran M F et al 1991 SH2 and SH3 domains: elements that control interactions of cytoplasmic signalling proteins. Science 252: 668–674 (Review)

Kyriakis J M, App H, Zhang X et al 1992 Raf-1 activates MAP kinase-kinase. Nature 358: 417–421

Lacal J C, McCormick F (eds) 1993 The Ras superfamily of GTPases. CRC Press, Florida (in press)

Leevers S J, Marshall C J 1992 Activation of extracellular signal-regulated kinase, ERK2, by p21^{ras} oncoprotein. EMBO J 11: 569–574

Li Y, Bollag G, Clark R et al 1992 Somatic mutations in the Neurofibromatosis 1 gene in human tumours. Cell 69: 275–281

Lowenstein E J, Daly R J, Batzer A G et al 1992 The SH2 and SH3 domain-containing protein GRB2 links receptor tyrosine kinases to Ras signalling. Cell 70: 431–442

McCormick F 1989 *ras* GTPase activating protein: signal transmitter and signal terminator. Cell 56: 5–8 (Minireview)

Marshall M S, Hill W S, Ng A S et al 1989 A C-terminal domain of GAP is sufficient to stimulate *ras* p21 GTPase activity. EMBO J 8: 1105–1110

Martegani E, Vanoni M, Zippel R et al 1992 Cloning by functional complementation of a mouse cDNA encoding a homologue of *CDC25*, a *Saccharomyces cerevisiae* RAS activation. EMBO J 11: 2151–2157

Martin G A, Viskochil D, Bollag G et al 1990 The GAP-related domain of the neurofibromatosis type 1 gene product interacts with *ras* p21. Cell 63: 843–849

Molloy C J, Bottaro D P, Fleming T P et al 1989 PDGF induction of tyrosine phosphorylation of GTPase activating protein. Nature 342: 711–714

Moran M F, Polakis P, McCormick F et al 1991 Protein-tyrosine kinases regulate the phosphorylation, protein interactions, subcellular distribution, and activity of p21[ras] GTPase-activating protein. Mol Cell Biol 11: 1804–1812

Pawson T, Gish G D 1992 SH2 and SH3 domains: from structure to function. Cell 71: 359–362 (Minireview)

Pelicci G, Lanfrancone L, Grignani F et al 1992 A novel transforming protein (SHC) with a SH2 domain is implicated in mitogenic signal transduction. Cell 70: 93–104

Reiss Y, Goldstein J L, Seabra M C et al 1990 Inhibition of purified p21[ras] farnesyl: protein transferase by Cys-AAX tetrapeptides Cell 62: 81–88

Reiss Y, Seabra M C, Armstrong S A et al 1991 Non-identical subunits of p21[H-ras] farnesyl transferase. J Biol Chem 266: 10672–10677

Schaber M D, O'Hara M B, Garsky V M et al 1990 Polyisoprenylation of *ras* in vitro by a farnesyl transferase. J Biol Chem 265: 14701–14704

Schafer W R, Trueblood C E, Yang C-C et al 1990 Enzymatic coupling of cholesterol intermediates to a mating pheromone precursor and to the Ras protein. Science 249: 1133–1139

Seabra M C, Reiss Y, Casey P J et al 1991 Protein farneysl transferase and geranylgeranyl transferase share a common α subunit. Cell 65: 429–434

Settleman J, Narasimhan Y, Foster L C et al 1992 Molecular cloning of cDNAs encoding the GAP-associated protein p190: implications for a signalling pathway from *ras* to the nucleus. Cell 69: 539–549

Shou C, Farnsworth C L, Neel B G et al 1992 Molecular cloning of cDNAs encoding a guanine-nucleotide-releasing factor for Ras p21. Nature 358: 351–354

Simon M A, Bowtell D D, Dodson G S et al 1991 Ras1 and a putative guanine nucleotide exchange factor perform crucial steps in signalling by the sevenless protein tyrosine kinase. Cell 67: 701–716

Sinensky M, Beck L A, Leonard S et al 1990 Differential inhibitory effects of lovastatin on protein isoprenylation and sterol synthesis. J Biol Chem 265: 19937–19941

Smith M R, DeGudicibus S J, Stacey D W 1986 Requirement for c-*ras* proteins during viral oncogene transformation. Nature 320: 540–543

Stacey D W, Feig L A, Gibbs J B 1991 Dominant inhibitory Ras mutants selectively inhibit the activity of either cellular or oncogenic Ras. Mol Cell Biol 11: 4053–4064

Thomas S M, DeMarco M, D'Arcangelo G et al 1992 Ras is essential for nerve growth factor- and phorbol ester-induced tyrosine phosphorylation of MAP kinases. Cell 68: 1031–1040

Trahey M, McCormick F 1987 A cytoplasmic protein stimulates normal N-*ras* p21 GTPase, but does not affect oncogenic mutants. Science 238: 542–545

Willumsen B M, Norris K, Papageorge A G et al 1984 Harvey murine sarcoma p21 *ras* protein: biological significance of the cysteine nearest the carboxy terminus. EMBO J 3: 2581–2585

Wong G, Muller O, Clark R et al 1992 Molecular cloning and nucleic acid binding properties of the GAP-associated tyrosine phosphoprotein p62. Cell 69: 551–558

Wood K W, Sarnecki C, Roberts T M et al 1992 *ras* mediates nerve growth factor receptor modulation of three signal-tranducing protein kinases: MAP kinase, Raf-1 and RSK. Cell 68: 1041–1050

Xu G F, O'Connell P, Viskochil D et al 1990 The neurofibromatosis type 1 gene encodes a protein related to GAP. Cell 62: 599–608

6

Cell adhesion in the hematopoietic system

M. W. Makgoba   A. Bernard

Cellular adhesion plays a central role in many biological processes (Edelman 1985) such as morphogenesis, cell migration, and direct cell–cell cooperation. The phenomenon has important clinical consequences involving, for instance, vascular thrombosis, the inflammatory process, tumour metastasis, bacterial and parasite infections. Cells of the hematopoietic system in man are the best understood, analysed and characterized in terms of adhesion molecules. At present there are 78 'cluster of differentiation' (CD) molecules on the surface of these cells, defined by monoclonal antibodies, and clarified in four International Leukocyte Workshops (Knapp et al 1988). Some mediate adhesion, but the majority do not. Thus the term adhesion molecules refers to those cell surface structures that directly play a decisive mechanical role in the binding of a cell to its environment, either to the extracellular matrix or to another cell.

The events of cellular adhesion are closely linked to the events of cellular signalling. It is clear that the inherent coupling of adhesion to signalling is not only due to cell stabilization by the adhesion molecules permitting other surface molecules to bind their ligands, but that adhesion molecules per se are also directly involved in the transduction of powerful signals controlling cell activation/proliferation. The adhesion process is rigorously controlled and time dependent, since attachment of cells to solid support or extracellular matrix is cell-cycle-dependent, and conjugate formation between lymphocytes, or lymphocytes and accessory cells is initially loose, and rapidly strengthens before the cells spontaneously dissociate. Cellular adhesion in man is mediated via multiple molecular pathways which involve specific intermolecular events. These pathways are made of multimolecular complexes, and each pathway may strongly influence the affinity of another.

In this chapter we will first describe the known adhesion pathways, and then discuss their importance in haematological function and disease.

ADHESION PATHWAYS

The concept of leukocyte adhesion pathways was developed by Shaw et al (1986) who demonstrated two distinct molecular adhesion mechanisms utilized by cytotoxic T-cell clones on antigen negative targets. This simple

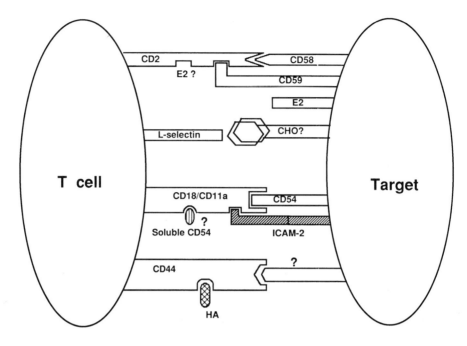

Fig. 6.1 Schematic, simplified model of the multiple adhesion/signalling molecules involved in T-cell/target interactions. HA, hyaluronic acid; CHO, carbohydrate; ?, uncertain site or molecule of interaction. These interactions are bidirectional. Reproduced with permission from Blackwell Scientific Publications.

model has since evolved to encompass an array of other pathways as more receptor–ligand pairs become defined (Fig. 6.1).

The CD2 adhesion pathway

CD2 was discovered as an important adhesion molecule when it was identified as the T-cell surface molecule mediating spontaneous rosettes with erythrocytes (Kamoun et al 1981). It is restricted to T-cells and natural killer (NK) cells, but its major ligand, CD58 (LFA-3), is present on most cell types (Selvaraj et al 1987) (Table 6.1). The CD2 pathway is involved in T-cell adhesion to most other cells. The extracellular segment of CD2 is made of two immunoglobulin-like domains (Sewell et al 1986). CD2 has a long intracellular segment, which is certainly involved in the transduction of activation signals (Bierer et al 1990). Indeed CD2 is the prototype of molecules displaying both adhesion and signalling activities. An important feature of CD2 is that its overall surface density, degree of sialylation and shape critically depend on T-cell differentiation and activation. This was demonstrated by the discovery of restricted epitopes ('CD2R') to thymocytes and activated T-cells, that can be induced after binding of certain CD2 monoclonal antibodies (mAbs) ('epitope modulation') (Bernard et al 1982,

Table 6.1 Molecules and pathways involved in adhesion/signalling

Receptor	Other name	Family	Tissue expression	Ligand (s)	Other name
CD2	T11 Sheep erythrocyte receptor LFA-2	Immunoglobulin	T- and NK cells	CD58 CD59	LFA-3 MEM-43
E-Selectin	ELAM-1	Selectin	Endothelial cells	Sialylated Lewis X	—
G-Selectin	GMP-140	Selectin	Endothelial cells and platelets	Lewis X	—
L-Selectin	LECAM-1	Selectin	Lymphocytes	Unknown	—
CDW49a	VLAα1 or VLA-1	β_1 Integrin	Activated T-cells	Laminin/collagen	—
CDW49b	VLAα2 or VLA-2	β_1 Integrin	Activated T-cells	Collagen/laminin	—
CDW49c	VLAα3 or VLA-3	β_1 Integrin	Lymphocytes	Laminin/fibronectin	—
CDW49d	VLAα4 or VLA-4	β_1 Integrin	Lymphocytes	VCAM-1, ICAM-2, fibronectin	—
CDW49e	VLAα5 or VLA-5	β_1 Integrin	Lymphocytes	Fibronectin	—
CDW49f	VLAα6 or VLA-6	β_1 Integrin	Lymphocytes	Laminin	—
CD18/CD11a	LFA-1	β_2 Integrin	All leukocytes	CD54, ICAM-2, others	ICAM-1
CD18/CD11b	MaC-1	β_2 Integrin	Monocytes/neutrophils	CD54, 3Cbi, fibrinogen	ICAM-1
CD18/CD11c	p150/95	β_2 Integrin	Neutrophils/T-cell clones	Unknown	—
CDW41a	gpIIb/IIIa	β_3 Integrin	Platelets	von Willebrand factor, vitronectin, fibrinogen	—
alpha$_v$/β_3	Vitronectin receptor	β_3Integrin	Osteoclasts	Vitronectin, osteopontin	—
CD44	HERMES PgP-1	Cartilage link protein	Ubiquitous	Hyaluronic acid	—

Reproduced with permission from Blackwell Scientific Publications.

Meuer et al 1984). Activated T-cells display high densities of CD2, which is poorly sialylated and displays epitopes not present on resting T-cells.

The discovery that pairs of CD2 mAbs in appropriate combinations can trigger T-cell activation as efficiently as — or even more efficiently than — mAb against the CD3–T-cell receptor (TCR), raised the question of whether T-cells could be activated independently from antigen recognition (Meuer et al 1984, Brottier et al 1985). It remains likely that engagement of the CD2 pathway serves to complement the primary signal transduced by the CD3–TCR complex (Yang et al 1986). Another striking aspect of CD2 is that it appears to be able to transduce, within T-cells, quite different activation signals according to the CD2 molecular arrangement (Springer et al 1987, Carrera et al 1988, Hahn et al 1991).

It was also observed that distinct CD2 mitogenic pairs of mAbs can induce distinct activation pathways in terms of the patterns of cytokines secreted and resulting T-cell functions (Huet et al 1986, Valentin et al 1990). This effect can be seen at the level of a single T-cell, as shown by using a potentially bifunctional T-cell clone (Eljaafari et al 1990). This finding does not exclude the possibility that distinct subsets of T-cells might also be recruited by these distinct CD2 pairs.

Several arguments, including the requirement for two mAbs to activate T-cells, suggested the possibility that CD2 could bind another ligand in addition to CD58 (Hunig et al 1987). Recent evidence has shown that CD59 — a glycophospho-inositol (GPI)-linked molecule also involved in protecting cells against attack by homologous C' — binds CD2 (Groux et al 1989, Deckert et al 1992). CD58 and CD59 molecules together have a synergistic effect on T-cell activation. But other molecular species are involved that strongly influence the CD2 pathway, such as the E2 molecule (Bernard et al 1988), a product of the *mic*-2 pseudoautosomal gene (Gelin et al 1990), and CD44 (Haynes 1989). Thus, the CD2 pathway is a multimolecular pathway playing a central and subtle role in T-cell adhesion/activation, to 'pilot' T-cells either in an unresponsive or an activated state.

Integrin-mediated adhesion pathways

The *integrin superfamily* of molecules forms the largest group of cell adhesion molecules in man (Table 6.1). They are transmembrane sialoglycoproteins consisting of non-covalently linked single alpha and beta subunits. They are classified into subfamilies according to the type of beta subunit (Hemler 1990). So far 11 alpha subunits and six beta subunits have been characterized in terms of their primary sequences. The integrin molecules mediate adhesion by three mechanisms of interaction: cell–cell, cell–matrix and cell–soluble factor. The characteristic of integrin-mediated adhesion is the absolute requirement for cations, especially magnesium, and temperature (Shaw et al 1986). They are the major mediators of cell–matrix interaction and cell migration out of the vascular compartment. Homologues of human integrins are conserved in evolution to the level of *Drosophila* and amoeba (MacKrell et al 1988, Mann et al 1991, Adams et al 1993). An emerging feature of integrin interaction is the multiplicity of ligands recognized by a single receptor, e.g. VLA-4 binding to VCAM, fibronectin and ICAM-2 (Springer 1990, Seth et al 1991) or the binding of LFA-1 to ICAM-1 and -2 (Springer 1990), and the ability of certain alpha subunits to complex with several different beta subunits. The classic example is the alpha-v subunit combining with either beta-3, beta-5 or beta-6 (Vogel et al 1990, Smith et al 1990). This multiplicity of interaction allows for diversity and specificity within this recognition system. Of great clinical interest is the observation that some of the ligands for integrins, such as ICAM-1, may occur in soluble forms in the circulation (Seth et al 1991, Rothlein et al 1991). Whether these soluble forms are distinct from the membrane-bound molecules or are the products of cell shedding, enzymatic cleavage or death, or whether they play any regulatory role in adhesion and/or signalling processes, remains to be determined. Their greatest impact is likely to come from their diagnostic and predictive potential in inflammatory and neoplastic diseases (Seth et al 1991, Rothlein et al 1991).

The expression of some integrins is known to be regulated during development. It is generally postulated that temporal expression of some of these molecules during development may be necessary for organogenesis as homologous structures in *Drosophila* have been shown to be critical to this process (MacKrell et al 1988). Some integrins such as the leukocyte integrins CD18/CD11a–c (LFA-1, Mac-1 and p150/95), the platelet and megakaryocyte integrin gpIIa/IIIb and the epithelial and epithelial tumor-specific integrin alpha-6/beta-4 (VLA-6) are expressed in a tissue specific pattern. A number of growth factors such as transforming growth factor-β may affect integrin expression (Heino et al 1989). Under normal physiological conditions integrins largely exist in an inactive form. This may be particularly important in haemopoietic cells, where univalent aggregation between activated integrins and their ligands would impair blood flow. Cell activation by a number of substances such as phorbol myriste acetate (PMA), lipopolysaccharide (LPS), tissue injury or inflammation leads to rapid activation of integrin binding. The ability to exist and rapidly change from an inactive, non-adherent state to an active and adherent/signalling state as a result of stimulus is a feature of integrin adhesion. The mechanisms underlying this change are poorly understood but are of immense interest in understanding the regulation of integrin-mediated adhesion/signalling.

Integrin recognition of ligands

Most integrin receptors recognize a tripeptide sequence RGD (arginine–glycine–aspartate) on their respective ligands with the exception of CD18/CD11a (LFA-1) (Ruoslahti & Pierschbacher 1987, Springer 1990). The precise mechanism of how this simple tripeptide is utilized by so many receptors for different adhesion and signalling processes is not known. Temporal and tissue-specific expression, inducible expression, the ability to exist as either active or inactive moieties are all mechanisms by which integrin-mediated function is regulated.

The *leukocyte integrins*, also known as the beta-2 integrins, CD18/CD11a–c are the main mediators of leukocyte diapedesis and homing by allowing cell binding to high endothelial venules. CD18/CD11a shows differential expression between naive and memory T-lymphocytes (Sanders et al 1988). CD18/CD11a is found mainly on lymphocytes, CD18/CD11b predominantly on monocytes and neutrophils and CD18/CD11c mainly on neutrophils. CD18/CD11a binds to the molecules ICAM-1 (CD54), ICAM-2 (Springer 1990) and possibly other undefined molecules. CD18/CD11b binds to CD54, iC3B and fibrinogen (Springer 1990). The cellular ligand for p150/95 remains undefined. The ligand ICAM-1 has become a very interesting adhesion molecule; it is highly inducible by various cytokines, associates with the interleukin-2 (IL-2) receptor, its expression correlates with T-cell infiltration into tumors and with autoimmune thyroiditis (Makgoba et al 1989), and it exists in several isoforms in the circulation (Seth et al 1991). It is a receptor for the rhinoviruses and falciparum malaria, and soluble ICAM-1 inhibits rhinovirus infection (Makgoba et al 1989, Springer 1990). The diversity of interaction found in the integrin molecules is also found in their ligands.

The *VLA beta-1* family of molecules are the major mediators of cell–extracellular matrix interactions and homing. T- and B-lymphocytes express different types of VLA molecules. B-cells express large amounts of VLA-4 but low amounts of VLA-2 and -3. They do not express VLA-1, -5 and -6. T-cells, on the contrary, express a combination of VLA molecules depending on the activation or differentiation state of the cells. Resting unactivated human T-cells express VLA-3, -4, -5 and -6. They do not express VLA-1 or -2 (Shimizu et al 1990). Following activation the level of expressed VLA-3, -4 and -5 increases, that of VLA-6 decreases and there is induced expression of VLA-1 and -2 (Saltini et al 1988). VLA-4 binds to fibronectin, laminin and VCAM. VLA-6 binds to laminin on platelets and lymphocytes to mediate adhesion. Platelet gpIIb/IIIa, a beta-3 integrin, binds fibronectin and vitronectin to mediate adhesion. This receptor also interacts with soluble factors such as fibrinogen. The integrin alpha-v/beta-3 found on osteoclasts binds to an RGD sequence found on osteopontin (Reinholt et al 1990). This mediates the adhesion of osteoclasts to bone.

Selectin-mediated adhesion pathways

Like integrins, selectins form a family of molecules which are structurally related and designed to mediate adhesion (see Table 6.1): they have an NH2-terminal mammalian lectin-like domain and they are highly conserved in evolution (Watson et al 1990). They also display common important functional features: they mediate adhesion of blood cells to vascular endothelium in privileged sites and their expression is strongly modulated after cell activation. ELAM-1, a selectin induced on the endothelial cells of postcapillary venules by IL-1, tumor necrosis factor (TNF) and bacterial LPS released during an inflammatory response (Stoolman 1989), mediates the adhesion of neutrophils and monocytes by binding the sialyl Lewis X determinant (a sialylated, fucosylated polylactosamine) (Springer 1990). ELAM-1 also mediates the adhesion of memory T-cells, but not virgin T-cells, to 'activated' endothelial cells (Shimizu et al 1991). These observations on privileged expression of an adhesion pathway on defined tissues and T-cells subsets were emphasized as an example of site-specific migration (Picker et al 1991).

The *LECAM-1, or LAM-1, molecule* was first described in mice as the Mel-14 antigen, allowing the homing of lymphocytes to lymph nodes by mediating their adhesion to high endothelial venule cells. LAM-1 binding to its ligand is specially inhibited by polysaccharides rich in mannose 6-phosphate, such as polyphosphomonoester core polysaccharide derived from the yeast *Hansenula* (PPME) (Brandley et al 1990). The affinity for PPME is increased when lymphocytes or neutrophils are activated (Spertini et al 1991). Yet LAM-1 expression disappears after lymphocytes have been activated and is no longer present on most memory T-cells (Tedder et al 1990). However, LAM-1 is present on cells that do not normally migrate into peripheral lymph nodes, namely hematopoietic progenitors, suggesting that its role encompasses homing of lymphocytes/monocytes into the periphery (Griffin et al 1990).

CD62, also called PADGEM or GMP-140 antigen, is an inducible granule-membrane protein of platelets and endothelial cells (Hsu-Lin et al 1984, McEver et al 1989). In resting platelets, it is located within the α-granules and is translocated onto the surface upon activation induced by thrombin, histamine, or the C5b–9 complex of complement. In endothelial cells it is present in Weibel–Palade (Bonfanti et al 1989) bodies and mobilized to their plasma membrane upon their activation. CD62 mediates adhesion of myelomonocytes to platelets or endothelial cells. CD62 binds to CD15 (fucosyl *N*-acetyllactosamine, Lewis X) (Larsen et al 1990) and also to sulfatides (heterogeneous 3-sulfated galactosylceramides).

CD44-mediated adhesion

The *CD44 molecule* has a wide tissue distribution. It is a single sialoglycoprotein of 80–90 kDa. The higher molecular forms are expressed differentially on cells (Haynes et al 1989). Unlike the integrins, selectins or the immunoglobulin-like adhesion receptors, CD44 has homology with chick and rat cartilage link proteins. Differential expression in mouse lymphocytes distinguishes the naive from memory T-lymphocyte subsets (Murakami et al 1990). CD44 mAbs have been shown to inhibit T-cell rosetting and B-cell adherence to stroma. Also CD44 mAbs have been shown to enhance T-cell proliferative responses. The ability of some CD44 mAbs to inhibit lympho-cyte adhesion to high endothelial venules has suggested that this molecule is important in the migration and homing of lymphoid cells from the vascular compartment into the lymph nodes (Berg et al 1989). Recent studies have shown that one ligand for CD44 is hyaluronic acid (Aruffo et al 1990). Binding of this molecule explains some but not all of the CD44 interactions, suggesting that other ligands may be involved.

ADHESION MOLECULES IN HEMATOLOGICAL FUNCTIONS

Hemopoiesis and *lymphopoiesis* in the bone marrow, liver, spleen, thymus and lymph nodes involve four processes for which cell adhesion molecules are essential. These processes are: anchorage or attachment, growth, differentia-tion and migration. Initial studies have shown the close interaction of macrophage plasma-membrane processes with bone marrow stroma and the involvement of adhesion receptors between these macrophages and prolifer-ating erythroid and myeloid cells. It was later observed that this interaction requires cations. Recent observations have shown that adherence of myeloid leukemic cells to bone marrow stroma is inhibited by mAbs to ICAM-1, the counter-receptor for CD18/CD11a–b (Makgoba et al 1989).

The migration of lymphocyte precursors from the bone marrow to primary lymphoid organs and finally into the periphery requires the participation of several adhesion molecules. This is illustrated by the interaction of maturing thymic lymphocytes via CD2–CD58 molecules. Other studies have demon-strated the involvement of a novel pathway mediated by CD44, antibodies which inhibit the differentiation of B-lymphocytes in long-term bone marrow culture. This adherence of B-cells to bone marrow stroma cells is mediated by CD44–hyaluronic acid binding (Miyake et al 1990). The essential role of hyaluronic acid in lymphocyte differentiation is underscored by the observa-tion that this extracellular matrix protein accounts for 40% of glycosaminoglycan synthesis by the thymic epithelium. Other studies have shown that peripheral blood T-lymphocytes grown in three-dimensional matrices generate stronger cytotoxic T-cells than those grown in conventional standard or collagen-coated plastic surfaces. Finally, the VLA, selectin and CD18 families of molecules have been shown to be essential for leukocyte homing and diapedesis (Shimizu & Shaw 1991).

Resting *platelets* do not appear to spontaneously aggregate or cluster. However, following activation by injury, inflammation, or exposure to ADP, collagen or adrenalin, platelets rapidly aggregate and also have the capacity to adhere to other cells such as endothelial cells or leukocytes. These activities are mediated by the integrin gpIIb/IIIa on the platelet surface membrane. gpIIb/IIIa binds to multivalent soluble factors such as von Willebrand factor and fibrinogen to mediate aggregation, while binding to fibronectin and vitronectin mediates adherence to other cells (Ginsberg et al 1988). Whether the soluble factors and the membrane-bound receptors bind the same epitopes is at present not clear. The regulation and manipulation of these events is of great therapeutic interest as platelet interactions are involved in a wide variety of common cardiovascular accidents such as ischaemic heart disease, stroke, pregnancy-induced hypertension and disseminated intravascular coagulation in shock. A number of therapeutic approaches have been suggested. For example, it has been shown that gpIIb/IIIa mAbs inhibit platelet aggregation. In addition, the finding that the gpIIb/IIIa protein and other integrins bind their counter-receptors by a specific tripeptide recognition sequence RGD has facilitated the design of therapeutic compounds which contain this or closely related sequences as potential therapies for many platelet disorders in which gpIIb/IIIa-mediated adhesion is involved. A number of reports have shown several such small peptides to inhibit platelet aggregation (Ginsberg et al 1988), and such compounds may be both specific and relatively cheap. It has also been known for a long time that certain snake venoms cause platelet defects that present as bleeding diatheses. Some of these have been shown to contain an active RGD site and are potent inhibitors of platelet aggregation. Unlike the synthetic peptides these are expensive, lack specificity and are less suitable as therapeutic reagents.

Immune functions

Adhesion is an essential event in almost every aspect of cellular immunity, including lymphocyte differentiation, immune cell cooperation and the development of inflammatory responses.

Cell cooperation

Direct physical interaction between cells in immune responses is central to antigen-specific recognition by T-cells. The T-cell receptor complex (TCR) can only recognize specific antigens in the context of HLA molecules. For both accessory and B-cells the processed antigen is presented in association with class II molecules. These specific interactions are by themselves of insufficient affinity for T-cell activation. Antigen-independent adhesion pathways are thus necessary to insure stability so that the appropriate signals can be transduced through the TCR complex (Makgoba et al 1989). The importance of both the CD2 and CD18/CD11a molecules in these stabilizing effects have been abundantly demonstrated. The engagement of the TCR in turn increases the affinity of CD18/CD11a for its ligands almost tenfold (Springer 1990). The CD2 pathway, in addition to providing mechanical stability, delivers strong accessory activation signals to the T-cell which are necessary to complement the primary signal transduced by the TCR. A defect in either of these pathways leads to inadequate T-cell activation by accessory-cells or B-lymphocytes. Effect or function is also dependent on these pathways since CD8 + cytotoxic T-cells require both CD2 and CD18/CD11a to kill their targets.

Leukocyte migration and the inflammatory process

Adhesion molecules dictate the pattern of circulation of lymphocytes. Virgin T-cells preferentially migrate to secondary lymph organs and return to the circulation via the thoracic duct. They express low levels of CD2, CD58, CD18, CD29 and CD44 and high levels of the selectin LAM-1 molecules. Memory cells in contrast express low levels of LAM-1 and high levels of CD2, CD58, CD18, CD29 and CD44. They do not migrate to lymph nodes but home to sites of inflammation.

Inflammatory mediators induce a rapid adherence of neutrophils to endothelium. This rapid, transient response is mediated by a change of affinity on the CD18/CD11a–b molecules for their ligands, most probably ICAM-1 and -2, both constitutively expressed by endothelial cells. Recently it has been suggested that selectin may play a major role in arresting cells in rolling motion while the integrins are necessary for cell migration.

The vascular endothelium plays an active role in controlling this leukocyte traffic, since it can be activated by various cytokines such as IL-1, TNFα and γ-interferon. Endothelial cells can also express an array of induced adhesion molecules such as ICAM-I and VCAM in addition to those they constitutively express. These cells are HLA class II positive and are reported to present antigens to T-cells. Endothelial cells can behave as full-fledged accessory cells in T cell-activation by providing costimulatory signals.

The identification of other tissue-specific adhesion molecules that direct the migration of cells into given tissues such as gut, skin and kidney, would provide more understanding into why cells migrate to where they are found.

ADHESION MOLECULES IN DISEASES

Leukocyte adhesion deficiency

The importance of beta-2 integrins in immune responses is highlighted by the generalized immunodeficiency observed in patients with a congenital defect of these integrins (Springer 1990). The clinical manifestations and age of presentation depend on the severity of the defect. The clinical manifestations include delayed umbilical cord separation, recurrent bacterial infections, leukocytosis, impaired wound healing and infectious lesions without pus formation. While surface expression of all three leukocyte integrins (CD18/ CD11a–c) is affected, the defect is in the gene encoding for CD18. Several precursor abnormalities of the beta-2 subunit have been described. These include a non-functional precursor, an aberrantly large or small precursor, and low-level detectable or undetectable precursor. In the absence of a functional molecule, neutrophil aggregation and chemotaxis are impaired and leukocytes fail to ingest complement-opsonized particles. Monocytes and neutrophils fail to adhere to a variety of substrates. Neutrophils in particular fail to migrate out of the vascular compartment into areas of inflammation.

Finally, a wide variety of CD18-mediated immune functions of lymphocytes such as cytotoxicity are also impaired. The advent of gene therapy offers a great opportunity to treat this condition.

Glanzmann's thrombasthenia

This is an autosomal recessive disorder characterized by a prolonged bleeding time, impaired platelet aggregation induced by ADP or other agents, reduced platelet adhesiveness and clot retraction in the presence of normal coagulation mechanism. The basic defect is an inherited deficiency of the gpIIb/IIIa protein (Ginsberg et al 1988).

Infections

A number of infectious agents of parasitic, bacterial (Isberg et al 1990), fungal or viral origin have been found either to use adhesion receptors for entry into cells, to have adherence receptors that share homology with human adhesion molecules, or to have recognition sequences on their cell-surface proteins that are identical with those recognized by human adhesion receptors. The rhinoviruses and falciparum malaria use ICAM-1 as the receptor to infect cells. *Chlamydia* and *Escherichia coli* have RGD sequences that are recognised by CD18/CD11b. The CD18/CD11a molecule is involved in HIV-induced syncytial formation in lymphocytes (Hildreth & Orentos 1989). *Entamoeba histolytica* has an adherence lectin that has homology with human integrins (Mann et al 1991). These findings are important in understanding the pathophysiological mechanisms of diseases and in the design of future therapeutic strategies.

Adhesion molecules in tumors

There is now increasing evidence that adhesion molecules contribute to tumor pathophysiology. Adhesion molecules are involved both in immune activity against malignant cells and in the metastatic spread of tumors. The clinical and experimental results obtained with IL-2 and other cytokines have focused considerable interest on the influence of the immune system on tumor growth. The importance of the CD18/CD11a pathway to both NK and antigen-specific cytotoxic T-cells in tumor control depends on the tumor target cells (Schmidt et al 1985, Shimonkevitz et al 1985). Activated NK cells express high levels of CD18/CD11b–c antigens while LAK cells in mice express high levels of beta-2 integrins and the selectin MEL-14 (Werfel et al 1991, Steen et al 1989). Macrophages, which are efficient in inducing tumor regression, also require CD18/CD11a to ingest tumor cells (Strassman et al 1986). The induction of ICAM-1 on tumor cells by T-cell-secreted cytokines increases their vulnerability to macrophage lysis (Webb et al 1991). In contrast, the induction of ICAM-1 on melanoma cells by infiltrating lymphocytes correlates with the risk for metastasis (Johnson et al 1989).

Modification of cell adhesion molecule expression may enhance the malignant potential of the cell. Some integrins appear to be modified upon transformation by the sarcoma virus, with resultant inability to adhere on extracellular matrix (Plantefaber & Hynes 1989). Low/defective expression of ICAM-1, CD18/CD11a and CD58 on Burkitt's lymphoma cells is associated with reduced susceptibility to cytotoxic killing (Gregory et al 1988). Accumulating evidence for the role of CD44 in tumor metastasis has come from studies in rat and man. In rat the metastatic potential of two tumor cell lines was linked to the expression of the heavy form of CD44 (Gunthert et al 1991), and in the human the two isoforms of CD44 might play distinct roles in tumor growth (Sy et al 1991).

KEY POINTS FOR CLINICAL PRACTICE

- Soluble circulating adhesion molecules such as ICAM-1 are important diagnostic markers of the inflammatory response to infections, neoplasia and autoimmune diseases. The development of sensitive immunoassays for circulating adhesion molecules is essential for this area.
- Recombinant ICAM-1 is known to inhibit rhinovirus infections.
- RGD peptides and gpIIb/IIIa mAbs inhibit platelet aggregation and have potential therapeutic value in the treatment of various thrombotic episodes.
- CD18 and CD54 mAbs inhibit myocardial reperfusion injuries, allograft rejection and HIV-induced syncytial formation. These examples illustrate the therapeutic potential of adhesion molecules.
- Differential expression of adhesion molecules on tumors may be useful as tumor markers, for diagnosis and classification, e.g. ICAM-1 expression on melanoma.
- Enhanced expression of adhesion molecules by cytokines may play a critical role in tumor lysis by cytolytic T-cells and macrophages.

ACKNOWLEDGEMENTS

M. W. Makgoba is supported by the MRC, the Wellcome Trust and the Royal Society. A. Bernard is supported by INSERM.

REFERENCES

Adams S A, Robson S C, Gathiriam V, Jackson T F H G et al 1993 Immunological similarity between 170 kD and amoebic adherence glycoprotein and human β_2 integrins. Lancet 341: 17–19
Aruffo A, Stamenkovic I, Melnick M et al 1990 CD44 is the principal cell surface receptor for hyaluronate. Cell 61: 1303–1313
Berg E L, Goldstein L A, Jutila M A et al 1989 Homing receptors and vascular addressins:

cell adhesion molecules that direct lymphocyte traffic. Immunol Rev 108: 5–18

Bernard A, Gelin C, Raynal B et al 1982 Phenomemon of human T-cells rosetting with sheep erythrocytes analyzed with monoclonal antibodies. 'Modulation' of a hidden epitope determining the conditions of interactions between T-cells and erythrocytes. J Exp Med 155: 1317

Bernard A, Aubrit F, Raynal B et al 1988 A T cell surface molecule different from CD2 is involved in spontaneous rosette formation with erythrocytes. J Immunol 140: 1802

Bierer B E, Bogart R E, Burakoff S J 1990 Partial deletions of the cytoplasmic domain of CD2 result in partial defect in signal transduction. J Immunol 144: 785–789

Bonfanti R, Furie B C, Furie B et al 1989 PADGEM (GMP 140) is a component of Weibel Palade bodies of human endothelial cells. Blood 73: 1109–1112

Brandley B K, Swiedler S J, Robbins P W 1990 Carbohydrate ligands of the LEC cell adhesion molecules. Cell 63: 861–863

Brottier P L, Boumsell L, Gelin C et al 1985 T-cell activation via CD2 (T:gp50) molecules. Accessory cells are required to trigger cell activation via CD2–D66 plus CD2–9.6/T111 epitopes. J Immunol 135: 1624

Carrera A C, Rincon M, De Landazuri M O et al 1988 CD2 is involved in regulating cyclic AMP levels in T cells. Eur J Immunol 18: 961–964

Deckert M, Kubar J, Bernard A 1993 CD58 and CD59 molecules exhibit potentializing effects in T cell adhesion and activation. J Immunol 148: 672–677

Edelman G M 1985 Cell adhesion and the molecular processes of morphogenesis. Annu Rev Biochem 54: 135–169

Eljaafari A, Vaquero C, Teillaud J L et al 1990 Helper or cytolytic functions can be selectively induced in bifunctional T cell clones. J Exp Med 172: 213–218

Gelin C, Aubrit F, Phalipon A et al 1980 The E2 antigen, a 32 kDa glycoprotein involved in T cell adhesion processes is the MIC2 gene product. EMBO J 8: 3253–3259

Ginsberg M H, Loftus J C, Plow E F 1988 Cytoadhesins, integrins and platelets. Thromb Haemost 59: 1–6

Gregory C D, Murray R J, Edwards C F et al 1988 Down-regulation of cell adhesion molecules LFA-3 and ICAM-1 in Epstein–Barr virus-positive Burkitt's lymphoma underlies tumor escape from virus-specific T cell surveillance. J Exp Med 167: 1811–1824

Griffin J D, Spertini O, Ernst T J et al 1990 Granulocyte macrophage colony stimulating factor and other cytokines regulate surface expression of the leukocyte adhesion molecule-1 on human neutrophils, monocytes and their precursors. J Immunol 145: 576–584

Groux H, Huet S, Aubrit F et al 1989 A 19-kDa human erythrocyte molecule H19 is involved in rosettes, present on nucleated cells and required for T-cell activation. J Immunol 142: 3013

Gunthert U, Hofmann M, Rudy W et al 1993 A new variant of glycoprotein CD44 confers metastatic potential to rat carcinoma cells. Cell 65: 13–24

Hahn W C, Rosenstein Y, Burakoff S J et al 1991 Interaction of CD2 with its ligand lymphocyte function associated antigen-3 induces adenosine 3′,5′ cyclic monophosphate production in T lymphocytes. J Immunol 147: 14–21

Haynes B F, Telen M J, Hale L P et al 1989 CD44-A molecule involved in leukocyte adherence and T cell activation. Immunol Today 10: 423

Heino J, Ignotz R A, Hemler M E et al 1989 Regulation of cell adhesion receptors by transforming growth factor-β. J Biol Chem 264: 380–388

Hemler M E 1990 VLA proteins in the integrin family: structures, functions, and their role on leukocytes. Annu Rev Immunol 8: 365–400

Hildreth J E K, Orentos R J 1989 Involvement of leukocyte adhesion receptor (LFA-1) in HIV-induced syncitium formation. Science 244: 1075–1078

Hsu-Lin S, Berman C L, Furie B C et al 1984 A platelet membrane protein expressed during platelet activation and secretion. Studies using a monoclonal antibody specific for thrombin-activated platelets. J Biol Chem 259: 9121–9126

Huet S, Wakasugi H, Sterkers G et al 1986 T-cell activation via CD2 (T,gp50): the role of accessory cells in activating resting T cells via CD2. J Immunol 137: 1420

Hunig T, Tierenthafer G, Meyer Zum Buschenfeld K H et al 1987 Alternative pathway activation of T cells by binding of CD2 to its cell-surface ligand. Nature 326: 298

Isberg R R, Leong J M 1990 Multiple β_1 chain integrins are receptors for invasin, a protein that promotes bacterial penetration into mammalian cells. Cell 60: 861–871

Johnson J P, Stade B G, Holzmann B et al 1989 De novo expression of intercellular adhesion molecule 1 in melanoma correlates with increased risk of metastasis. Immunology 86: 641–644

Kamoun M, Martin P J, Hansen J A et al 1981 Identification of a human T lymphocyte surface receptor protein associated with the E-rosette receptor. J Exp Med 153: 207

Knapp W, Dorken D, Gilks W R, Rieber E P et al (eds) 1989 Leucocyte typing IV: white cell differentiation antigens. OUP, Oxford

Larsen E, Palabrica T, Sajer S et al 1990 PADGEM dependent adhesion of platelets to monocytes and neutrophils is mediated by a lineage specific carbohydrate, LNFIII (CD15). Cell 63: 467–474

McEver R P, Beckstead J H, Moore K L et al 1989 GMP-140, a platelet alpha granule membrane protein is also synthesized by vascular endothelial cells and is localized in Weibel Palade bodies. J Clin Invest 84: 92–99

MacKrell A, Blumberg B, Haynes S et al 1988 The lethal mysospheroid gene of *Drosophila* encodes a membrane protein homologous to vertebrate integrin β subunits. Proc Natl Acad Sci USA 85: 2633–2637

Makgoba M W, Sanders M E, Shaw S 1989 The CD2–LFA-3 and LFA-1–ICAM pathways: relevance to T-cell recognition. Immunol Today 10: 417–422

Mann B J, Torian B E, Veduick T S et al 1991 Sequence of a cysteine-rich galactose-specific lectin of *Entamoeba histolytica*. Proc Natl Acad Sci USA 88: 3248–3252

Meuer S C, Hussey R E, Fabbi M et al 1984 An alternative pathway of T-cell activation: a functional role for the 50 kD T11 sheep erythrocyte receptor protein. Cell 36: 897

Miyake K, Medina K L, Hayashi S I et al 1990 Monoclonal antibodies to Pgp-1/CD44 block lympho-hemopoiesis in long-term bone marrow cultures. J Exp Med 171: 477–488

Murakami S, Miyake K, June C H et al 1990 IL-5 induces a Pgp-1 (CD44) bright B cell subpopulation that is highly enriched in proliferative and Ig secretory activity and binds to hyaluronate. J Immunol 145: 3618–3627

Picker L J, Kishimoto T K, Wayne Smith C et al 1991 ELAM-1 is an adhesion molecule for skin-homing T cells. Nature 349: 796–799

Plantefaber L C, Hynes R O 1989 Changes in integrin receptors on oncogenically transformed cells. Cell 56: 281–290

Reinholt F P, Hultenby K, Oldberg A et al 1990 Osteopontin: a possible anchor of osteoclasts to bone. Proc Natl Acad Sci USA 87: 4473–4475

Rothlein R, Mainolfi E A, Czajkowski M et al 1991 A form of circulating ICAM-1 in human serum. J Immunol 147: 3788–3793

Ruoslahti E, Pierschbacher M D 1987 New perspectives in cell adhesion: RGD and integrins. Science 238: 491–497

Saltini C, Hemler M E, Crystal R G 1988 T lymphocytes compartmentalized on the epithelial surface of the lower respiratory tract express the very late activation antigen complex VLA-1. Clin Immunol Immunopathol 46: 221–233

Sanders M E, Makgoba M W, Shaw S 1988 Human naive and memory T-cells: reinterpretation of helper–inducer and suppressor–inducer subjects. Immunol Today 9: 195–200

Schmidt R E, Bartley G, Levine H et al 1985 Functional characterization of LFA-1 antigens in the interaction of human NK clones and target cells. J Immunol 135: 1020–1025

Selvaraj P, Plunkett M L, Dustin M et al 1987 The T lymphocyte glycoprotein CD2 binds the cell surface ligand LFA-3. Nature 326: 400–403

Seth R, Raymond F D, Makgoba M W 1991 Circulating ICAM-1 isoforms: diagnostic prospects for inflammatory and immune disorders. Lancet 338: 83–84

Seth R, Salcedo R, Patarroyo M et al 1991 ICAM-2 peptides mediate lymphocyte adhesion by binding to CD11a/CD18 and CD49d/CD29 integrins. FEBS 282: 193–196

Sewell W A, Brown M H, Dunne J et al 1986 Molecular cloning of the human T lymphocyte surface CD2 (11) antigen. Immunology 83: 9718–9722

Shaw S, Ginther Luce G E, Quinones R et al 1986 Two antigen-independent adhesion pathways used by human cytotoxic T-cell clones. Nature 323: 262–264

Shimuzu Y, Shaw S 1991 Lymphocyte interactions with extracellular matrix. FASEB J 5: 2292–2299

Shimizu Y, Van Seventer G A, Horgan K J et al 1990 Regulated expression and binding of three VLA (β_1) integrin receptors on T cells. Nature 345: 250–253

Shimizu Y, Shaw S, Graber N et al 1991 Activation independent binding of human memory T cells to adhesion molecule ELAM-1. Nature 349: 799–802

Shimonkevitz R, Cerottini J C, Robson McDonald H 1985 Variable requirement of murine lymphocyte function-associated antigen-1 (LFA-1) in T cell mediated lysis depending upon the tissue origin of the target cells. J Immunol 135 (3): 1555

Smith J W, Vestal D J, Irwin S V et al 1990 Purification and functional characterization of integrin $\alpha_V\beta_5$. An adhesion receptor for vitronectin. J Biol Chem 265: 11008–11013

Spertini O, Kansas G S, Munro J M et al 1991 Regulation of leukocyte migration by activation of the leukocyte adhesion molecule-1 (LAM-1) selectin. Nature 349: 691–694

Springer T A 1990 Adhesion receptors of the immune system. Nature 346: 425–434

Springer T A, Dustin M L, Kishimoto T K et al 1987 The lymphocyte function associated LFA-1, CD2, and LFA-3 molecules: cell adhesion receptors of the immune system. Annu Rev Immunol 5: 223–252

Steen P D, McGregor J R, Lehman C M et al 1989 Changes in homing receptor expression on murine lymphokine activated killer cells during IL-2 exposure. J Immunol 143 (12): 4324–4330

Stoolman L M 1989 Adhesion molecules controlling lymphocyte migration. Cell 56: 907–910

Strassmann G, Springer T A, Sommers S D et al 1986 Mechanisms of tumor cell capture by activated macrophages: evidence for involvement of lymphocyte function associated (LFA)-1 antigen. J Immunol 136 (11): 4328

Sy M S, Guo Y J, Stamenkovic I 1991 Distinct effects of two CD44 isoforms on tumors growth in vivo. J Exp Med 174: 859–866

Tedder T F, Matsuyama T, Rothstein D et al 1990 Human antigen specific memory T cells express the homing receptor (LAM 1) necessary for lymphocyte recirculation. Eur J Immunol 20: 1351–1355

Valentin H, Groux H, Gelin C et al 1990 Modulation of lymphokine release and cytolytic activities by activating peripheral blood lymphocytes via CD2. J Immunol 144: 875–882

Vogel B E, Tarone G, Giancotti F G et al 1990 A novel fibronectin receptor with an unexpected subunit composition ($\alpha_V\beta_1$). J Biol Chem 265: 5934–5937

Watson M L, Kingsmore S F, Johnston G I et al 1990 Genomic organization of the selectin family of leukocyte adhesion molecules on human and mouse chromosome 1. J Exp Med 172: 263–272

Webb D S A, Mostowski H S, Gerrard T L 1991 Cytokine induced enhancement of ICAM-1 expression results in increased vulnerability of tumor cells to monocyte mediated lysis. J Immunol 146 (10): 3682

Werfel T, Witter W, Gotze O 1991 CD11b and CD11c antigens are rapidly increased on human natural killer cells upon activation. J Immunol 147 (7): 2423

Yang S Y, Chouaib S, Dupont B 1986 A common pathway for T lymphocyte activation involving both the CD3-TI complex and CD2 sheep erythrocyte receptor determinants. J Immunol 137: 1097

7

Immunotherapy of leukemia

M. K. Brenner

Although historical attempts to use immunotherapy to improve the outcome of leukemia have proved largely barren, a number of recent advances have begun to raise hopes that enhancement or modification of immune effector mechanisms may represent a useful supplement to conventional therapy and may be of particular value in the eradication of minimal residual disease.

That the immune system has the *potential* to eradicate residual leukemia in man is no longer in doubt. This statement can be confidently made largely because of results from allogeneic bone marrow transplantation, in which the presence of the incoming donor immune system generates a readily detectable graft-versus-leukemia (GVL) effect. This activity has been shown in three ways (Barrett et al 1989, Bortin et al 1979, International Bone Marrow Transplant Registry 1989, Horowitz et al 1990a,b). First, patients who suffer from graft-versus-host disease (GVHD) are less likely to relapse than those who do not have this complication (Horowitz et al 1990b, Apperley et al 1988, Weiden et al 1979, 1981, Ferrara & Deeg 1991, Weisdorf et al 1987). Secondly, patients receiving T-lymphocyte depleted bone marrow transplant — in whom the risk of GVHD is very low — may have a higher risk of relapse (Horowitz et al 1990b, Goldman et al 1988); and finally, recipients of syngeneic (identical twin) allograft have a higher risk of relapse than recipients of HLA-identical sibling grafts (International Bone Marrow Transplant Registry 1989, Horowitz et al 1990a). Taken together, these results indicate that the incoming graft may contribute to the eradication of residual leukemia. However, they also strongly imply that the GVL effect may simply be another aspect of GVHD; since residual leukemia cells are of host origin, they too are susceptible to the damage inflicted on the normal tissues of skin, gut, and liver during GVHD. The challenge now facing would-be immunotherapists of leukemia is to discover whether GVL and GVHD really are manifestations of the same phenomenon, or whether they can be separated, thereby freeing the immune system's potential for disease eradication from its capacity to cause damage (Bortin et al 1979, Truitt et al 1986, Prentice & Brenner 1989). If GVL mechanisms can be separated from GVHD, it might be possible to generate this immunotherapeutic effect, not only in allograft recipients, but also in patients receiving autologous bone marrow transplantation or indeed chemotherapy alone. If, on the other hand,

GVL and GVHD are in reality inseparable, then the future of immuno-therapy in leukemia treatment is limited at best; using one disease to treat another is rarely a successful stratagem.

This chapter begins by describing the potential mechanisms by which the host immune system may recognize leukemia independently of an allogeneic 'GVHD' effect. We will then describe current efforts to exploit these discriminatory abilities and conclude by describing future approaches which it is hoped will further improve immunotherapy.

HOW DOES THE IMMUNE SYSTEM DISCRIMINATE BETWEEN NORMAL AND LEUKEMIC CELLS?

Two main types of cellular effector mechanisms are available to the immune system and may be important in GVL action: MHC restricted antigen specific T-lymphocytes and MHC unrestricted effector cells (superantigen specific or antigen non-specific killer cells). While antibodies to tumor specific antigens might make an additional therapeutic contribution, there is no evidence that the humoral immune response contributes to any naturally occurring GVL effect.

Leukemia specific killing by MHC restricted T-cells that recognize leukemia specific antigens

A number of models have shown that MHC restricted antigen specific T-lymphocytes can protect animals against transplantable (usually lymphoid) leukemias (Cheever et al 1986). For these effects to be relevant to the successful eradication of human leukemia, it is probably necessary to show not only that leukemic cells universally express unique antigens, but that these antigens are critical to the leukemic behavior of the cell. Expression of leukemia specific antigens per se may not be sufficient. For example, the one certain example of a leukemia specific antigen is the unique immunoglobulin idiotype expressed by many leukemia/lymphomas derived from mature B-cells. Although anti-idiotypic antibody responses can be generated against these unique tumor epitopes, they rarely succeed in eradicating the malig-nancy, since subclones are generated which either express Ig of modified idiotype or no Ig at all (Sosman et al 1990). Similar clonal escape from specific cytotoxic T-cells might also occur were the specific antigenic structure dispensable in terms of the malignant process.

Fortunately, a substantial number of leukemias have been found to produce proteins which are both unique and apparently important in the leukemic process. These include the fusion proteins formed following gene translocations and the abnormal oncogenes produced following point muta-tions in the encoding genes (Ben-Neriah et al 1986, Chan et al 1987, Browett & Norton 1989, Ridge et al 1990, De The et al 1990, Platsoucas 1991, Moller et al 1988). Both types of protein contain unique peptide sequences and thereby provide the *potential* for the leukemic cells to be recognized by antigen specific T-lymphocyte clones. However, since these leukemia specific products are all internal proteins, it is not obvious why they should be recognized by antigen specific T-cells. This difficulty may be more apparent than real, since many internal proteins are processed to peptides in the pre-Golgi compartment, where they become associated with nascent MHC molecules (Fig. 7.1). The complex of processed peptide and MHC antigen subsequently appears on the cell surface. It is this complex of specific peptide and specific MHC polymorphism which is recognized by the CD3 specific T-cell receptor complex on the classical MHC restricted T effector cell (Fig. 7.2A). Since the existence of leukemia specific proteins is not in doubt, the relevant questions therefore become:

1. Are point mutated or fusion peptides processed and presented by leukemic cells?
2. Can T-cells distinguish such mutants from the wild-type peptides?

The past year has produced evidence favoring a positive response to both questions. Although relatively little is known about antigen processing and presentation by leukemic cells, data from Sosman et al (1989) suggest that leukemia specific antigens appear on leukemia cell surfaces. They described the generation of CD3+, CD4+ T-cell clones reacting with allogeneic ALL (acute lymphoblastic anemia) cells which do not react with remission

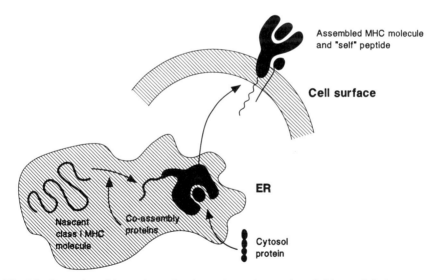

Fig. 7.1 Processing of internal proteins: internal proteins are degraded intracellularly to peptide fragments; in the endoplasmic reticulum these are helped by a variety of co-assembly proteins to associate with newly formed Class I MHC molecules. The peptide is enfolded in the binding cleft of the MHC molecule and the peptide – MHC complex moves to the cell surface where it can be recognized by a (non-tolerant) T-lymphocyte. It is postulated that proteins unique to malignant cells, such as mutant oncogenes and fusion proteins, behave in the same way.

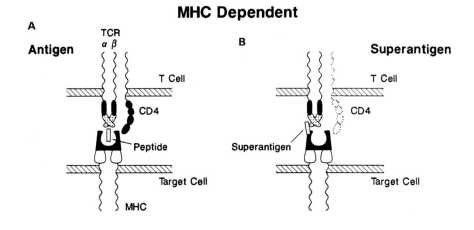

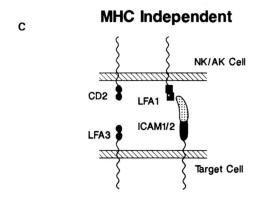

Fig. 7.2 Recognition of antigen by immune system cells: Antigen may be recognized in an MHC-restricted or unrestricted fashion. **A** Classical antigen-specific T-cells recognize the MHC peptide complex, formed as described in Fig. 7.1. Recognition is stabilized by a variety of accessory molecules, such as CD4 in T helper cell–target cell interaction. Anti-tumor MHC-restricted interactions may occur on the surface of professional antigen-presenting cells which may derive the presented antigen from the breakdown of tumor cells or they may occur on the tumor cell surface itself, if these cells express Class I and/or Class II MHC molecules. **B** Superantigen recognition: superantigens bind to non-polymorphic regions of MHC molecules (usually Class II), and are then recognized by T-cell receptor *families*, rather than by T-cell receptors of unique specificity. Superantigens may or may not be processed internally by the cell. Superantigen recognition may be considered a 'half-way house' between the classical antigen specific recognition described in **A** and MHC-independent recognition described in **C**. **C** MHC independent recognition: binding to and destruction of tumor cell targets may come about independently of MHC by recognition of a number of different receptor and ligands on the effector–target cell surface. Two such receptor–ligand interactions are illustrated: CD2 and its ligand LFA-3 (CD58), and LFA-1 (CD11/18) and its ligand ICAM-1 (CD54)/2.

lymphocytes from the same patient, implying that these clones recognize an antigen expressed on leukemic but not on normal cells. This evidence, of course, is not definitive, but active efforts are being made by a number of groups to consolidate the issue.

There is less doubt that, if mutant proteins are presented by leukemic cells, they can be distinguished from the wild-type products by antigen specific T-cells. Jung & Schluesner (1991) synthesized a *ras*-derived peptide in which valine was substituted for glycine at residue 12, a substitution associated with transforming ability in the intact protein. They were able to generate an MHC restricted CD4 T-cell line which proliferated only in response to mutant peptide and had no response to stimulation with wild-type peptide. Mutant specific responses may also be generated in vivo. Peace et al (1991) used a similar ras peptide — but now with arginine substituted at residue 12 — to immunize C57BL/6 mice. Again MHC restricted CD4+ specific T-cells were generated in vivo which recognized both mutant peptide and mutant ras protein processed by antigen presenting cells, but did not respond to wild-type peptide or protein. Using a similar approach, the bcr–abl junctional peptide has subsequently been shown to recruit specific T-cells when injected into mice. These observations may mean that a specific antileukemia effect can be generated against a range of acute and chronic leukemias and imply that the previously discredited concept of leukemia specific vaccines may be gaining a new legitimacy.

Leukemia selective but MHC-unrestricted killing (superantigen specific or antigen non-specific)

Whether or not MHC restricted, antigen specific recognition of leukemia blast cells genuinely exists, an alternative mechanism of antileukemia effector function may be relevant (Karre et al 1980). Natural killer (NK) cells are MHC unrestricted effector cells (Herberman & Ortaldo 1981) which can inhibit clonogenic leukemia growth in vitro and which are particularly numerous and active (activated killer (AK) cells) for the first few weeks following both autologous and allogeneic bone marrow transplant (BMT) (Karre et al 1980, Brenner et al 1986) or following administration of cytokines such as interleukin 2 (IL-2) (Rosenberg et al 1988, Anderson et al 1988, Gottlieb et al 1989a, Smith 1988). Although these cells inhibit leukemic growth in vitro, it was uncertain whether or not they could discriminate between normal and leukemic progenitors to produce a selective antileukemia effector function in vivo. Many cells with NK/AK function are CD3– and therefore lack the only known antigen specific receptor present on cytotoxic lymphocytes. Therefore, even if leukemic cells do express specific antigens, it is unclear how these CD3– effectors would recognize them. Even though a subpopulation of NK/AK cells are in fact CD3+, there has still been a problem in understanding how these T-cell receptor positive cells could distinguish normal from malignant cells. One functional definition of NK and AK lymphocytes is that they are MHC unrestricted. Since the CD3 receptor classically only recognizes specific antigen complexed with a specific MHC polymorphism (Fig. 7.2a), the MHC unrestricted killing of CD3+ AK cells had been thought to mean that target cell recognition could not involve the antigen specific CD3+ receptor and therefore by definition could not be antigen specific.

It has now been demonstrated that both CD3− and CD3+ AK cells may in fact selectively kill leukemic blasts despite their lack of a conventionally functioning MHC restricted antigen specific CD3 receptor.

Leukemia specific killing by MHC unrestricted but CD3+ AK cells

Although conventional protein antigens are processed within the cell and are recognized following association with newly synthesized MHC molecules, antigens also exist which by-pass this route. Although these 'superantigens' may be processed, they associate directly with a range of non-polymorphic determinants on the cell surface where they bind a family of T-cell receptors (see below). Since these products are not limited to specific MHC molecules, CD3 receptor binding occurs in a MHC unrestricted manner (Fig. 7.2B).

Although bacterial products were the first superantigens described, a number of cellular products can behave in the same way, including proteins of the heat shock family. Fisch et al (1990a,b) were able to generate CD3+ T-cell lines using Vγ9 and Vδ2 T-cell receptor proteins which could recognize ligands homologous to heat shock superantigens on the surface of Daudi, a Burkitt lymphoma line. Cross-reactive antisera to GroEL — a protein from *Escherichia coli* homologous to mycobacterial heat shock proteins — blocked the proliferative response of these lines, but antibody to MHC products had no effect. In other words, proliferation was antigen specific (to the heat shock superantigens), but was also MHC unrestricted. If other leukemia/lymphoma cells express qualitatively or even quantitatively different superantigens to their normal equivalents, then the CD3+ MHC unrestricted AK cells appearing after BMT or during cytokine infusion could contribute to leukemia specific killing.

Killing by the CD3− subset

In order to kill their target cells effectively, CD3− AK lymphocytes must first bind to them, an effect achieved by a variety of cell adhesion molecules (CAM) (Fig. 7.2C) (Davignon et al 1981, Simmons et al 1988, Timonen 1990). Oblakowski et al (1991) showed that normal and malignant CD34+ myeloid progenitor cells may express different patterns of CAM. Normal CD34+ cells express LFA-3 (CD58) the ligand for LFA-2 (CD2) but no detectable ICAM-1 (CD54), a ligand for a second AK cell adhesion molecule LFA-1 (CD11a/18). Killing of normal progenitors by CD3− AK cells is therefore largely dependent on the interaction of CD2–CD58 ligand – receptor pathway and monoclonal antibodies to CD58 block cytotoxicity. By contrast, CD34+ myeloid blasts express large quantities of the ligands CD54 *and* CD58, so that binding of effectors may occur through both the CD11a/18–CD54 and CD2–CD58 pathways. As a consequence, killing of malignant blasts is not prevented by monoclonal antibody to the CD58 ligand alone. The authors postulate that because of in vivo competition from erythrocytes — which express high levels of CD58 — AK cells will preferentially bind to and therefore preferentially kill malignant blasts. Whether this suggestion is true or not, differences in patterns of CAM expression clearly provide the opportunity for selectivity of killing by CD3– AK subsets (Anichini et al 1990). As we learn more about the other target cell surface molecules recognized by NK cells, we may well discern other differences in the pattern of their expression which permit selective recognition and killing (Ciccone et al 1990a,b).

ENHANCEMENT OF ANTILEUKEMIC MECHANISMS

Methods of producing immunomodulation

A variety of approaches have been used in the past, most notably BCG immunization (Reizenstein 1990). At present, however, three approaches to immunostimulation are favored: cytokines such as IL-2; orally active drugs such as linomide; and induction/promotion of GVHD with the hoped-for by-product of increased GVL activity.

Cytokines

Although a number of cytokines and cytokine antagonists are being evaluated in clinical studies for their antileukemic activity, most appear to act by an antiproliferative mechanism. At present IL-2 — and perhaps α-interferon — are the only cytokines to be used clinically as antileukemic immuno-modulators (Rosenberg et al 1988, Gottlieb et al 1989a,b, Blaise et al 1990). In animal and human preclinical models, IL-2 increases antigen specific cytotoxic effector function and also induces and enhances MHC unrestricted NK/AK function (Farrar et al 1982). IL-2 also induces release of a number of other cytokines including TNF (tumor necrosis factor) and γ-interferon which themselves may have an antileukemic effect (Heslop et al 1989a,b). α-Interferon probably produces its therapeutic effects by antiproliferative mechanisms (Heslop et al 1990) but may also recruit AK function or increase the sensitivity of leukemic cells to immune effector mechanisms.

Pharmacological agents

An alternative approach to producing activation of T-cell independent effector mechanisms after BMT is to use immunostimulatory drugs. One recent addition to this group is roquinimex (Linomide), a drug related in structure to the quinoline antibiotics. This agent was found to have antileukemic properties in mice and was subsequently shown to augment NK activity, to induce AK function, and to enhance cytokine release, including TNF and γ-interferon (Bengtsson et al 1990). This drug has now been given in pilot studies in patients recovering from autologous bone marrow transplantation chemotherapy for myeloid leukemia where it was reasonably well tolerated in doses which induced considerable modulation of NK/AK function and of cytokine release, and a randomized double-blind study is in progress.

Immunostimulation by induction of GVHD

Since GVL and GVHD are so closely linked, attempts have been made to induce GVHD after allogeneic BMT in patients at high risk of relapse, by giving them donor buffy-coat infusions after engraftment (Sullivan et al 1989a,b). Although these studies succeeded in their primary aim of exacerbating GVHD, there was no evidence that relapse rates were reduced. Instead, there was high mortality from the complications of the therapy.

A similar line of reasoning forms the basis for attempts to induce 'mild' GVHD in recipients of autologous bone marrow transplants (Jones et al 1989). These patients have a relapse risk above that of age- and disease-matched patients receiving allogeneic transplant, although overall survival is often little different because of lower procedure related mortality (Gorin et al 1986). It had been shown in a rat model that administration of cyclosporine A following autologous BMT could induce mild GVHD like responses, which could be exacerbated by sudden reduction of cyclosporine A administration (Grazier et al 1983). This autologous GVHD probably relates to a requirement for IL-2 during thymic processing of immature T-lymphocytes. In rodents, at least, IL-2 appears to be essential for selection of 'self-unreactive' T-cell clones (Jenkins et al 1988). If IL-2 is prevented from stimulating T-cells during their passage through the thymus, then the organ is no longer able to remove autoreactive T-cell clones. Instead, clones emerge into the peripheral circulation which have the ability to recognize self antigens as foreign. Since the quantity of marrow returned for an autologous BMT contains only a tiny portion of the T-lymphocytes required to repopulate the patient, substantial T-cell regeneration is required. Although this need may in part be met by expansion of mature T-cell clones — which will already have been selected for non-autoreactivity — it may also be met by expansion of prethymic progenitor cells. These will require thymic processing to remove autoreactive precursors offering a window for intervention.

Cyclosporine A produces its immunosuppressive effects by blocking the release of autocrine growth factors, including IL-2, which are normally produced after T-lymphocyte stimulation (Elliot et al 1984, Espevik et al 1990). Cyclosporine A achieves this by binding to a cell receptor, cytophilin. Although this protein is a peptidyl isomerase (Fischer et al 1989, Takahashi et al 1989), its natural ligand is not yet known. The receptor – cyclosporine A complex is then internalized, binds to DNA and blocks production of cytokine transcripts. Thus, in the presence of cyclosporine A, production of IL-2 is impaired. The IL-2-dependent thymic selection procedure may therefore be less rigorous than normal, permitting the emergence of new, autoreactive T-cell clones with 'GVHD' inducing potential.

Regardless of the underlying mechanism, this approach has successfully produced mild GVHD in patients with lymphoma who are treated with ABMT autologous bone marrow transplant. Autologous GVHD has also been induced in AML (acute myeloid leukemia) patients receiving autografts (Talbot et al 1990, Yeager et al 1992). Overall, toxicities have been low.

Immunomodulation by genetically modified tumor cells

In mouse models, transfer of cytokine genes into tumor cells renders them highly immunogenic. Not only are the injected gene modified tumor cells rejected but a response is generated which allows the animal to reject unmodified tumor cells — in some cases even if these have already established themselves as sizable tumors. Transfer of a number of different cytokine genes (including IL-1, IL-2, IL-4, IL-7, TNF, γ-interferon and GM-CSF) can produce this tumor-vaccine-like effect, and the modified cells may recruit T-lymphocytes, NK cells, monocytes and eosinophils to produce tumor rejection (Asher et al 1991, Blankenstein et al 1991, Connor et al 1991, Storb et al 1990, Gansbacher et al 1990). This approach is now being investigated clinically in adults and children with a number of different solid tumors and may well have a future contribution to make to the immunotherapy of leukemia.

INDICATIONS AND CONTRAINDICATIONS FOR ENHANCING ANTILEUKEMIC EFFECTOR MECHANISMS

Minimal residual disease

Most attempts at immunomodulation have occurred in the setting of minimal residual disease. The evidence that the immune system may contribute to leukemia eradication after BMT makes this procedure an obvious first choice for immunomodulation; not only is the tumor burden lowest at this time and the ratio of effector: target cells therefore greatest, but many patients with active leukemia may have severely impaired cytotoxic effector function (Foa et al 1991a). However, attempts to augment GVL after *allogeneic* BMT using cytokines such as IL-2 or pharmacological agents such as linomide, have been constrained by a concern that these efforts would simply augment the growth of alloreactive donor T-lymphocytes and so exacerbate GVHD — the phenomenon deliberately exploited in the Seattle study (Sullivan et al 1989b). To date, therefore, clinical immunomodulation has predominantly been attempted in patients following *autologous* BMT or after chemotherapy alone (Gottlieb et al 1989a,b, Blaise et al 1990), although low-dose IL-2 may be safely administered to patients after allogeneic BMT (Soiffer et al 1992). An approach has been described, however, which may allow even high-dose

IL-2-mediated enhancement of antileukemic effector function after allo-BMT without exacerbating GVHD.

If lethally irradiated mice receiving allogeneic T-cell-replete BMT are also given IL-2 post grafting, then GVHD is both accelerated and intensified (Malkovsky et al 1986). But if the mice are simultaneously given syngeneic T-cell-depleted marrow, then GVHD is absent — even when donor and recipient are MHC disparate, and even though there is full donor engraftment (Sykes et al 1990a). Moreover, the new graft retains 'GVL' activity since it can eradicate leukemic cells given at the same time (Sykes et al 1990b). Although the mechanism for this effect has not been established, it is likely that the proliferating mature T-cells in the incoming graft are anergized by exposure to recipient immune system cells and high doses of IL-2. That this anergy is specific is demonstrated by the capacity of T-cells in the incoming immune system to prevent engraftment of a transplantable leukemia.

If this approach can be demonstrated to be safe and effective in larger animals, it is reasonable to hope that we may be able to prevent GVHD even after MHC non-identical BMT and yet retain or even enhance both the MHC restricted and non-restricted GVL effects we have described.

Following BMT and chemotherapy

One concern about using IL-2 in minimal residual disease is that patients have been exposed to high-dose chemotherapy and may also have been given supralethal chemotherapy/radiation as a preparative regimen if they are to receive a BMT. Such intensive treatment carries a significant morbidity and mortality. Similarly, infusion of a cytokine such as IL-2 in immuno-modulatory doses produces its own morbidity and occasional mortality, since it is toxic to many of the same target organs damaged by preparative regimens (Rosenberg et al 1988, Smith 1988). It has therefore been questioned whether it would be possible to combine cytokine infusion with BMT/intensive chemotherapy or whether the combined toxicity would make it impossible to administer immunomodulatory doses of the drug.

Leukemia subtypes

It should be noted that differential sensitivity to cytotoxic effector mechanisms may not be shown by all types of leukemia. For example, while myeloid blasts are more sensitive than normal myeloid progenitors to MHC unrestricted killing, this differential effect is somewhat harder to demonstrate when acute lymphoblastic leukemia blast cells are the target cells (Oblakowski et al 1991, Archimbaud 1991). Similarly, antigen specific T-cell-mediated killing may be more important in leukemias, such as CML (chronic myelocytic leukemia), where a clear-cut phenotypic difference (bcr-abl) is present between normal and malignant cells. Effective immunotherapy may therefore be limited in applicability.

Presence of IL-2 receptors on malignant target cells

The potential benefits of IL-2 on potentiation of immune system effector mechanism could be neutralized if the agent also acted as a growth factor for leukemic cells. To demonstrate that IL-2 is a direct growth factor requires two criteria to be fulfilled. The first is that receptors for the cytokine should be present on the malignant cell, and the second is that the cell should proliferate in the presence of the factor, or at least transduce the signal provided by the binding of the cytokine and enter the cell cycle. There seems little doubt that a proportion of patients with ALL and lymphoma have malignant clones whose progeny fulfil both these requirements — although the precise proportion remains controversial (Foa et al 1990a).

For AML, there is much less certainty. While cells from some patients — particularly those with the Fab M4/5 subtypes — have been shown to express either the low-affinity p55 component of the IL-2 receptor (Armitage et al 1986) or the intermediate-affinity p75 chain (Rosolon et al 1989), there is no convincing evidence that AML blasts express both IL-2 receptor chains. Since both chains need to be expressed to form a high-affinity binding site, it is unlikely that AML blasts would effectively compete for IL-2 at the low systemic concentrations achieved during infusion. Moreover, there is no evidence to suggest that receptor expressing AML blasts can respond in any way to IL-2 even at concentrations substantially higher than can be achieved by administration in vivo. Nonetheless it is possible to show in vitro that some AML blasts will undergo a degree of DNA synthesis in the presence of IL-2 at high concentrations (Carron & Cawley 1990, Tanaka 1991). Even in these cases it is possible that much of the apparent response may be explained by lymphocyte contamination. In short, IL-2 may act as a growth factor for a proportion of ALL cells, but it is much less certain that it has an equivalent effect on AML blasts.

IMMUNOMODULATION AFTER AUTOLOGOUS BMT AND CHEMOTHERAPY

If we accept that immunomodulation is optimal when patients are in a state of minimal residual disease post therapy, a number of treatment options are available.

IL-2

Most studies of IL-2 in patients with minimal residual leukemia have administered the drug to the patients themselves, although efforts have also been made to use the cytokine to treat marrow ex vivo as a form of immunological purging (Charak et al 1991, Gambacorti-Passerini et al 1991). Starting in January 1987, we undertook a phase I–II trial of IL-2 infusion in individuals with AML in remission after chemotherapy or autologous BMT. The aim was to see if the drug could be tolerated in doses which would produce measurable immunomodulation. In general IL-2 was well tolerated when given as 5-day courses repeated twice, at doses between 200 and 800 μg/m^2/day (Gottlieb et al 1989a).

Almost all patients developed fever >38°C and nausea and about half became significantly, but transiently, hypotensive. No patient needed treatment in intensive care. The first two patients, however, were treated by longer infusions, continuing over 10 days. This was poorly tolerated; both patients developed hypotension, one patient developed severe bronchospasm, and the other developed an interstitial pneumonitis that progressed to a fatal outcome despite withdrawal of the IL-2.

Fortunately, even the well-tolerated doses of IL-2 produced a high level of immune modulation, characterized by increased numbers of CD56+, CD16+ or CD8+ AK cells (Gottlieb et al 1989b). There was increased direct cytotoxicity against cells infected with Epstein–Barr virus but not against target cells infected with another member of the herpes group, cytomegalovirus (Duncombe et al 1992). More importantly, perhaps, there was a substantial increase in the number and activity of cells able to inhibit the clonogenic growth of leukemic blasts (Gottlieb et al 1989b). Leukemic colony and cluster formation was inhibited by up to 95%. It was also possible to augment production of the antileukemic/antiviral cytokines TNF and γ-interferon (Heslop et al 1989b). Serum levels of γ-interferon rose sharply during infusion of IL-2, and although a rise in serum TNF could not be detected, CD16+ and CD3+ lymphocytes cultured from these patients showed a greatly increased production of TNF in vitro if they were obtained during IL-2 infusion.

One residual concern about IL-2 infusion was that the cytokines induced, particularly TNF and γ-interferon, would not only inhibit the growth of malignant myeloid progenitor cells but would also damage the engrafting normal progenitor cells: although these cytokines may be preferentially cytotoxic to malignant cells, their selectivity is relative, not absolute (Heslop et al 1989b). In fact, the neutrophil count rose significantly during IL-2 infusion, an effect that could not be attributed entirely to demargination. Instead, IL-2 also induced hematopoietic growth factors. IL-3 and GM-CSF could both be detected in circulating lymphoid cells as transcripts and as proteins; there was also a rise in serum GM-CSF during infusion (Heslop et al 1991). Despite production of IL-3, however, platelet levels fell during IL-2 infusion, perhaps due to increased consumption mediated by the effects of TNF on vascular endothelium (Bauer et al 1989).

Other studies

Subsequent studies of IL-2 infusions in AML have produced comparable safety and immunologic efficiency data (Blaise et al 1990, Soiffer et al 1992,

MacDonald et al 1991, Foa et al 1991b, Olive et al 1991, Lotzova et al 1991, Higuchi et al 1991). Only when IL-2 is given in high dose immediately after BMT is there an unacceptably high level of toxicity. More recently, it has been shown that subcutaneous low-dose IL-2 was well tolerated when given alone (Soiffer et al 1992) or after high-dose IL-2 infusion (Higuchi et al 1991). In both cases significant increases in cytotoxic effector function were shown. In addition, therapy with low-dose IL-2 alone was well tolerated after allogeneic BMT (Soiffer et al 1992), and did not induce GVHD. Low-dose, long-term administration (3 months) of IL-2 may therefore allow the potentially beneficial effects of IL-2 to be produced and maintained with minimal adverse effects.

Conclusions of phase I–II studies

Overall, these investigations show that IL-2 can be given safely after autologous BMT and will induce or enhance effector mechanisms that would be predicted to exert a GVL effect and reduce relapse rates; however, there have been too few patients to allow firm conclusions to be drawn about clinical benefit.

Does any form of immunomodulation translate to clinical benefit?

This question cannot yet be answered. One basic assumption made about both T-cell-mediated and T-cell-independent GVL mechanisms is that they will be effective only in an environment of minimal residual disease. The assumption is made, because it is in minimal residual disease, that the ratio of effectors to malignant targets would most favor the effector cells, providing the optimum setting for a successful immunologic assault. In bulky disease, where normal and malignant cells are numerically matched, or where the numerical advantage may even be with the malignant cells themselves, success is much less likely. Indeed most attempts to use IL-2 − the most potent of the immunomodulators − in the treatment of relapsed leukemia have failed, although reports from Italy suggest that it is able to induce remission in some patients with relapsed AML, provided it is given when the percentage of marrow blasts is low (Foa et al 1990b).

Unfortunately, it is exceedingly difficult to study the efficacy of any putative antineoplastic drug in the setting of minimal residual disease. No immediate feedback of the effect of different doses or dose regimens is available, and the study has to be large, randomized and long term before any beneficial effects can be assessed with certainty. But, for the reasons explained, these minimal residual disease studies are essential, since approaches using immunomodulatory agents to treat bulky disease are likely to be disappointing.

Randomized studies of IL-2 and linomide are now in progress, and the next year should begin to reveal whether this immunomodulatory approach is of benefit. Designing a randomized trial to analyze an alternative method of producing an antileukemic effector function — 'auto-GVHD' — is considerably more demanding.

IMPROVING THE IMMUNOLOGICAL EFFICACY OF IMMUNOSTIMULATORS

Although the clinical efficacy of IL-2 or other immunomodulators is not yet established, it is still worthwhile to attempt to improve the immunologic efficacy of these agents while minimizing their toxicity. One way to achieve this aim may be to use long-term low dosage as already described (Soiffer et al 1992, Higuchi et al 1991). Another route is to manipulate those mechanisms responsible for the down-regulation of lymphocyte activation. For example, IL-4 is a cytokine induced during IL-2 infusion, and contributes to the homeostatic regulation of IL-2 induced effects. If endogenous IL-4 activity is neutralized by monoclonal antibody, then the half-life of AK function is greatly prolonged in patients receiving IL-2 (Bello-Fernandez et al 1991). Moreover, neutralization of endogenous IL-4 augments secretion of antileukemic/antiviral cytokines such as TNF and γ-interferon 100-fold or more. It might therefore be possible to reduce IL-2 dosage and simplify IL-2 treatment regimens if infusion of IL-2 were combined with injection of antibody to IL-4 or its receptors. This approach is being investigated.

KEY POINTS FOR CLINICAL PRACTICE

- Studies of the graft versus leukemia effect following allogeneic bone marrow transplantation show that the immune system has the ability to eradicate residual leukemia.
- As more mutations are identified in leukemic cells, more targets for immunotherapy may become available.
- Clinical studies with immunostimulators such as interleukin 2 and linomide have shown that patient immunocompetence can be augmented even after intensive chemotherapy or bone marrow transplantation.
- Randomized controlled trials are currently in progress to assess the value of immunomodulation in preventing relapse of acute myeloblastic leukemia.
- Substances which enhance immune system activity may also enhance the growth of leukemias originating from lymphoid cells.

ACKNOWLEDGMENTS

This work was supported by NIH grant CA 21765 (CORE) and by the American Lebanese Syrian Associated Charities (ALSAC).

REFERENCES

Anderson P M, Bach F H, Ochoa A C 1988 Augmentation of cell number and LAK activity in peripheral blood mononuclear cells activated with anti-CD3 and interleukin-2. Preliminary results in children with acute lymphocytic leukemia and neuroblastoma. Cancer Immunol Immunother 27: 82–88

Anichini A, Mortarini R, Spino R et al 1990 Human melanoma cells with high susceptibility to cell-mediated lysis can be identified on the basis of ICAM-1 phenotype, VLA profile and invasive ability. Int J Cancer 46: 508–513

Apperley J F, Mauro F R, Goldman J M 1988 Bone marrow transplantation for chronic myeloid leukemia in first chronic phase: importance of a graft versus leukemia effect. Br J Haematol 69: 239–245

Archimbaud E, Thomas X, Compos L et al 1991 Susceptibility of adult acute lymphoblastic leukemia blasts to lysis by lymphokine-activated killer cells. Leukemia 5: 967–971

Armitage R J, Lai A P, Roberts P J et al 1986 Certain myeloid cells possess receptors for interleukin-2. Br J Haematol 64: 799–807

Asher A L, Mule J J, Kasid A et al 1991 Murine tumor cells transduced with the gene for tumor necrosis factor alpha. J Immunol 146: 3227–3234

Barrett A J, Horowitz M M, Gale R P 1989 Marrow transplantation for acute lymphoblastic leukemia: factors affecting relapse and survival. Blood 74: 862–871

Bauer K A, ten Cate H, Barzegar S 1989 Tumor necrosis infusions have a procoagulant effect on the hemostatic mechanism of humans. Blood 74: 165–172

Bello-Fernandez C, Bird C, Heslop H E et al 1991 Homeostatic action of interleukin 4 on endogenous and rIL2 induced activated killer cell function. Blood 77: 1283–1289

Bengtsson M, Simonsson B, Smedmyr B et al 1990 Immunostimulation post autologous bone marrow transplantation (ABMT) with the novel drug linomide: augmentation of T- and NK-cell functions. Fifth International Symposium on Autologous Bone Marrow Transplantation Omaha, Nebraska, 113: 234

Ben-Neriah Y, Daley G Q, Mes-Massom A M et al 1986 The chronic myelogenous leukemia-specific p210 protein is the product of the *bcl/abl* hybrid gene. Science 233: 212–214

Blaise D, Olive D, Stoppa A M et al 1990 Hematologic and immunologic effects of recombinant interleukin-2 after autologous bone marrow transplantation. Blood 76: 1092–1097

Blankenstein T, Qin Z, Uberla K et al 1991 Tumor suppression after tumor cell-targeted tumor necrosis factor alpha gene transfer. J Exp Med 173: 1047–1052

Bortin M J, Truitt R L, Rimm A A et al 1979 Graft-versus-leukemia rectivity induced by alloimmunisation without augmentation of graft-versus-host reactivity. Nature 281: 490–491

Brenner M K, Reittie J E, Grob J-P et al 1986 The contribution of large granular lymphocytes to B cell activation and differentiation after T cell depleted allogeneic bone marrow transplantation. Transplantation 42: 257–261

Browett P J, Norton J D 1989 Analysis of *ras* gene mutations and methylation state in human leukemias. Oncogene 4: 1029–1036

Carron J A, Cawley J C 1990 IL2 and myelopoiesis: IL2 induces blast cell proliferation in some cases of acute myeloid leukemia. Br J Haematol 73: 168–172

Chan L C, Karhi K K, Rayter S I 1987 A novel abl protein expressed in Philadelphia chromosome positive acute lymphoblastic leukemia. Nature 325: 635–637

Charak B S, Agah R, Gray D et al 1991 Interaction of various cytokines with interleukin 2 in the generation of killer cells from human bone marrow: application in purging of leukemia. Leuk Res 15: 801–810

Cheever M A, Britzmann Thompson D, Klarnet J P et al 1986 Antigen driven long term cultured T cells proliferate in vivo, distribute widely, mediate specific tumor therapy, and persist long-term as functional memory T cells. J Exp Med 163: 1100–1112

Ciccone E, Pende D, Viale O et al 1990a Specific recognition of human CD3– CD16+ natural killer cells requires the expression of an autosomic recessive gene on target cells. J Exp Med 172: 47

Ciccone E, Colonna M, Viale O et al 1990b Susceptibility or resistance to lysis by alloreactive natural killer cells is governed by a gene in the human major histocompatibility complex between BF and HLA-A. Proc Natl Acad Sci USA 87: 9794

Connor J P, Gansbacher B, Cronin K et al 1991 A new approach to the immunotherapy of bladder cancer using IL-2 gene transfer into MBT-2 cells. Proc Annu Meet Am Assoc Cancer Res 32: A1475

Davignon D, Martz E, Reynolds T et al 1981 Lymphocyte function-associated antigen 1 (LFA-1): a surface antigen distinct from Lyt 2,3 that participates in T lymphocyte-mediated killing. Proc Natl Acad Sci USA 78: 4535–4539

De The H, Chomienne C, Lanotte M et al 1990 The t(15;17) translocation of acute promyelocytic leukaemia fuses the retinoic acid receptor alpha gene to a novel transcribed locus. Nature 347: 558–561

Duncombe A S, Grundy J E, Oblakowski P 1992 Bone marrow transplant recipients have defective MHC-unrestricted cytotoxic responses against cytomegalovirus in comparison with Epstein-Barr virus: the importance of target cell expression of lymphocyte function-associated antigen 1 (LFA1). Blood 79: 3059–3066

Elliot J F, Lin Y, Mizel S B 1984 Induction of interleukin-2 messenger RNA inhibited by cyclosporin A. Science 226: 1439–1441

Espevik T, Figari I S, Shalaby M R et al 1990 Inhibition of cytokine production by cyclosporin A and transforming growth factor B. J Exp Med 166: 571–576

Farrar J J, Benjamin W R, Hilfiker M L et al 1982 The biochemistry, biology and role of interleukin 2 in the induction of cytotoxic T cell and antibody-forming B cell responses. Immunol Rev 63: 129–166

Ferrara J L M, Deeg H G 1991 Graft-versus-hot disease. N Engl J Med 324: 667–674

Fisch, P, Weil-Hillman G, Uppenkamp M et al 1990a Antigen-specific recognition of autologous leukemia cells and allogeneic Class-I MHC antigens by Il-2-activated cytotoxic T cells from a patient with acute T-cell leukemia. Blood 74: 343–353

Fisch P, Malkowsky M, Kovats S et al 1990b Recognition by human V9 and V2 T cell of a GroEL homolog on Daudi Burkitt's lymphoma cells. Science 250: 1269–1273

Fischer G, Wittman-Liebold B, Lang K et al 1989 Cyclophilin and peptidyl-prolyl cis–trans isomerase are probably identical proteins. Nature 337: 476–478

Foa R, Caretto P, Fierro M T et al 1990a Interleukin 2 does not promote the in vitro and in vivo proliferation and growth of human acute leukemia cells of myeloid and lymphoid origin. Br J Haematol 75: 34–40

Foa R, Meloni G, Tosti S et al 1990b Treatment of residual disease in acute leukemia patients with recombinant interleukin 2 (IL2); clinical and biological findings. Bone Marrow Transplant 6 (Suppl 1): 98–102

Foa R, Fierro M T, Cesano A et al 1991a Defective lymphokine-activated killer cell generation and activity in acute leukemia patients with active disease. Blood 78: 1041–1046

Foa R, Guarini A, Gillio T A et al 1991b Peripheral blood and bone marrow immunophenotypic and functional modifications induced in acute leukemia patients treated with interleukin 2: evidence of in vivo lymphokine activated killer cell generation. Cancer Res 51: 964–968

Gambacorti-Passerini C, Rivoltini L, Fizzotti M et al 1991 Selective purging by human interleukin-2 activated lymphocytes of bone marrows contaminated with a lymphoma line or autologous leukaemic cells. Br J Haematol 78: 197–205

Gansbacher B, Zier K, Daniels B et al 1990 Interleukin 2 gene transfer into tumor cells abrogates tumorigenicity and induces protective immunity. J Exp Med 172: 1217–1224

Goldman J M, Gale R P, Horowitz M M et al 1988 Bone marrow transplantation for chronic myelogenous leukemia in chronic phase. Increased risk for relapse associated with T-cell depletion. Ann Intern Med 108: 806–814

Gorin N C, Herve P, Aegerter P et al for the Working Party on Autologous Bone Marrow Transplantation of the European Bone Marrow Transplantation Group 1986 Autologous bone marrow transplantation for acute leukemia in remission. Br J Haematol 64: 385–395

Gottlieb D J, Brenner M K, Heslop H E et al 1989a A Phase I trial of recombinant interleukin 2 following high dose chemoradiotherapy for haematological malignancy: applicability to the elimination of minimal residual disease. Br J Cancer 60: 610–615

Gottlieb D J, Prentice H G, Heslop H E et al 1989b Effects of recombinant interleukin 2 administration on cytotoxic effector function following intensive chemoradiotherapy. Blood 74: 2335–2342

Grazier A, Tutschka P J, Farner E R et al 1983 Graft-versus-host disease in cyclosporin A-treated rats after syngeneic and autologous reconstitution. J Exp Med 158: 1–8

Herberman R B, Ortaldo J R 1981 Natural killer cells: their role in defenses against disease. Science 214: 24–30

Heslop H E, Gottlieb D J, Reittie J E et al 1989a Spontaneous and interleukin 2 induced secretion of tumour necrosis factor and gamma interferon following autologous marrow transplantation or chemotherapy. Br J Haematol 72: 122–126

Heslop H E, Gottlieb D J, Bianchi A C M et al 1989b In vivo induction of gamma interferon and tumour necrosis factor by interleukin 2 infusion following intensive chemotherapy or autologous marrow transplantation. Blood 74: 1374–1380

Heslop H E, Bianchi A C M, Cordingley F T et al 1990 Effects of alpha-interferon on autocrine growth factor loops in B lymphoproliferative disorders. J Exp Med 172: 1729–1734

Heslop H E, Duncombe A S, Reittie J E et al 1991 Interleukin 2 infusion after autologous bone marrow transplantation accelerates hemopoietic regeneration. Transplant Proc 23: 1704–1705

Higuchi C M, Thompson J A, Petersen F B et al 1991 Toxicity and immunomodulatory effects of interleukin-2 after autologous bone marrow transplantation for hematologic malignancies. Blood 77: 2561–2568

Horowitz M M, Gale R P, Sondel P M 1990 Graft-versus-leukemia reactions after bone marrow transplantation. Blood 75: 555–562

International Bone Marrow Transplant Registry 1989 Transplant or chemotherapy in acute myelogenous leukemia. Lancet i: 1119–1122

Jenkins M K, Schwartz R H, Pardoll D M 1988 Effects of cyclosporin A on T cell development and clonal deletion. Science 241: 1655–1658

Jones R J, Vogelsang G B, Hess A D et al 1989 Induction of graft-versus-host disease after autologous bone marrow transplantation. Lancet i: 754–757

Jung S, Schluesner H J 1991 Human T lymphocytes recognize a peptide of single point-mutated, oncogenic ras proteins. J Exp Med 173: 273–276

Karre K, Klein G O, Kiessling R et al 1980 Low natural in vivo resistance to syngeneic leukemias in natural killer-deficient mice. Nature 284: 624–626

Lotzova E, Savary C A, Schachner J R et al 1991 Generation of cytotoxic NK cells in peripheral blood and bone marrow of patients with acute myelogenous leukemia after continuous infusion with recombinant interleukin-2. Am J Hematol 37: 88–99

MacDonald D, Jiang Y Z, Swirsky D et al 1991 Acute myeloid leukaemia relapsing following interleukin-2 treatment expresses the alpha chain of the interleukin-2 receptor. Br J Haematol 77: 43–49

Malkovsky M, Brenner M K, Hunt R et al 1986 T-cell depletion of allogeneic bone marrow prevents acceleration of graft-versus-host disease induced by exogenous interleukin 2. Cell Immunol 103: 476–480

Moller D R, Konishi K, Kirby M et al 1988 Bias toward use of a specific T cell receptor beta-chain variable region in a subgroup of individuals with sarcoidosis. J Clin Invest 82: 1183–1191

Oblakowski P, Bello-Ferandez C, Reittie J E et al 1991 Possible mechanisms of selective killing of myeloid leukaemic blast cells by lymphokine-activated killer cells. Blood 77: 1996–2001

Olive D, Lopez M, Blaise D et al 1991 Cell surface expression of ICAM-1 (CD54) and LFA-3 (CD58), two adhesion molecules, is up-regulated on bone marrow leukemic blasts after in vivo administration of high-dose recombinant interleukin-2. J Immunother 10: 412–417

Peace D J, Chen W, Nelson H et al 1991 T cell recognition of transforming proteins encoded by mutated *ras* proto-oncogenes. J Immunol 146: 2059–2065

Platsoucas CD 1991 Human autologous tumor-specific T cells in malignant melanoma. Cancer Metastasis Rev 10: 151–176

Prentice H G, Brenner M K 1989 Donor marrow T-cell depletion for prevention of GVHD without loss of the GVL effect. Current results in acute myeloblastic leukaemia and future directions. In: Gale R P (ed) Bone marrow transplantation: current controversies. Alan R Liss, New York, pp 117–128

Reizenstein P 1990 Adjuvant immunotherapy with BCG of acute myeloid leukemia: a 15-year follow-up. Br J Haematol 75: 288–289

Ridge S A, Worwood M, Oscier D et al 1990 FMS mutations in myelodysplastic, leukemic, and normal subjects. Proc Natl Acad Sci USA 87: 1377–1380

Rosenberg S A, Lotze M T, Mule J J 1988 New approaches to the immunotherapy of cancer using interleukin-2. Ann Intern Med 108: 853–864

Rosolen A, Nakanishi M, Poplack D G et al 1989 Expression of interleukin-2 receptor B subunit in hematopoietic malignancies. Blood 73: 1968–1972

Simmons D, Makgoba M W, Seed B 1988 ICAM, an adhesion ligand of LFA-1, is homologous to the neural cell adhesion molecule NCAM. Nature 331: 624–627

Smith K A 1988 Interleukin-2: inception, impact and implications. Science 240: 1169–1176

Soiffer R J, Murray C, Cochran K et al 1992 Clinical and immunologic effects of prolonged infusion of low-dose recombinant interleukin-2 after autologous and T-cell-depleted allogeneic bone marrow transplantation. Blood 79: 517–526

Sosman J A, Oettel K R, Hank J A et al 1989 Specific recognition of human leukemic cells by allogeneic T cell lines. Transplantation 48: 486–495

Sosman J A, Oettel K R, Smith S D et al 1990 Specific recognition of human leukemic cells by allogeneic T cells: II. Evidence for HLA-D restricted determinants on leukemic cells that are crossreactive with determinants present on unrelated nonleukemic cells. Blood 75: 2005–2016

Storb R, Pepe M, Anasetti C et al 1990 What role for prednisone in prevention of acute graft-versus-host disease in patients undergoing marrow transplants? Blood 76: 1037–1045

Sullivan K M, Weiden P L, Storb R et al 1989a Influence of acute and chronic graft-versus-host disease on relapse and survival after bone marrow transplantation from HLA-identical siblings as treatment of acute and chronic leukemia. Blood 73: 1720–1728

Sullivan K M, Storb R, Buckner C D et al 1989b Graft-versus-host disease as adoptive immunotherapy in patients with advanced hematologic neoplasms. N Engl J Med 320: 828–834

Sykes M, Romick M L, Hoyles K A et al 1990a In vivo administration of interleukin 2 plus T cell-depleted syngeneic marrow prevents graft-versus-host disease mortality and permits alloengraftment. J Exp Med 171: 645–658

Sykes M, Romick M L, Sachs D H 1990b Interleukin 2 prevents graft-versus-host disease while preserving the graft-versus-leukemia effect of allogeneic T cells. Proc Natl Acad Sci USA 87: 5633–5637

Takahashi N, Hayano T, Suzuki M 1989 Peptidyl-prolyl cis–trans isomerase is the cyclosporin A-binding protein cyclophilin. Nature 337: 473–475

Talbot D C, Powles R L, Sloane J P et al 1990 Cyclosporine-induced graft-versus-host disease following autologous bone marrow transplantation in acute myeloid leukaemia. Bone Marrow Transplant 6: 17–20

Tanaka M 1991 Growth of certain myeloid leukemic cells can be stimulated by interleukin-2. Growth Factors 5: 191–199

Timonen, T 1990 Characteristics of surface proteins involved in binding and triggering of human natural killer cells. In: Schmidt R E (ed) Natural killer cells: biology and clinical application. 6th International Natural Killer Cell Workshop, Goslar. Karger, Basel, pp 18–23

Truitt R L, Shih C C-Y, LeFever A V 1986 Manipulation of graft-versus-host disease for a graft-versus-leukemia effect after allogeneic bone marrow transplantation in AKR mice with spontaneous leukemia/lymphoma. Transplantation 41: 301–310

Weiden P L, Flournoy N, Thomas E D et al 1979 Antileukemic effect of graft-versus-host disease in human recipients of allogeneic-marrow grafts. N Engl J Med 300: 1068–1073

Weiden P L, Sullivan K M, Flournoy N et al 1981 Seattle marrow transplant team: antileukemic effect of chronic graft-versus-host disease. Contribution to improved survival after allogeneic marrow transplantation. N Engl J Med 304: 1529–1533

Weisdorf D J, Nesbit M E, Ramsay N K C et al 1987 Allogeneic bone marrow transplantation for acute lymphoblastic leukemia in remission: prolonged survival associated with acute graft-versus-host disease. J Clin Oncol 5: 1348–1355

Yeager A M, Vogelsang G B, Jones R J et al 1992 Induction of cutaneous graft-versus-host disease by administration of cyclosporine to patients undergoing autologous bone marrow transplantation for acute myeloid leukemia. Blood 79: 3031–3035

8

Bone marrow transplantation for hemoglobinopathy and sickle cell disease

M. Walters   D. Matthews   K. M. Sullivan

Marrow transplantation is an effective curative therapy for certain non-malignant disorders. Initially, allogeneic marrow transplantation was reserved for application in the treatment of rapidly fatal disorders such as aplastic anemia and immunodeficiency syndromes. More recently it has been utilized increasingly in the treatment of inborn errors of metabolism, Fanconi anemia, and thalassemia major. Much of the recent success in these uses of transplantation has resulted from improved prevention and treatment of transplant-related complications such as graft-versus-host disease (GVHD), graft failure and infection (Storb et al 1992, Sullivan et al 1992).

We have recently embarked upon a study of the use of marrow transplantation as curative therapy in the treatment of young patients with sickle cell disease, who have evidence of early organ dysfunction (Sullivan & Reid 1991). With the advent of prophylactic antibiotics and early identification of patients with sickle cell disease through newborn screening and enrollment into comprehensive clinical settings, early mortality in this disorder has been significantly reduced (Vichinsky et al 1988; Gaston et al 1986). Nonetheless, significant morbidity is commonly observed and 10–15% of patients with sickle cell disease do not survive past the second decade of life (Leikin et al 1989). One challenge facing investigators is to identify patients at risk for early complications in order to target them for consideration of allogeneic marrow transplantation.

SICKLE CELL DISEASE: MORBIDITY AND MORTALITY

Sickle cell disease results from the substitution of a single nucleotide in the β-globin coding sequence, which in turn results in the replacement of glutamic acid with valine in the sixth position of the β-globin polypeptide chain (Platt & Nathan 1987). This creates a 'sticky' patch on the β-globin chain which, in the deoxygenated state, promotes the formation of long polymers of globin chains. Sickle globin polymerization deforms red cells and alters red cell membrane properties, leading to occlusion of small blood vessels. There are multiple clinical ramifications of the vasculopathy resulting from these molecular and cellular events. Vaso-occlusive events which cause painful crises are the most common consequences. Patients with the highest

119

number of vaso-occlusive painful events appear to be at increased risk for early mortality. Platt and colleagues reporting from the Cooperative Study of Sickle Cell Disease found that among 66 patients with three or more vaso-occlusive episodes per year, the survival rate to age 40 was 40%, compared with an 80% survival to age 40 among 614 patients free of frequent painful events ($P = 0.009$) (Platt et al 1991).

Stroke affects 6–12% of all patients with sickle cell disease and sickle disease is the most common cause of stroke in childhood (Powars et al 1978). Hypertransfusion programs to maintain Hb S below 30% have been shown to be effective in preventing recurrence of stroke in the majority of cases (Sarnaik et al 1979, Sarnaik & Lusher 1982, Portnoy & Herier 1975, Ohene-Frempong 1991, Wilimas et al 1980). Unfortunately, it remains unclear when, if ever, hypertransfusion can be safely discontinued. One prospective study in a small group of patients who had evidence of persistent intracranial vascular occlusion showed a stroke recurrence rate of 50% in patients discontinuing chronic transfusion programs given for 6–12 years (Wang et al 1991). Hypertransfusion carried on indefinitely carries the risk of infection, red blood cell antigen alloimmunization, and iron overload. Moreover, transfusion therapy may not protect against the late complication of intracranial hemorrhage. Microvascular neurologic damage may be responsible for the substantial cognitive deficits apparent in neuropsychologic evaluation of children with sickle cell disease (Swift et al 1989).

Sickle lung disease has been recognized as a major contributor to early morbidity and mortality (Powars et al 1988). There is evidence that development of restrictive pulmonary disease early in life portends a poor outcome. Acute chest syndrome consists of a clinical syndrome of fever, hypoxia, chest pain, and pulmonary infiltrate (Charache et al 1979; Davies et al 1984). Recurrent episodes appear to contribute to progressive chronic pulmonary disease, which later in life lead to cor pulmonale and death. Sickle nephropathy is another manifestation of sickle cell vasculopathy (Allon 1990, Falk et al 1992). While this is seldom a problem in childhood, patients with nephrotic syndrome have a 2-year survival of only 50% (Bakir et al 1987).

Taken together, these data confirm the magnitude of morbidity and mortality of sickle cell disease. The need, therefore, is to identify young patients with signs of early organ dysfunction who are likely to have disabling and fatal complications of sickle cell disease. In these patients, the benefits of transplantation may be judged to outweigh the risks of the procedure. The following will analyze this consideration of risks versus gains in light of experience of marrow transplantation for other non-malignant disorders.

MARROW TRANSPLANTATION FOR APLASTIC ANEMIA

Aplastic anemia is a disease characterized by pancytopenia and severe marrow hypoplasia. Allogeneic marrow transplantation remains the most effective treatment for this disease. Improved outcome following marrow transplantation occurred through improvements in acute GVHD prophylaxis, prevention of graft rejection, and improved treatment of chronic GVHD. A total of 322 patients with severe aplastic anemia were conditioned for transplantation with cyclophosphamide, 200 mg/kg divided in four consecutive daily doses, and received marrow from histocompatibility locus antigen (HLA) matched siblings in Seattle between 1970 and 1990 (Loughran & Storb 1990; Storb et al 1984, 1991, 1992). Before 1975, graft rejection accounted for most of the treatment failures and appeared to result from sensitization to minor histocompatibility antigens as a consequence of blood product transfusions given prior to marrow transplantation. By avoiding pretransplantation transfusions, outcome was improved due to a reduced incidence of graft rejection (Fig. 8.1) (Storb et al 1991). Another apparent contribution to this improvement was the use of antithymocyte globulin as a component of the conditioning regimen. This was first evaluated in a group of patients with aplastic anemia receiving second marrow transplants for graft rejection (Storb et al 1991, 1992). Sustained engraftment was demonstrated in 15 of 18 evaluable patients. Subsequently, this conditioning regimen of alternating cyclophosphamide and antithymocyte globulin has been applied to patients with aplastic anemia receiving first marrow transplants. In a recent consecutive series of 29 patients, 28 had sustained engraftment and 27 of the 29 are currently surviving (Storb et al 1992). These results suggest that the use of antithymocyte globulin may reduce the incidence of graft rejection, and improve survival.

The development of acute GVHD has been associated with decreased survival in patients with aplastic anemia. Among patients who received methotrexate alone for GVHD prophylaxis, 35% developed grade II–IV acute GVHD. This had an adverse effect on survival, with only 40–45% of patients having long-term survival (Storb et al 1991). In comparison, 85% of patients with grade 0–I acute GVHD were long-term survivors. The administration of cyclosporine alone did not decrease the incidence of acute GVHD below that

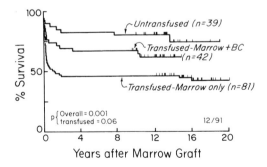

Fig. 8.1 HLA-identical marrow grafts for cyclophosphamide in patients with aplastic anemia. Survival of untransfused (n = 39) versus transfused patients given marrow only (n = 81) versus transfused patients given marrow and buffy-coat (BC) cells (n = 42). All patients were given methotrexate post grafting. Deaths at 10.5 and 14.5 years are from cancer.

seen in patients receiving methotrexate only. However, the combination of methotrexate and cyclosporine reduced the incidence of acute GVHD to <20% and no patient developed grade IV GVHD (Fig. 8.2) (Storb et al 1991). As a result, the survival of patients who received methotrexate and cyclosporine was significantly better than those receiving methotrexate alone. In Figure 8.3 the survival of a group of 21 patients less than 18 years of age who received methotrexate and cyclosporine prophylaxis was compared to a group of 81 children given methotrexate only for GVHD prophylaxis. The overall survival in the former group was 94% (Storb et al 1991). These data suggest that in children receiving HLA-identical marrow, the combination of methotrexate and cyclosporine represents potent therapy for prevention of GVHD and results in excellent long-term survival.

The main determinant of late morbidity and mortality following allogeneic marrow transplantation for non-malignant disorders is chronic GVHD. Among 212 patients with aplastic anemia, 30% of patients developed chronic GVHD. The adverse effect on survival in 212 patients transplanted for aplastic anemia is illustrated in Figure 8.4 (Sullivan et al 1991). Recipients of HLA-matched marrow who survived beyond 150 days had the following probability of developing chronic GVHD: 13% in patients aged 1–9 years; 28% in those 10–19 years; and 42–46% in those over the age of 20 (Fig. 8.5) (Atkinson et al 1990, Storb et al 1983, Niederwieser et al 1989). Additional predictive factors for developing chronic GVHD include receiving HLA-non-identical or unrelated donor marrow, prior acute GVHD, and administration of unirradiated donor buffy-coat transfusions.

In patients with standard- and high-risk chronic GVHD, prolonged immunosuppression with prednisone and/or cyclosporine has improved outcome (Sullivan et al 1988, 1990). Approximately 80% of surviving patients have treatment successfully discontinued within 2 years and fewer than 8% of

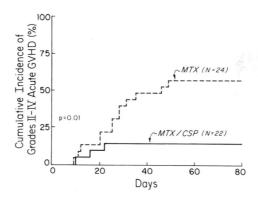

Fig. 8.2 HLA-identical transplantation for aplastic anemia following conditioning with cyclophosphamide. Probability of grades II–IV acute GVHD in a cohort of mostly adult patients given methotrexate (MTX) versus methotrexate plus cyclosporine (MTX/CSP) for GVHD prophylaxis. (Reproduced with permission from Storb et al 1992.)

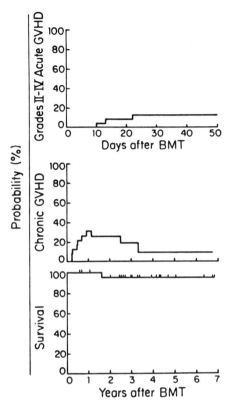

Fig. 8.3 HLA-identical transplantation in children with aplastic anemia. A cohort of 23 patients 18 years old and younger following conditioning with cyclophosphamide. Incidence of acute GVHD (top), chronic GVHD (center panel) and survival (bottom) are shown. BMT, bone marrow transplantation.

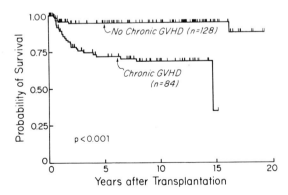

Fig. 8.4 Probability of survival in 212 patients with severe aplastic anemia transplanted through August 1990 who survived at least 150 days after marrow transplantation from HLA-identical siblings. Patients were prepared for transplant with cyclophosphamide and were analyzed in relation to the presence or absence of clinical extensive chronic GVHD.

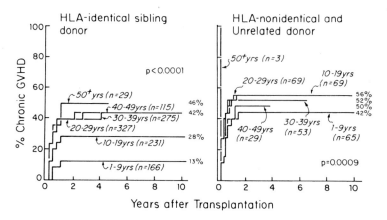

Fig. 8.5   Probability of developing clinical extensive chronic GVHD in patients with hematologic malignancies transplanted through December 1989 who survived at least 150 days after marrow transplantation from HLA-identical siblings (left panel) and HLA-non-identical family members or unrelated donors (right panel). Results are displayed in relation to patient age at the time of transplantation.

long-term survivors have Karnofsky performance scores of less than 70%. However, infections remain a frequent complication and contribute to a 15–20% mortality in standard-risk patients and a 35–40% mortality of high-risk chronic GVHD (Sullivan et al 1991).

MARROW TRANSPLANTATION FOR THALASSEMIA

The experience with bone marrow transplantation in patients with thalassemia has relevance in designing marrow transplantation trials for sickle cell disease. The first successful marrow transplant from an HLA-identical sibling for thalassemia was performed in December 1982 (Thomas ED et al 1982). This child received dimethylbusulfan (5 mg/kg) and cyclophosphamide (200 mg/kg) for cytoreductive therapy and remains entirely well 10 years later. Lucarelli and colleagues in Pesaro have subsequently performed over 500 marrow transplants in patients with homozygous β-thalassemia. All were prepared with busulfan (14 mg/kg) and cyclophosphamide (200 mg/kg) and received cyclosporine alone for prevention of GVHD. Overall survival was 84%, with graft rejection occurring in 12% (Fig. 8.6) (Lucarelli et al 1990, Lucarelli 1991).

Outcome was influenced by the clinical state of the patient at the time of transplantation, which in turn reflected primarily the duration and nature of transfusion therapy. The level of 'clinical wellness' appeared to be inversely proportional to the number of transfusions received, due to the increasing degree of iron overload with subsequent organ damage, compounded in part by transmission of infectious agents through transfusion. This was well supported by hepatic histopathology: portal fibrosis developed in 10% of

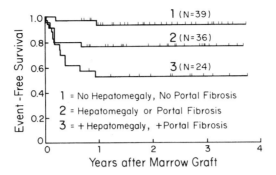

Fig. 8.6 Marrow grafting in patients with thalassemia after busulfan/cyclophosphamide. Shown are the event-free survivals in three risk groups of patients with thalassemia major where an event is defined as rejection, death, or recurrence of thalassemia.

patients under 4 years of age; in 25% between ages 4 and 7; in 50% between 8 and 11; in 60% between 12 and 16; and in 85% of patients over age 16. Patients were retrospectively classified according to the degree of hepatic damage present prior to transplantation: class 1 patients had no hepatomegaly and no portal fibrosis; class 2 patients had either hepatomegaly or portal fibrosis; and class 3 patients had both hepatomegaly and portal fibrosis (Lucarelli et al 1990, 1991b). The outcome based on this patient stratification is illustrated in Figure 8.7. Patients in class 1 had a 98% probability of survival and a 94% probability of disease-free survival (*n* = 50). Patients in class 2 had an 86% probability of survival and 83% disease-free survival. Patients in class 3 experienced a mortality rate of 46%.

Based on this outcome, the preparative regimen for class 3 patients was revised, with the reduction of cyclophosphamide to 120 mg/kg, and the

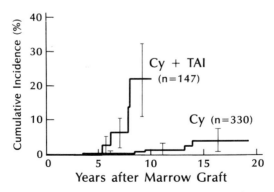

Fig. 8.7 Rates of secondary malignancy in patients with severe aplastic anemia following marrow grafting. Cumulative incidence of secondary malignancy in 330 patients with aplastic anemia in Seattle prepared with cyclophosphamide alone compared with 147 patients with aplastic anemia in Paris prepared with cyclophosphamide (cy) and thoracoabdominal irradiation (TAI). (Reproduced with permission from Storb et al 1992.)

addition of antithymocyte globulin given as 10 mg/kg from day −5 pre transplant through day +5 post transplant. On the revised protocol, overall survival in advanced-stage patients has improved to 91%, with 60% disease-free survival, and a graft rejection rate of 37% ($n = 34$) (Lucarelli 1991). More recently, outcome in adults aged 17–26 years has been presented by investigators from Pesaro (Lucarelli et al 1991a). This group of 20 adults had a survival of 80% at 2 years, with five of five class 2 patients and 11 of 15 class 3 patients surviving with donor engraftment.

Taken together, these data illustrate the outcome one might anticipate in sickle cell disease provided marrow transplantation is performed in young patients before development of extensive organ damage.

BONE MARROW TRANSPLANTATION FOR SICKLE CELL DISEASE

Nearly 40 patients with sickle cell disease have been successfully treated with marrow transplantation. The published results to date are summarized in Table 8.1. The first reported case was an 8-year-old girl with sickle cell disease who developed acute myelogenous leukemia (Johnson et al 1984). Her preparative regimen consisted of cyclophosphamide and total body irradiation. She developed chronic GVHD following transplantation, but remains alive, without evidence of sickle cell disease or leukemia over 9 years following transplant. Another patient with sickle cell disease and Morquio's disease was transplanted successfully (Mentzer et al 1990). This patient rejected the first marrow transplant following preparation with busulfan (15 mg/kg) and cyclophosphamide (120 mg/kg), but was successfully engrafted following a second marrow transplant using total body irradiation in the cytoreductive regimen. Another patient had sickle cell and acute leukemia and was prepared with total body irradiation and died of transplant-related complications (Milpied et al 1988). The largest published series of sickle cell disease is a series of 12 Belgian patients (Vermylen et al 1988, 1991). They

Table 8.1 Marrow transplantation for sickle cell disease (published results 1 March 1992)

	Europe			USA	
Factor	Vermylen	Ferster	Milpied	Johnson	Mentzer
No. of patients	12	5	1	1	1
Disease	SCD	SCD	SCD/ALL	SCD/AML	SCA/MD
Regimen (mg/kg)	BU (16)	BU (14)	CY (120)	CY (120)	BU/CY/ATG
	+ CY (200)	+ CY (200)	+ TBI	+ TBI	CY/ATG/TBI
Graft rejection	1	0	1	0	1
GVHD	2	1	0	1	0
No. surviving	12	5	0	1	1
Follow-up (months)	9–51	8–28	–	101	29

Abbreviations: ALL, acute lymphocytic leukemia; ATG, antithymocyte globulin; BU, busulfan; CY, cyclophosphamide; GVHD, graft-versus-host disease; MD, Morquio's disease; SCA, sickle cell anemia; SCD, sickle cell disease; TBI, total body irradiation.

ranged in age from 11 months to 23 years. Their families were from Zaire or Cameroon, and parents were students in Brussels. They were selected for transplantation mostly because of concern for transfusion support and medical care in Africa. This group of patients had a median of 4 (range 1–6) vaso-occlusive episodes per year. None had evidence of chronic organ damage. The oldest patient had osteonecrosis of multiple joints, and a history of bilateral hip replacements. All patients received busulfan 16 mg/kg and cyclophosphamide 200 mg/kg administered in four doses over 4 days. Patients over 12 years were given 750 cGy thoracoabdominal irradiation with lung shielding. All received cyclosporine for GVHD prophylaxis, and patients over 12 years of age were given methotrexate in addition to cyclosporine. In one patient, a second marrow transplant was performed at day 62 due to graft rejection. This patient received cyclophosphamide, antithymocyte globulin, and thoracoabdominal irradiation as preparation for the second marrow transplant. All 12 patients are well 9–51 (median 27) months following transplantation. In 11 of 12 patients, hemoglobin electrophoresis following transplantation confirmed donor engraftment and one patient had a small amount of Hb S present 36 months after transplantation, consistent with mixed chimerism. Four patients developed grade I–II acute GVHD. One patient developed thrombocytopenia thought to be a sign of chronic GVHD, which resolved after treatment with steroids, intravenous immunoglobulin, azathioprine, and splenectomy. Seven of the 12 patients have subsequently returned home to Africa. Another series of five patients has also been recently reported by another group in Belgium, and outcomes have been very similar (Table 8.1) (Ferster et al 1992).

A growing number of recent European reports of marrow transplants in patients with sickle cell disease has been noted. A total of 25 patients (including the 17 noted above) have been successfully transplanted by groups in Brussels and Paris (Vilmer 1991). Experience in the USA has been more limited. A patient with a history of stroke received a marrow transplant in Cincinnati, and remains well (Morris et al 1992). Another patient with recurrent painful crises (14 hospitalizations in 2 years) and acute chest syndrome was recently transplanted in Charleston (Aboud et al 1992).

We have developed a collaborative national protocol for marrow transplantation for patients with symptomatic sickle cell disease, and have recently enrolled a patient from Seattle. She is a 10-year-old with a past history of stroke. She had been maintained on a chronic hypertransfusion program, and had an elevated ferritin at the time of her transplant but no evidence of chronic organ damage. She received busulfan (14 mg/kg), cyclophosphamide (200 mg/kg), and antithymocyte globulin (90 mg/kg) for cytoreductive therapy. Cyclosporine and methotrexate were administered for GVHD prophylaxis, and she was placed in a laminar air flow environment, given prophylactic antibiotics and weekly intravenous immunoglobulin to prevent infections. She is well with evidence of donor engraftment more than 6 months following marrow transplantation. Her course was complicated by the development of grade I–II acute GVHD which was treated with a short course of prednisone. The post-transplant course was also complicated by the development of seizures. The symptomatology suggested an epileptiform focus in the distribution of her previous cerebral infarction, but no interval change was noted on magnetic resonance imaging. Based on this finding and our concern that similar epileptogenic foci in patients with silent cerebral infarction may develop, we routinely administer dilantin prophylaxis throughout cyclosporine prophylaxis.

LATE EFFECTS OF MARROW TRANSPLANTATION

While these initial reports are encouraging, several concerns remain. Detailed information is needed about the resistance of sickle cell marrow to the marrow ablative effects of cyclophosphamide and busulfan. Similarly, little detailed information exists about how African-Americans process busulfan and high-dose cyclophosphamide. In Caucasians, busulfan pharmacokinetics differ in children compared with adults (Grochow et al 1990).

In addition, the late effects of marrow transplantation in children, with regard to subsequent growth, sexual maturation, and intellectual development, are now being studied in long-term survivors. Children with aplastic anemia who have been transplanted using high-dose cyclophosphamide alone have experienced normal growth rates and thyroid function following transplantation (Sanders et al 1991). Similarly, patients who have received busulfan and cyclophosphamide cytoreductive therapy have had normal growth rates, although children who developed chronic GVHD demonstrated decreased growth velocity while they had active GVHD. Catch-up growth occurs once the chronic GVHD resolves and corticosteroid therapy is discontinued.

Gonadal hormone production and germ cell survival may be adversely affected by the cytoreductive agents. In prepubertal boys who received high-dose cyclophosphamide (200 mg/kg), elevated follicle stimulating hormone (FSH) and abnormal testicular histology were observed. However, cyclophosphamide given in doses ≤200 mg/kg has been associated with minimal alteration in spermatogenesis. Similarly, cumulative doses exceeding 500 mg/kg in girls have been associated with primary ovarian failure. Little data are currently available regarding the effects of busulfan on gonadal function. In a small number of prepubertal boys who received high-dose busulfan (16 mg/kg) and cyclophosphamide (200 mg/kg), approximately one-half have shown delayed sexual maturation.

The administration of high-dose alkylating agents after puberty has resulted in significant impairment in gonadal function (Sanders et al 1991). In 14 women who received high-dose busulfan and cyclophosphamide for marrow transplantation in the treatment of thalassemia or hematologic malignancy, all have amenorrhea, elevated levels of gonadotropins, and low estradiol. Only four men have been evaluated for gonadal function post puberty after receiving busulfan and cyclophosphamide for marrow ablative purposes. Normal luteinizing hormone and testosterone levels with minimally elevated FSH levels have been noted 1 year following transplant. Two of the four patients had evidence of sperm on semen analysis. Thus, although additional follow-up and further study are required, it appears that the combination of high-dose busulfan and cyclophosphamide does not result in growth or thyroid function abnormalities. However, sexual maturation and fertility may be adversely affected by this combination, and patients may require gonadal hormone supplementation.

The development of secondary malignancy following bone marrow transplantation is a rare but serious late complication (Witherspoon et al 1989). Among 320 patients with aplastic anemia and 1926 patients with hematologic malignancy who underwent allogeneic, syngeneic, and autologous marrow transplantation in Seattle, 35 of the 2246 patients developed secondary malignancies (16 non-Hodgkin's lymphoma, six leukemia, and 13 solid tumors). The development of secondary neoplasms occurred at a median of 1.0 year following transplantation (range 0.1–13.9 years). The age-adjusted incidence of secondary malignancy was 6.69 times that reported for primary malignancy in the general population. Risk factors for developing secondary malignancy included the administration of total body irradiation, and the treatment of acute GVHD with antithymocyte globulin or anti-CD3 monoclonal antibody. Thus, by the avoidance of total body irradiation in preparative regimens and effective prevention of acute GVHD, the incidence of secondary malignancy may be decreased in recipients of marrow transplants for non-malignant disorders. These findings can be illustrated by comparing rates of secondary malignancies in patients with aplastic anemia (including Fanconi anemia). In a series of French patients given cyclophosphamide and thoracoabdominal irradiation, the cumulative incidence of secondary neoplasms was 25% at 8 years (Socié et al 1991) compared with an incidence of 1.4% at 10 years in recipients of cyclophosphamide alone (Fig. 8.7) (Witherspoon et al 1990, 1992).

INDICATIONS FOR TRANSPLANTATION IN SICKLE CELL DISEASE

Controversy surrounds the issue of marrow transplantation in the treatment of sickle cell disease. This stems in part from the fact that, in most instances, this disorder is not a rapidly fatal condition. With improved supportive care, a significant fraction of patients are surviving into middle age. Who, then, should be considered for transplantation? To address this issue, a symposium was convened in August 1990 in Seattle, in hopes of arriving at a consensus regarding inclusion criteria for bone marrow transplantation (Sullivan & Reid 1991). One strategy proposed was to identify patients at risk for subsequent morbidity and mortality while still young, before they develop complications from their disease that preclude a favorable outcome after marrow transplantation. Data from β-globin gene haplotypes were presented, suggesting that patients carrying the CAR/CAR haplotype may be at increased risk for early mortality (Powars 1991). If these data are confirmed, haplotype identity may become a very useful selection criterion for marrow transplantation.

Most in attendance at the symposium agreed that stroke patients represent a population to be considered for marrow transplantation. The cost of conventional medical care for these patients is considerable. One analysis estimated the annual cost of transfusion and iron chelation with desferrioxamine in a 30-kg child at $31 986/year, or a 5-year cost of $159 930 (Kirkpatrick et al 1991). Given the estimated cost for bone marrow transplant at $150 000, its cost-effectiveness is not in question. Stroke appears to be only a late, most severe manifestation of neurologic disease in the sickle cell patient. Radiographic and neuropsychologic screening of asymptomatic sickle cell patients have suggested that stroke patients may represent only a fraction of those with significant neuropathy (Vichinsky 1991). In one study, five out of 55 sickle cell patients with no history of stroke had previously undetected cerebral infarction documented on magnetic resonance imaging (Pavlakis et al 1988). Another study evaluated asymptomatic sickle cell patients with a battery of cognitive assessment tests. While normal intellectual ability was found, a majority of patients demonstrated neuropsychologic deficits, such as a shortened attention span, and impaired visual–spatial reasoning (Chapar 1988). Thus, it would appear that a pervasive vasculopathy develops in patients with sickle cell disease, which may cause microvascular lesions as well as large vessel occlusion. A case can therefore be made for intervening early before further damage occurs.

Other indications for marrow transplantation were considered. Lung disease was recognized as a major cause of death in young adults with sickle cell disease (Vichinsky 1991). Moreover, as the general sickle cell population has aged, the incidence of chronic lung disease appears to be rising (Powars 1991). Chronic renal failure may occur in as many as 18% of adults with sickle cell disease (Thomas A et al 1982). Of course, one would like to identify these patients early, before end-stage renal insufficiency develops. While renal allograft transplantation is feasible, long-term outcome for these patients is poor (Gonzalez-Carillo et al 1982).

Pain is another potential selection factor. It is the most common reason for hospitalization among patients with sickle cell disease. A recent study commented upon the great variability between individuals with sickle cell disease who experience painful episodes, but suggested that increased disease severity and early mortality was associated with increased numbers of painful events (Platt et al 1991). While one in three patients rarely have vaso-occlusive episodes, 5% of patients experience as many as 40 episodes per year. For these individuals in whom pain is so debilitating, consideration of marrow transplantation appears warranted.

A set of selection criteria for marrow transplantation for sickle cell anemia have been developed (Table 8.2). While there may be debate as to individual

Table 8.2   Sickle cell patients for marrow transplantation

Inclusions
1. Homozygous SS disease < 16 years old
2. One of the following complications:
    a. Stroke or central nervous system hemorrhage
    b. Sickle pulmonary disease/recurrent acute chest syndrome
    c. Sickle nephropathy
    d. Chronic debilitating pain

Exclusions
1. Age > 15 years old
2. HLA-non-identical donor
3. Glomerular filtration rate (GFR) < 30% predicted
4. Active hepatic disease
5. Severe residual central nervous system impairment
6. Severe sickle lung disease

---

factors, these characteristics are felt to reflect significant disease morbidity and, in some instances, predictors of early mortality. In addition, we have established criteria that would currently exclude adults or patients with progressive end-organ damage, which would increase the risk of regimen-related toxicity or GVHD.

A recent publication explored the issue of the willingness of families to consider allogeneic marrow transplantation (Kodish et al 1991). Parental attitudes were assessed through interviews regarding the level of an acceptable risk of death given the benefit of cure for their children with sickle cell disease. It was found that 54% of parents questioned were willing to accept some risk of short-term mortality, and 37% were willing to accept at least a 15% risk of mortality.

Many questions remain regarding the role of marrow transplantation in the treatment of sickle cell disease (Beutler 1991). Will vasculopathy reverse after transplantation? Will neurologic damage incurred prior to transplantation remain static, progress, or resolve over time? Will marrow transplantation have any effect on subsequent risk of intracranial hemorrhage? Will splenic function return? Will other end-organ damage improve? What will be the quality of life and cost of care? How will marrow transplantation compare to other treatment modalities such as chronic transfusion therapy, or hydroxyurea administration?

KEY POINTS FOR CLINICAL PRACTICE

- Children with aplastic anemia receiving HLA-identical marrow transplants and methotrexate/cyclosporine prophylaxis have experienced 94% long-term survival.
- HLA-identical marrow transplantation in children with thalassemia free of organ damage has resulted in 94% event-free survival.
- Similar results might be observed following marrow transplantation in

young children with symptomatic sickle disease.
- Transplantation results to date in a small number of patients with sickle cell disease have been encouraging.
- Patients with neurologic problems should have highest priority, followed by those with lung and renal lesions.
- A multi-institutional clinical trial to investigate the role of marrow transplantation in sickle cell disease is currently in progress to more fully define the risks and rewards of this treatment.

ACKNOWLEDGMENT

Supported in part by grants CA 09351, CA 09645, CA 18221, CA 18029, CA 15704, CA 09515 and HL 36444 from the National Institutes of Health, DHHS.

REFERENCES

Aboud M, Jackson S, Barredo J et al 1992 Bone marrow transplantation for recurrent pain crises in patients with sickle cell disease from the 17th Annual National Sickle Cell Disease Conference, Nashville, TN, p 14a
Allon M 1990 Renal abnormalities in sickle cell disease. Arch Intern Med 150: 501–504
Atkinson K, Horowitz M M, Gale R P et al 1990 Risk factors for chronic graft-versus-host disease after HLA-identical sibling bone marrow transplantation. Blood 75: 2459–2464
Bakir A, Hathiwala S, Anis H et al 1987 Prognosis of the nephrotic syndrome in sickle glomerulopathy. Am J Nephrol 7: 110–115
Beutler E 1991 Bone marrow transplantation for sickle cell anemia: summarizing comments. Semin Hematol 28: 263
Chapar G N 1988 Chronic diseases of children and neuropsychologic dysfunction. J Dev Behav Pediatr 9: 221–222
Charache S, Scott J, Charache P 1979 Acute chest syndrome in adults with sickle cell anemia. Arch Intern Med 139: 67–69
Davies S, Luce P, Winn A et al 1984 Acute chest syndrome in sickle cell disease. Lancet 1: 36–38
Falk R, Scheinman J, Phillips G et al 1992 Prevalence and pathobiologic features of sickle cell nephropathy and response to inhibition of Angiotensin-converting enzyme. N Engl J Med 326: 910–915
Ferster A, DeValck C, Azzi N et al 1992 Bone marrow transplantation for severe sickle cell anemia. Br J Haematology 80: 102–105.
Gaston M, Verter J, Woods G et al 1986 Prophylaxis with oral penicillin in children with sickle cell anemia. A randomized trial. N Engl J Med 314: 1593–1599
Gonzalez-Carillo M, Rudge C, Parsons V et al 1982 Renal transplantation in sickle cell disease. Clin Nephrol 18: 209–210
Grochow L, Krivit W, Whitley C et al 1990 Busulfan disposition in children. Blood 75: 1723–1727
Johnson L, Look A, Cockerman J et al 1984 Bone marrow transplantation in a patient with sickle cell anemia. N Engl J Med 312: 780–783
Kirkpatrick D V, Barrios N J, Humbert J H 1991 Bone marrow transplantation for sickle cell anemia. Semin Hematol 28: 240–243
Kodish E, Lantos J, Stocking C et al 1991 Bone marrow transplantation for sickle cell disease: a study of parent's decisions. N Engl J Med 325: 1349–1353
Leikin S, Gallagher D, Kinney T et al 1989 Mortality in children and adolescents with sickle cell disease. Pediatrics 84: 500–508
Loughran T P, Jr., Storb R 1990 Treatment of aplastic anemia. In: Hematology/Oncology Clinics of North America Vol. 4. Saunders, Philadelphia, PA, pp 559–575

Lucarelli G, Galimberti M, Polchi P et al 1990 Bone marrow transplantation in patients with thalassemia. N Engl J Med 322: 417–421

Lucarelli G 1991 For debate: bone marrow transplantation for severe thalassemia (1) the view from Pesaro. Br J Haematol 78: 300–303

Lucarelli G, Galimberti M, Polchi P et al 1991a Bone marrow transplantation in adults with thalassemia. Blood 78 (Suppl.1): 197a

Lucarelli G, Galimberti M, Polchi P et al 1991b Bone marrow transplantation in thalassemia. Hematol Oncol Clin North Am 5: 549–556

Mentzer W C, Packman S, Wara W et al 1990 Successful bone marrow transplant in a child with sickle cell anemia and Morquio's disease. In: Pathobiology and clinical management of sickle cell disease: recent advances, p 79

Milpied N, Harrouseau J L, Garand R et al 1988 Bone-marrow transplantation for sickle-cell anaemia. Letter to the editor. Lancet ii: 328–329

Morris C, Kalinyak K, Cooney P et al 1992 Bone marrow transplantation in a patient with homozygous sickle cell anemia and stroke, from the 17th Annual National Sickle Cell Conference, Nashville, TN, p 30a.

Niederwieser D, Pepe M, Storb R et al 1989 Factors predicting chronic graft-versus-host disease and survival after marrow transplantation for aplastic anemia. Bone Marrow Transplantation 4: 151–156

Ohene-Frempong K 1991 Stroke in sickle cell disease: demographic devices and therapeutic considerations. Semin Hematol 28: 213–219

Pavlakis S, Bello J, Prokovnik I et al 1988 Brain infarction in sickle cell anemia: magnetic resonance imaging correlates. Ann Neurol 23: 123–125

Platt O, Nathan D 1987 Sickle cell disease. In: Hematology of Infancy and Childhood. Saunders, Philadelphia, PA, pp 655–699

Platt O, Thorington B, Brambilla D et al 1991 Pain in sickle cell disease. N Engl J Med 325: 11–16

Portnoy B, Herier J 1975 Neurologic manifestations in sickle cell disease with a review of the literature and emphasis on the prevalence of hemiplegia. Ann Intern Med 76: 643–652

Powars D 1991 Sickle cell anemia: β^s gene cluster haplotypes as prognostic indicators of vital organ failure. Semin Hematol 28: 202–208

Powars D, Wilson B, Imbus C et al 1978 The natural history of stroke in sickle cell disease. Am J Med 65: 461–470

Powars D, Weidman J A, Odom-Mayon T et al 1988 Sickle cell chronic lung disease: prior morbidity and the risk of pulmonary failure. Medicine 67: 66–76

Storb R, Sanders J, Pepe M et al 1991 Graft-vs-host disease with methotrexate/cyclosporine in children with severe aplastic anemia treated with cyclophosphamide and HLA-identical marrow grafts [letter] Blood 78: 1144–1145

Sanders J E and the Seattle Marrow Transplant Team 1991 The impact of marrow transplant preparative regimens on subsequent growth and development. Semin Hematol 28: 244–249

Sarnaik A, Lusher J 1982 Neurological complications of sickle cell anemia. Am J Pediatr Hematol Oncol 4: 386–394

Sarnaik S, Soorya D, Kim J et al 1979 Periodic transfusion for sickle cell anemia and CNS infarction. Am J Dis Child 133: 306–394

Socié G, Henry-Amar M, Cosset J M et al 1991 Increased incidence of solid malignant tumors after bone marrow transplantation for severe aplastic anemia. Blood 78: 277–279

Storb R, Longton G, Anasetti C et al 1992 Changing trends in marrow transplantation for aplastic anemia. Bone Marrow Transplantation 10(S1): 45–52

Storb R, Prentice R L, Sullivan K M et al 1983 Predictive factors in chronic graft-versus-host disease in patients with aplastic anemia treated by marrow transplantation from HLA-identical siblings. Ann Intern Med 98: 461–466

Storb R, Thomas E D, Buckner C D et al 1984 Marrow transplantation for aplastic anemia. Semin Hematol 21: 27–35

Storb R, Anasetti C, Appelbaum F et al 1991 Marrow transplantation for severe aplastic anemia and thalassemia major. Semin Hematol 28: 235–239

Sullivan K M, Reid C D 1991 Introduction to a symposium on sickle cell anemia: current results of comprehensive care and the evolving role of bone marrow transplantation. Semin Hematol 28: 177–179

Sullivan K M, Witherspoon R P, Storb R et al 1988 Alternating-day cyclosporine and prednisone for treatment of high-risk chronic graft-v-host disease. Blood 72: 555–561

Sullivan K M, Mori M, Witherspoon R et al 1990 Alternating-day cyclosporine and prednisone (CSP/PRED) treatment of chronic graft-vs-host disease (GVHD): Predictors of survival. Blood 76: 568a(Abstract)

Sullivan K M, Mori M, Sanders J et al 1992 Late complications of allogeneic and autologous marrow transplantation. Bone Marrow Transplantation 10(S1): 127–134

Sullivan K M, Agura E, Anasetti C et al 1991 Chronic graft-versus-host disease and other late complications of bone marrow transplantation. Semin Hematol 28: 250–259

Swift A, Cohen M, Hynd G et al 1989 Neuropsychologic impairment in children with sickle cell anemia. Pediatrics 84: 1077–1085

Thomas A, Pattison C, Serjeant G 1982 Causes of death in sickle cell disease in Jamaica. Br Med J 285: 633–635

Thomas E D, Buckner C D, Sanders J E et al 1982 Marrow transplantation for thalassaemia. Lancet ii: 227–229

Vermylen C, Fernandez-Robles E, Ninone J, Cornu G 1988 Bone marrow transplantation in five children with sickle cell anaemia. Lancet i: 1427–1428

Vermylen C, Cornu G, Phillips M et al 1991 Bone marrow transplantation in sickle cell anemia. Arch Dis Child 66: 1195–1198

Vichinsky E 1991 Comprehensive care in sickle cell disease: its impact on morbidity and mortality. Semin Hematol 28: 220–226

Vichinsky E, Hurst D, Earles A et al 1988 Neuron screening for sickle cell disease. Effect on mortality. Pediatrics 81: 749–755

Vilmer E 1991 Personal communication

Wang W, Kornar E, Tonkin I et al 1991 High risk of recurrent strokes after discontinuance of five to twelve years of transfusion therapy in patients with sickle cell disease. J Pediatr 377: 382

Wilimas J, Goff J, Anderson J et al 1980 Efficacy of transfusion therapy for one to two years: patients with sickle cell disease and cerebrovascular accidents. J Pediatr 96: 205–208

Witherspoon R P, Fisher L D, Schoch G et al 1989 Secondary cancers after bone marrow transplantation for leukemia or aplastic anemia. N Engl J Med 321: 784–789

Witherspoon R P, Fisher L D, Sullivan K M et al 1990 Secondary cancers after bone marrow transplantation. N Engl J Med 322: 853

Witherspoon R P, Storb R, Pepe M et al 1992 Cumulative incidence of secondary solid malignant tumors in aplastic anemia patients given marrow grafts after conditioning with chemotherapy alone (Letter). Blood 79: 289–290

9

The management of HIV infection

M. C. I. Lipman   M. A. Johnson

The first reports of acquired immunodeficiency syndrome (AIDS) appeared a decade ago (Centers for Disease Control (CDC) 1981) and already it is clear that AIDS and its infectious cause, human immunodeficiency virus (HIV), are responsible for a devastating global pandemic. This review will concentrate on the practical management of adult HIV-1 infection, though so far HIV-2 (isolated mainly in West Africa) appears to have a similar, though rather slower, clinical picture.

BACKGROUND

It is estimated that there are 10 million HIV infected adults worldwide, of whom at least 6 million are in Africa, 1 million each in North America, South America and Asia, and 500 000 in Europe (World Health Organization 1991); 1 million adults and 500 000 children are thought to have AIDS. Approximately 60% of the infected population are men, and over 75% of infections were acquired through sexual intercourse (the vast majority heterosexually). Other risks for HIV seropositivity are intravenous drug use and perinatal transmission (each accounting for 10% of the total), and the use of infected blood or blood products (responsible for 5% of all infections).

It seems likely that eventually most HIV positive individuals will develop AIDS (Rutherford et al 1990). Thus a strategy is needed that will control the spread of HIV. To be successful this requires information and education, functioning health and social services, and a supportive social environment (Zwi & Cabral 1991). For example, one important cofactor increasing the transmission of HIV in Africans appears to be the presence of sexually transmitted disease (Cameron et al 1989). Hence treatment of genital infection and the advocation of condom usage would appear to be a logical strategy. However the latter requires a widespread change in sexual practice which may be resisted at a local level. Equally within the developed world, if HIV is to be controlled, advice on safe sex, access to clean needles and self-exclusion from blood donations by high-risk groups are imperative.

As only an estimated 10% of infected individuals have AIDS, there is a large reservoir of asymptomatic unknown infection within the community. An increased public awareness of this issue, as well as the demonstration that infected individuals can benefit from early intervention and treatment, has led to more people coming forward for voluntary HIV antibody testing. The provision of an open access service is important, and same-day testing — where an individual is counselled (Bor et al 1991) and tested in the morning, and then receives the result that afternoon — has further increased uptake (Squire et al 1991).

LABORATORY MARKERS AND STAGING CLASSIFICATIONS OF DISEASE

The median time between infection and development of AIDS has been estimated as 10 years (Rutherford et al 1990). Over this period changes in laboratory markers can be used to predict the likelihood of developing AIDS. Currently the most useful tests are either T-lymphocyte based (fall in absolute and relative CD4 count, reduced CD4/CD8 ratio) or measure increased systemic viral (HIV antigenaemia) or 'immune activation' (e.g. rising serum β_2-microglobulin (β2M) — which presumably reflects increased cell destruction) and rising serum neopterin — (a marker of increased macrophage turnover). Taken together these have a relatively good predictive value (Moss & Bachetti 1989) though more accurate methods are needed: for example, using the phenotypic properties of the HIV isolate to measure T-cell reactivity or viral load.

HIV antigenaemia is present early in disease in only about 15% of cases. However its persistence increases the relative risk of progression to AIDS two to four times in the common subgroup of individuals with CD4 counts $>200 \times 10^6/l$ and B2M <5 mg/l (Moss & Bachetti 1989).

The frequency with which one measures T-lymphocyte subsets, B2M and HIV antigen is subject to debate. The 'average' rate of decline of CD4 counts is 11% per 6 months (Aledort et al 1992), though variation can occur through stress, exercise, time of day, intercurrent infection and laboratory measurement. Thus, in an asymptomatic seropositive, it is probably wise to measure immune markers at least twice a year, though more frequently if a patient has evidence of marked immunosuppression (CDC 1992).

Staging of HIV infection is useful as it enables one to make prognoses, select treatments and define trial end-points before clinical progression has occurred. Early classifications were based on clinical criteria (Table 9.1 — CDC classification) though there is now an increasing tendency to incorporate immune markers into HIV staging (Royce et al 1991). It is likely that, by the time of publication, a CD4 T-lymphocyte cell count $<200 \times 10^6/l$ or CD4 $<14\%$ in the absence of clinical findings will be regarded as an AIDS defining condition.

THE NEWLY DIAGNOSED HIV SEROPOSITIVE PATIENT

An HIV antibody test may have been performed for a number of different reasons. These include recent or long-standing 'high-risk' activity, the

Table 9.1 Centers for Disease Control Classification of HIV infections (1985)

Group I	Acute infection
Group II	Asymptomatic infection
Group III	Persistent generalized lymphadenopathy
Group IV	Other disease

Subgroup A	Constitutional disease
	e.g. weight loss > 10% body wt or > 4.5 kg
	      fevers > 38°
	      diarrhoea > 2 weeks

Subgroup B	Neurological disease
	e.g. HIV encephalopathy
	      myelopathy
	      peripheral neuropathy

Subgroup C	Secondary infectious diseases
	
	C1 — AIDS defining secondary infectious disease
	e.g. *Pneumocystis carinii* pneumonia
	      cerebral toxoplasmosis
	      cytomegalovirus retinitis
	C2 — Other specified secondary infectious diseases
	e.g. oral candida
	      pulmonary tuberculosis
	      multidermatomal varicella zoster

Subgroup D	Secondary cancers e.g. Kaposi's sarcoma non-Hodgkin's lymphoma
Subgroup E	Other conditions e.g. lymphoid intestitial pneumonitis

development of symptoms attributable to HIV, or as part of routine screening (e.g. through the blood transfusion service or an insurance medical). Time must be spent with new seropositive patients dealing with the considerable psychological and social problems generated (e.g. who to tell, what to do about jobs/pensions/mortgages, contemplating thoughts of death and suffering).

The important medical points are:

1. Confirming the HIV antibody test, using different assays on a second blood sample;
2. Ascertaining the individual's stage of disease through history, examination and laboratory tests;
3. Performing baseline screening for other potentially important diseases;
4. Establishing a good rapport with the patient which will encourage him/her to return for regular review;
5. Educating the individual about risk reduction, lifestyle management and the role of therapeutic interventions;
6. Considering issues of relevance to the individual's specific risk group (e.g. cervical smears in women or rehabilitation programmes in intravenous drug users).

Table 9.2   Baseline investigations of a new HIV seropositive patient

Virology	Reason
HIV antibody*	Confirmation
HIV (p24) antigen	Prognostic marker
CMV antibody	? Cofactor; future disease
Hepatitis screen (A, B, C)	1. If HBs Ab negative consider immunization
	2. May develop chronic disease
	3. ? Cofactor
Immunology	
T-lymphocyte subsets	Prognostic marker
β_2-Microglobulin/neopterin	Prognostic marker
Microbiology	
Syphilis serology (VDRL/TPHA/FTA)	? Occult/latent disease
Toxoplasma serology (dye test)	Future disease
Biochemistry	
Urea, electrolytes and creatinine	Assess disease state
Liver function tests	Abnormal with infection or drugs/therapy
Calcium	Malnourishment
Creatinine phosphokinase	May increase on zidovudine/with HIV
Amylase	May increase on ddI
Haematology	
Full blood count	HIV-related haematological abnormalities
Differential	(plus effect of treatment)
Film	

*HIV-1 antibody may take up to 3 months (and very rarely longer) to become positive from time of last risk; if in doubt repeat testing is advised and check HIV antigen (may be present before antibody).

The help of a counsellor who can advise on social issues and benefits, as well as provide support for the individual and partner/family in the long term, is essential.

Baseline investigations are summarized in Table 9.2.

Tuberculin testing and a careful history of BCG immunization should be undertaken at diagnosis. In America prophylactic antituberculous chemotherapy such as isoniazid has been advocated for all HIV seropositive individuals with either a positive skin reaction (Mantoux, 5 tuberculin units ≥5 mm of induration) and no previous treatment, or who come from a population with a high prevalence of tuberculosis (>10%) (CDC 1990). Recent guidelines from the British Thoracic Society further recommend that all patients with a CD4 count $<200 \times 10^6$/l, a negative Mantoux (10 tuberculin units, induration <5 mm) and no response to at least two other recall antigens, should be given isoniazid chemoprophylaxis irrespective of previous BCG immunization (British Thoracic Society 1992).

PRIMARY HIV INFECTION

In the majority of cases primary HIV-1 infection is symptomatic but is usually not correctly diagnosed. A wide variety of symptoms and signs have been described, the most common of which are fever, malaise, diarrhoea, myalgia, arthralgia, sore throat, headaches, lymphadenopathy and a maculopapular rash (De Jong et al 1991). The most common neurological manifestation is an aseptic meningoencephalitis (presenting with headache, fever, photophobia and confusion).

The time from infection with HIV-1 to clinical disease seems to vary between 1 and 4 weeks for the 'flu-like' illness and up to 6 weeks for neurological disease. The acute illness is self-limiting, though there is evidence that the duration of symptoms (>14 days) predicts early progression to AIDS (Pedersen et al 1989).

During symptomatic primary HIV-1 infection, specific HIV antibodies are usually detectable in serum. However HIV antigenaemia is an earlier feature of infection and there may be a window period when no antibody is detectable though the patient is in fact highly infectious. Repeat HIV antibody testing 6–12 weeks later may be needed to establish the diagnosis.

There is no evidence at present that antiretroviral therapy given at the time of infection alters either the course of the seroconversion illness or the natural history of HIV. Occasionally seroconversion may produce such a profound (but transient) fall in immunity that the patient may develop oesophageal candidiasis. This should not be regarded as AIDS defining as, once treated, immunity will return towards normal.

ASYMPTOMATIC HIV INFECTION

The proportion of seropositives who will progress to AIDS is unknown. A San Francisco cohort study of gay men revealed that 11 years after seroconversion 19% of the population had no clinical symptoms or signs, and 3% had asymptomatic generalized lymphadenopathy (Rutherford et al 1990). However it was also clear that the likelihood of developing AIDS was related to the duration of HIV-1 infection, with an estimated 11-year cumulative incidence of AIDS of 54%. Thus, although the majority of seropositives may ultimately develop AIDS, a large proportion will remain well for several years.

Asymptomatic seropositives may see friends and partners progress to AIDS and die. Thus a large part of their management involves adequate counselling, support and education. They should be encouraged to self-report symptoms, and should feel that they have easy access to clinics if necessary. Typically patients are reviewed 3 monthly at which time full clinical examination and laboratory monitoring is performed (i.e. CD4 counts, HIV antigen and $\beta2M$).

Persistent generalized lymphadenopathy (PGL), histologically a follicular hyperplasia, is often a worry for patients as it marks them out as having obvious signs of 'disease'. However, the prognosis in this subgroup is the same as that for clinically asymptomatic seropositives. Indications for investigation of lymphadenopathy in HIV are: development of lymph nodes associated with symptoms, e.g. night sweats, weight loss; rapidly enlarging or painful nodes, and markedly asymmetrical nodes. Mediastinal adenopathy is unlikely to be due to PGL and a further cause should be sought, e.g. lymphoma or mycobacterial disease.

EARLY SYMPTOMATIC HIV INFECTION

In practice, many 'asymptomatic' seropositives will have early symptoms or signs of HIV infection. These, however, may be non-specific or represent a worsening of a previous condition. Examples include folliculitis, molluscum contagiosum, seborrhoeic dermatitis, psoriasis and viral warts. The development of some conditions, though, indicates advancing disease and marked immunosuppression. These are often known as AIDS-related complex (ARC) and are summarized in Table 9.3. The presence of ARC is associated with an increased risk of AIDS; for example, without antiretroviral therapy 75% of patients with oral hairy leukoplakia will develop AIDS in 2–3 years.

Table 9.3 Components of AIDS-related complex (ARC)

Persistent fever	Persistent or recurring fever > 38°C for at least 2 weeks
Fatigue	Persistent fatigue for at least 2 weeks
Diarrhoea	Diarrhoea for at least 2 weeks
New rash	New skin rash that lasts for at least 2 weeks
Worse herpes	More frequent, more severe, longer duration
Bullous impetigo	By physical examination or self-report
Oral hairy leukoplakia	By physical examination or self-report
Oral thrush	By physical examination (may be confirmed by KOH testing) or self-report
Varicella zoster	Shingles (uni- or multidermatomal)
Unintentional weight loss	Unintentional weight loss of at least 10 lb (4.5 kg) unrelated to dieting
Night sweats	Sweating at night for at least 2 weeks

LATE SYMPTOMATIC HIV INFECTION

With advancing immunosuppression (CD4 count $<200 \times 10^6/l$) patients become prey to a wide variety of infectious, neoplastic and infiltrative disorders. These correspond to CDC stage IV disease and often represent an AIDS diagnosis (Table 9.1). Therapeutic intervention has improved post-AIDS median survival (currently 18 months), yet may also have altered the natural history of HIV: there is less early and survivable *Pneumocystis carinii* pneumonia (PCP) and more fatal lymphoma. The following section will deal with the management of common symptoms in the different organ systems and will conclude with a section on HIV-related tumours.

Respiratory disease

Pneumocystis carinii pneumonia (PCP)

Respiratory disease is the most common AIDS presentation. The typical picture is several weeks of breathlessness, dry cough, fevers, and malaise with few respiratory signs. This is often due to PCP which occurs in more than 70% of AIDS patients. Thus any seropositive at risk of PCP (in practical terms this means CD4 $<200 \times 10^6/l$) (Graham et al 1991) who presents with a history of breathlessness should be assumed to have this until proven otherwise.

Certain clinical features may suggest other respiratory pathogens (e.g. purulent sputum, pleuritic chest pain and focal signs imply a bacterial pneumonia; pleural effusions are usually due to mycobacterial disease or Kaposi's sarcoma), though it should be remembered that dual infection occurs in up to 30% of AIDS patients.

The vigour with which the diagnosis is pursued will vary from centre to centre, though it is mandatory to perform a chest radiograph and either resting and exercise oxygen saturation (via a pulse oximeter) or arterial blood gases. In early disease these investigations may be normal, but typically the chest radiograph reveals bilateral alveolar and interstitial shadowing predominantly lower zone with absence of Kerley 'B' lines. Often the patient is either hypoxic at rest or markedly desaturates when exercised (e.g. oximetry 97% at rest, falls to 90% after 'step ups' for 5–10 min). When doubt remains, thoracic computed tomography (CT) scans and radionuclear uptake methods (e.g. 99^mTc, DTPA) can provide further information.

For a definitive diagnosis, sputum, bronchoalveolar washings or lung parenchyma must be examined by histological, cytological or microbiological techniques. The methods employed are listed in Table 9.4. None of the procedures are without risk or discomfort to the patient, which may be important when considering the quality of an AIDS patient's life. Indeed the chance of PCP in a high-risk individual is so great that simple scoring systems have been devised that attempt to dispense with the need for first-line invasive investigations (Smith et al 1992).

As mentioned earlier, PCP is the most likely diagnosis, though similar presentations are found with viral (e.g. cytomegalovirus (CMV), Herpes simplex virus), protozoal (toxoplasma), fungal (candida, histoplasma, cryptococcus), bacterial and mycobacterial infections — all of which occur with increased frequency in HIV disease. In practical terms, if someone is suspected of having PCP they should be started on therapy as soon as possible, with a diagnostic procedure planned for an appropriate time within the next few days (pneumocystis can still be recovered after several weeks of treatment).

The standard therapy for PCP is either trimethoprim–sulphamethoxazole (cotrimoxazole) or pentamidine isethionate. There is little to choose between

Table 9.4 Diagnostic investigations in HIV-related respiratory disease

Investigation	Method	Comment
Induced sputum production	Hypertonic saline via ultrasonic nebulizer with postural drainage	Unpleasant, time-consuming, poor yield without prior experience of technique
Fibreoptic bronchoscopy with bronchoalveolar lavage	180–240 ml buffered isotonic saline into right middle lobe or area of focal change	Requires sedation, intra/post procedure hypoxia well documented. May cause acute deterioration in sick patient. Good diagnostic yield
Fibreoptic bronchoscopy with transbronchial biopsy	Multiple biopsies of right lower lobe or area of focal change	High risk of complication in HIV, e.g. pneumothorax, bleeding. Good diagnostic yield
Open lung biopsy		Requires general anaesthetic. Often ITU care postoperatively. Useful if all else fails (and patient can tolerate procedure)

the two: they are equally efficacious (80% response rate), both are prescribed for an initial 21 days and each has a large number of disadvantages. Cotrimoxazole causes adverse effects (nausea, rash, fever and neutropenia) in 40–80% of AIDS patients, whilst pentamidine will induce hypotension, hypoglycaemia and worsening renal function in up to 70% of AIDS patients. The response to either drug is slow and often clinical improvement is not obvious until day 5 of therapy.

In most departments cotrimoxazole (trimethoprim 20 mg/kg/day and sulphamethoxazole 100 mg/kg/day) is favoured as first-line drug as patients can receive oral therapy once stabilized or, with mild disease, be commenced on tablets at the outset. If the patient continues to deteriorate after 5 days of treatment one can switch to pentamidine (4 mg/kg/day) overlapping the two drugs by at least 48 h. In some patients cotrimoxazole is effective but causes marked adverse effects of uncontrolled nausea and vomiting. In this case the second-line combination of trimethoprim (20 mg/kg/day) and dapsone (100 mg/day) may be more appropriate. Surprisingly 70% of patients who experience side-effects from cotrimoxazole tolerate this combination. Folinic acid (15 mg every 3 days) should be given when high-dose folate antagonists are used. Regular haematological and biochemical monitoring is necessary for all anti-PCP drugs.

Other drugs may have a role in 'salvage therapy' of PCP, where first-line treatments have failed. These include trimetrexate, eflornithine, primaquine and clindamycin combination, and the promising new drug 566C80. The results from the few studies that have been performed suggest that at best these drugs are effective in only about 50% of cases, though it must be remembered that often they have been used where standard therapy has failed (Hughes 1991).

Prophylaxis against PCP relies heavily on either oral cotrimoxazole or nebulized pentamidine. There is benefit in both primary (no previous PCP, but CD4 $<200 \times 10^6/l$ or CDC IV disease) and secondary prophylaxis (started immediately after the high-dose induction course). The San Francisco Community Prophylaxis Trial (Leoung et al 1990) established the standard pentamidine dose of 300 mg every 4 weeks via a jet nebulizer (Respirgard II). Recent (yet unpublished) work from the American AIDS Clinical Trials Group (ACTG 021) demonstrated the superiority of cotrimoxazole (960 mg o.d.) over pentamidine (300 mg/month via Respirgard II) in secondary prophylaxis (1-year estimated recurrence rate of 3.5% versus 18.5%). There was also a suggestion of cross-prophylaxis against toxoplasma and bacterial infections in the cotrimoxazole group. However, there were a large number of adverse reactions to cotrimoxazole reported. On balance most clinicians now favour the use of cotrimoxazole as first-line prophylaxis and would use pentamidine in patients who are sulphonamide intolerant. Other drugs (e.g. dapsone and Fansidar) have been explored as possible prophylactic agents. At present there are few efficacy data to recommend their use (CDC 1992).

The first episode mortality rate of PCP has fallen from 20% to 7% whilst postventilation survival has risen from 14% to 55%. This is due to a number of factors including earlier detection of disease, aggressive PCP management and use of antiretroviral/prophylactic drugs. Some of the therapeutic strategies that seem to be important include the early use of systemic glucocorticoids (dose at least 60–80 mg prednisolone per day reducing after day 5) in moderate to severe PCP [$P_aO_2 < 70$ mmHg (9.3 kPa); O_2 saturation $< 90\%$ on air; or alveolar–arterial gradient > 35 mmHg (4.7 kPa)] (McGowan et al 1992), and appropriate selection of patients for either continuous positive pressure airway circuits, where the patient is breathing spontaneously, and/or intubation with formal mechanical ventilation (Wachter et al 1992).

Mycobacterial disease

Since 1985 the number of cases of mycobacterium tuberculosis (MTB) reported annually in the USA has risen by 16%. This is mainly due to coexistent HIV infection (Snider & Roper 1992). Globally the situation is similar with an estimated 4 million people coinfected with HIV and MTB. A large proportion of these individuals will have extrapulmonary disease (e.g. pleural, pericardial, lymphatic, central nervous system or genitourinary system involvement), whilst pulmonary MTB may itself be anatomically atypical (Elliot et al 1990). MTB can present at any stage of HIV disease and normally responds to standard quadruple drug therapy. However, long-term relapse (especially in the developing world) appears very common and so many physicians will maintain patients on lifelong isoniazid.

Multidrug-resistant MTB is seen increasingly frequently in the USA. Clinical features that suggest its presence include continued fever, worsening pulmonary infiltrates, sputum smear positivity and extrapulmonary MTB cultures whilst on standard treatment. It is extremely difficult to treat, has a high mortality and has been implicated in several outbreaks of nosocomial MTB.

The opportunist pathogen *Mycobacterium avium intracellulare* complex (MAIC) is a much later finding in HIV disease, presenting as disseminated infection usually 7–15 months after AIDS diagnosis. Its clinical features are often non-specific, e.g. fever, night sweats, malaise, anorexia and weight loss. Occasionally it may present in a specific organ system, e.g. gut infiltration or within the lung parenchyma. The presence of MAIC reduces patient survival probably via general malnutrition and cachexia. It can be diagnosed on the basis of culture from any normally sterile site (e.g. blood, bone marrow). Treatment remains a problem due to widespread drug resistance, though there is some optimism that rifabutin, amikacin and the new macrolides (e.g. clarithromycin) may be more effective (Scoular et al 1991). The current recommended regimen is combination therapy with clarithromycin, ethambutol and rifabutin. Rifabutin has also been used with moderate success as a primary prophylactic agent in patients with CD4 $< 200 \times 10^6/l$ and AIDS. An important point to consider, however, is that drug therapy may do little to help the patient long term yet markedly reduce the quality of the life that remains.

Gastrointestinal disease

The three common presentations of disease are oral disease, difficulty in swallowing and diarrhoea.

Oral disease

Seropositive individuals should be encouraged to see their own (or a hospital recommended) dentist on a regular basis as gingivitis and periodontitis are common. An acute attack of gingivitis will usually respond rapidly to metronidazole and penicillin, though the antibiotics may cause oral thrush.

Patients with oral candidiasis may complain of loss of taste, a dry mouth or the unappealing look of the fungus. The presence of oral thrush should prompt enquiry regarding any difficulty or discomfort swallowing as the patient may also have oesophageal candidiasis. If there is no indication of this, then a short course of an imidazole antifungal (e.g. fluconazole or ketoconazole) will be effective. Cheaper alternatives (e.g. nystatin pastilles or amphotericin lozenges) are unfortunately not so successful, though are worth trying in the first instance.

Mouth ulcers may result from a variety of causes and should always be swabbed for microbiological, mycobacterial and virological culture. Painful ulcers are usually due to Herpes simplex virus (HSV) and respond to acyclovir 400 mg q.d.s. for 5 days or until the ulcer has healed, though any ulcer that does not clear or increases in size may need biopsy for histological diagnosis. Acyclovir-resistant herpes is now more commonly seen, and here topical trifluridine appears to be effective. Giant aphthous ulceration is also well recognized in HIV disease, and is treated with thalidomide which can be prescribed on a named-patient basis.

Oral hairy leukoplakia (OHL) appears as a whitish lesion on the lateral border of the tongue. It represents heaped up hyperparakeratotic epithelium which is presumed to have proliferated in response to Epstein–Barr virus stimulation. It is often asymptomatic though its prognostic significance has been mentioned earlier. Some cases may respond to either high-dose acyclovir (800 mg q.d.s.) or topical retin-A.

Difficulty swallowing

Difficulty swallowing is an important symptom as it may indicate an AIDS diagnosis. Commonly it is due to candidal oesophagitis, but it may result from CMV or HSV oesophagitis (both usually more painful), or obstruction from tumour, e.g. Kaposi's sarcoma. Endoscopy rather than barium swallow tends to be the investigation of choice as here there is little risk of perforation. Endoscopy also enables biopsies to be taken which should be sent to cytology/histopathology, microbiology and virology. Treatment is as necessary (e.g. candida: fluconazole 200–400 mg/day for 14 days), though if this is a first AIDS diagnosis consideration should be given to antiretroviral/prophylactic therapy.

Diarrhoea

Diarrhoea occurs in 30–50% of North American and European patients with AIDS, and in nearly 90% of those from the developing world (often with marked cachexia — 'slim disease') There is increasing evidence that protracted diarrhoea (i.e. > 3 liquid or semiformed stools most days per week for > 4 weeks) will usually have a specific pathogenic cause, though not always a specific treatment (Quinn et al 1992).

Diarrhoea may be profuse, watery and associated with crampy abdominal pains and dehydration as seen with cryptosporidium or *Isospora belli* and microsporidial species. It may be more dysenteric with fever, malaise, abdominal pain and blood and pus in the motion (e.g. CMV colitis, salmonella dysentery), or it may be associated with malabsorption and weight loss, e.g. giardiasis. Stepwise investigations are summarized in Table 9.5.

CMV colitis occurs in about 13% of AIDS patients. The diagnosis should be based strictly on either histology or culture as treatment involves 2–3 weeks of ganciclovir or foscarnet, both of which are currently only available intravenously and both of which have serious side-effects (neutropenia and

Table 9.5 Stepwise investigation of HIV-related diarrhoea

1. Stools and stool chart (one divided sample on $\geq$ 3 consecutive days)	Microscopy, culture for dysenteric pathogens Ova, cysts, parasites Mycobacterial culture *Clostridium difficile* toxin (drug-induced pseudomembranous colitis) Viral culture (CMV, HSV, adenovirus)
2. Sigmoidoscopy and rectal biopsy	Histology Bacteriology Mycobacteriology Virology
3. Colonoscopy and biopsy	Histology Bacteriology Mycobacteriology Virology
4. Duodenoscopy, duodenal brushings and duodenal juice aspiration	'HIV Villous atrophy' Ova, cysts, parasites Biopsy macroscopic lesions
5. Electron microscopy of tissue samples	Microsporidia species

renal impairment, respectively). At present there is no consensus on maintenance therapy for isolated CMV gastrointestinal disease.

CMV has been implicated in the pathogenesis of both HIV cholangiopathy (similar radiologically to sclerosing cholangitis) and HIV pancreatitis. So too have cryptosporidium species which are isolated in the stool of up to 25% of AIDS patients. Cryptosporidium can cause profound malabsorption which may not respond at all to treatment. Therapeutic strategies include macrolide antibiotics (e.g. azithromycin) and imidazoles (e.g. fluconazole), though often symptomatic therapy (fluids and antidiarrhoeals) is all that can be offered.

Diarrhoea may be due to gut wall infiltration by tumours such as Kaposi's sarcoma or lymphoma, which may be revealed at endoscopic examination.

General measures

Nutrition is an important part of general AIDS/HIV management. The mechanisms promoting malabsorption and cachexia are not clearly understood, though the precipitous weight loss in AIDS seems to be related to infection (low serum albumin, normal or raised metabolic rate) (Editorial 1991). In early disease general 'healthy eating' guidelines are probably adequate, whilst in advanced HIV infection specialist dietetic help is needed to advise on enteral and parenteral feeding.

Neurological disease

Direct HIV infection

HIV may cause direct neurological disease, affecting the brain ('HIV encephalopathy'), the spinal cord (presenting as a vacuolar myelopathy with long tract signs and a sensory level) and the peripheral nervous system (e.g. symmetrical peripheral neuropathy, mononeuritis multiplex, autonomic neuropathy). HIV encephalopathy is characterized by abnormalities of cognition, motor function and behaviour. It is the AIDS defining illness in less than 5% of cases yet is a common histological finding at autopsy. There is some evidence that antiretroviral therapy may slow down the progressive deterioration (Schmitt et al 1988) though in practice most patients with HIV encephalopathy require supportive care within weeks to months.

Opportunist central nervous system disease

Opportunistic infection is the most common cause of neurological dysfunction. Toxoplasma encephalitis (the most common AIDS defining neurological disease) may present either as a space-occupying lesion with or without focal signs, as a seizure or as a depressed level of consciousness. In 95% of cases toxoplasma encephalitis is a reactivation of old disease. The diagnosis is made by the history, examination and CT brain scan appearance which will show one or more areas of hypodense oedema often with contrast ring-enhancement signifying abscess formation. Treatment is started for toxoplasmosis on a presumptive basis as toxoplasma encephalitis is common and will respond to therapy whereas the other likely causes of this picture have a uniformly poor outlook. Indications for brain biopsy include failure of therapy (after about 2 weeks), atypical CT findings and negative toxoplasma serology (Barker & Holliman 1992).

Standard treatment is 4–8 weeks of sulphadiazine 6–8 g/day with pyrimethamine 75 mg/day plus folinic acid supplements. Clindamycin is an effective substitute for sulphadiazine if there is sulphonamide intolerance. Lower dose maintenance therapy needs to be life-long. Recent work suggests that primary prophylaxis with dapsone and pyrimethamine may prevent toxoplasma reactivation (and hence disease). This needs further confirmation but may be important for patients who are toxoplasma IgG positive.

Other causes of focal neurological dysfunction include primary central nervous system lymphoma, progressive multifocal leucoencephalopathy (a degenerative disease due to a papova virus, also carrying a poor prognosis), then much more rarely tuberculoma, bacterial abscess (usually in drug addicts) and viral and fungal infections.

Diffuse central nervous dysfunction may present as drowsiness, confusion or behavioural changes. It is important to exclude metabolic (e.g. systemic infection, hyponatraemia) and hypoxic causes (undiagnosed chest infection). Drugs can also be a potent cause of confusion (e.g. opiates for pain relief). Infections that produce this sort of picture include cryptococcal meningitis (which may have minimal associated meningism) and respond in only 40–50% of cases to either amphotericin B or the less toxic fluconazole (200–400 mg/day) (Saag et al 1992). Bacterial and mycobacterial meningitis may also present in this way, as may CMV/HSV encephalitis in the immunosuppressed. Recent reports have stressed the danger of missing active neurosyphilis and thus it is important that routine 'work-up' includes magnetic resonance imaging/CT brain scan and then lumbar puncture with cerebrospinal fluid analysis by cytology (lymphoma, fungi), microbiology, mycobacteriology, serology laboratory, virology and biochemistry.

Retinal involvement is usually due to CMV disease. This presents as floaters or loss of vision and is a fairly late AIDS event. To save the eye, treatment should be started as soon as possible and again maintenance therapy will need to be given indefinitely. A recent trial compared the benefits of foscarnet and ganciclovir and appeared to show a survival advantage for the former (median 12.6 versus 8.5 months) (Studies of Ocular Complications of AIDS (SOCA) Research Group 1992). However, oral maintenance ganciclovir may soon be available, reducing the need for permanent indwelling lines — which would be a considerable advance as patients invariably develop septicaemia requiring frequent line changes.

Haematological disease

The haematological manifestations of HIV are protean and may result from HIV infection per se, opportunist disease (e.g. anaemia from disseminated MAIC, bone marrow infiltration by lymphoma), or the drug therapy used in treating these conditions (Costello 1990). Cytopenias may be due to either increased destruction or failure of production. Any form of cytopenia can be present, though typically HIV will cause more thrombocytopenia than either drugs or opportunist infections, whilst drugs such as cotrimoxazole, zidovudine and ganciclovir produce neutropenia and anaemia. Zidovudine (AZT) also frequently causes a macrocytosis irrespective of the haemoglobin level. The presence of malaise, fever and falling haematological indices should suggest opportunist infection or neoplasm. Often, however, direct HIV infection appears to be responsible for the haematological disorder, and a trial of antiretroviral therapy as 'treatment' is justified.

Cytokine therapy is becoming increasingly important in the management of HIV-associated haematological disease. Fischl's work in 1990 demonstrated that recombinant erythropoietin both corrected the anaemia and reduced the transfusion requirements of AIDS patients who had AZT-induced anaemia and low or normal endogenous erythropoietin levels at the start of treatment (Fischl et al 1990a). Promising results have also been found with both granulocyte colony-stimulating factor (G-CSF) and granulocyte–macrophage colony-stimulating factor (GM-CSF) in reversing AZT induced and HIV-related leucopenia (Mitsuyasu 1991). Given that G-CSF may influence the development of the earliest red blood cell precursors, trials of combination G-CSF and erythropoietin have been undertaken. A phase I/II trial of 22 patients demonstrated that AZT-associated neutropenia and anaemia could both be reversed, but that the latter recurred with reintroduction of AZT (Miles et al 1991). However, AZT-induced anaemia is a dose-related phenomenon, and is clinically much less of a problem with current reduced dosage regimens.

Apart from the anticipated side-effects of flu-like symptoms, and high cost, there is a potential disadvantage with GM-CSF in particular in that it can stimulate macrophages which may lead to increased HIV replication within these retroviral reservoirs. Fortunately this has not been borne out in clinical practice.

HIV-related neoplastic disease

Kaposi's sarcoma (KS) is the main non-infectious AIDS complication. It is more common in homosexual than heterosexual men, and is rare in Caucasian women. It can behave as a benign solitary tumour or rapidly develop multicentrically to involve the gut, lungs and lymph nodes. It is commonly found on the skin and palate and resembles at first a bruise which then becomes a purplish nodule. Treatment can be expectant, or if required local radiotherapy or cryotherapy is often effective for skin KS. Intralesional chemotherapy can also be used, though if KS is extensive or involves the viscera, systemic chemotherapy (currently vincristine and bleomycin with AZT if possible) is advocated. Median survival time with extensive disease is 8–10 months. α-Interferon exerts an antiproliferative action on KS. It appears to be most successful if given with AZT to an individual with a relatively intact immune system (CD4 $> 200 \times 10^6$/l) (Fischl et al 1991), and thus it should be considered early in patients with KS.

Non-Hodgkin's lymphoma is an AIDS defining condition which can be either primary central nervous or systemic. The former appears to be associated with Epstein–Barr virus and carries a dismal prognosis (median survival under 2 months) whilst the latter responds to chemotherapy, though often relapses several months later (Levine 1992).

It is likely that improving post-AIDS survival will lead to an increased recognition of HIV-related tumours. Examples already include cervical carcinoma (Maiman et al 1990) and squamous cell carcinoma of the anus.

ANTIRETROVIRAL THERAPY

In the long term, antiretroviral therapy is the only hope of eradicating established HIV infection. At present the licensed agents can only inhibit HIV reverse transcriptase (suppressing HIV replication by blocking the synthesis of viral DNA) and thus are not curative. These drugs need to be taken lifelong and so questions of short- and long-term toxicity and sustained effect become paramount. Zidovudine (azidothymidine, AZT) is the only agent of proven efficacy (prolonged survival, reduction in opportunistic infections and improved quality of life) for the treatment of AIDS (Fischl et al 1987, Vella et al 1992). In America, in addition, the dideoxynucleoside analogue didanosine (ddI) is licensed for use. Drug trials with these agents have been hampered by the length of time required for clinical end-points (e.g. death, development of AIDS), and thus ddI has been deemed efficacious on the basis of favourable changes in surrogate immune markers (e.g. CD4 count and HIV antigen) (Lambert et al 1990) which appear to predict short-term risk for clinical progression rather than survival (Jacobson et al 1991).

The value of treatment in patients who are less symptomatic (Fischl et al 1990b) or even asymptomatic (Volberding et al 1990) is not as yet clearly defined. Placebo controlled studies to date have only demonstrated a reduction in rate of fall of CD4 count, and a delayed progression to AIDS. In a recent observational study Graham showed AZT reduced mortality by slowing the progression to AIDS. However, this survival advantage had disappeared after the second year of follow-up (Graham et al 1992). The results of the Veterans Affairs Cooperative Study suggest that 'early versus late' AZT use may be a trade-off between a longer pre-AIDS symptom-free period or a presumably improved quality and quantity of life once AIDS has developed (Hamilton et al 1992). AZT is at present licensed for use at the onset of symptoms, or when the CD4 count is persistently $<200 \times 10^6/l$, or is rapidly declining from $500 \times 10^6/l$. We believe that in the latter case treatment should be discussed with the patient who should then make his/her own decision regarding therapy.

AZT is a toxic drug. It can cause bone marrow suppression, nausea, vomiting, myositis, headache and insomnia. These effects are dose-related and can be severe enough to warrant stopping the drug. Fortunately much smaller doses than first used seem equally efficacious (Volberding et al 1990, Nordic Medical Research Councils' HIV Therapy Group 1992) and the standard prescribed regimen is now 400–600 mg/day in divided doses. AZT also appears to be safe during pregnancy (Sperling et al 1992), though there are no data to show that it will influence vertical transmission of HIV from mother to infant.

AZT appears to have a limited clinical duration of effect, which may correspond to in vitro resistance (Tudor-Williams et al 1992). This can be demonstrated after as little as 6 months of therapy (Larder et al 1989) and is present in all AIDS/ARC patients at 18 months. No cross-resistance has been found with other antiretrovirals, and dideoxynucleoside analogues may be of value in these situations. For example, the recent ACTG 116B/117 trial comparing AZT 600 mg/day with two doses of ddI (500 mg/day and 750 mg/day) in patients who had tolerated AZT for more than 16 weeks revealed a significant decrease in the number of opportunist infections in the 500 mg ddI group. This effect, however, was only seen in those entering the study with ARC or asymptomatic disease, and there was no difference in survival between any treatment arm.

AZT sensitivity may return when the drug is stopped (St Clair et al 1991). This, plus the different toxicity profiles of AZT and the dideoxynucleoside analogues (ddI — pancreatitis and peripheral neuropathy; ddC — peripheral neuropathy), has led to trials of combination chemotherapy with some encouraging early results (Meng et al 1992). On the basis of this, the American FDA recently licensed ddC for use in combination with AZT.

At present there are no other licensed antiretroviral agents. Several clinical trials of non-nucleoside analogue reverse transcriptase inhibitors, e.g. TIBO derivatives (active almost solely against HIV-1 and responsible for profound single agent resistance), and of retroviral protease inhibitors are underway. Soluble CD4 has generated interest, though doubts remain whether this fluid phase intervention can limit in vivo cell-to-cell spread. Cytokines and interferons are also under investigation, though whether they are useful as pure antiretroviral agents remains unclear. A recent study in asymptomatic HIV positive individuals demonstrated that α-interferon could maintain CD4 lymphocyte percentages, decrease the frequency of peripheral blood virus isolation and over a 24-month mean follow-up period reduce the incidence of opportunistic infections. However, all patients taking interferon had flu-like symptoms and 35% of the sample withdrew because of toxicity (Lane et al 1990).

Vaccines against HIV are now being tested for safety and immunogenicity in several clinical trials. Most vaccines are based on HIV envelope proteins, e.g. gp 160 (Dolin et al 1991), though some use whole killed virus. Results so far suggest that a cellular but not a humoral immune response is generated and sustained over at least a 2-year period. The clinical significance of this remains unclear.

It seems unlikely that a cure for HIV will be found in the next few years, though in the long term vaccines and immunotherapy may hold some promise. However, if a drug is found to be effective in preventing HIV, the paradox remains that the developing nations who need a cure the most will be those least able to afford it.

KEY POINTS FOR CLINICAL PRACTICE

- HIV infection is increasing worldwide.
- Surrogate markers (e.g. CD4 lymphocyte count) can predict risk of progression to AIDS and should be monitored regularly.
- Median time from seroconversion to AIDS is currently 10 years.
- Effective intervention (e.g. antiretroviral and prophylactic agents) are available which increase quality and length of life. However, the optimum time for intervention is not as yet determined.
- Since 1981 median survival with AIDS has increased from 9 to 18 months.

REFERENCES

Aledort L M, Hilgartner M W, Pike M C et al 1992 Variability in serial CD4 counts and relation to progression of HIV-1 infection to AIDS in haemophilic patients. Br Med J 304: 212–216

Barker K F, Holliman R E 1992 Laboratory techniques in the investigation of toxoplasmosis. Genitourin Med 68: 55–59

Bor R, Miller R, Johnson M A 1991 A testing time for doctors: counselling patients before an HIV test. Br Med J 303: 905–907

British Thoracic Society, Subcommittee of the Joint Tuberculosis Committee 1992 Guidelines on the management of tuberculosis and HIV infection in the United Kingdom. Br Med J 304: 1231–1233

Cameron D W, Simonsen J N, D'Costa L J et al 1989 Female to male transmission of human immunodeficiency virus type 1: risk factors for seroconversion in men. Lancet 2: 403–407

Centers for Disease Control 1981 Pneumocystis pneumonia — Los Angeles. MMWR 30: 250–252

Centers for Disease Control 1990 The use of preventive therapy for tuberculous infection in the United States: recommendations of the Advisory Committee for Elimination of Tuberculosis. MMWR 39: 9–12

Centers for Disease Control 1992 Recommendations for prophylaxis against pneumocystis carinii pneumonia for adults and adolescents infected with human immunodeficiency virus. MMWR 41: 1–11

Costello C (ed) 1990 Haematology in HIV disease. Clin Haematol 3: 1–218

De Jong M D, Hulsebosch H J, Lange J M A 1991 Clinical, virological and immunological features of primary HIV-1 infection. Genitourin Med 67: 367–373

Dolin R, Graham B S, Greenberg S B et al 1991 The safety and immunogenicity of a human immunodeficiency virus type 1 (HIV-1) recombinant gp 160 candidate vaccine in humans. Ann Intern Med 114: 119–127

Editorial 1991 Nutrition and HIV. Lancet 338: 86–87

Elliot A M, Luo N, Tembo G et al 1990 Impact of HIV on tuberculosis in Zambia: a cross sectional study. Br Med J 301: 412–415

Fischl M A, Richman D D, Grieco M H et al 1987 The efficacy of azidothymidine (AZT) in the treatment of patients with AIDS or AIDS related complex: a double-blind placebo-controlled trial. N Engl J Med 317: 185–191

Fischl M A, Galpin J E, Levine J D et al 1990a Recombinant human erythropoietin for patients with AIDS treated with zidovudine. N Engl J Med 322: 1488–1493

Fischl M A, Richman D D, Hansen N et al 1990b The safety and efficacy of zidovudine (AZT) in the treatment of subjects with mildly symptomatic human immunodeficiency virus type 1 (HIV) infection. Ann Intern Med 112: 727–737

Fischl M A, Uttamchandani R B, Resnick L et al 1991 A phase 1 study of recombinant human interferon-α or human lymphoblastoid interferon α and concomitant zidovudine in patients with AIDS-related Kaposi's sarcoma. J Acquir Immune Defic Syndr 4: 1–10

Graham N M H, Zeger S L, Park L P et al 1991 Effect of zidovudine and pneumocystis carinii pneumonia prophylaxis on progression of HIV-1 infection to AIDS. Lancet 338: 265–269

Graham N M H, Zeger S L, Park L P et al 1992 The effects on survival of early treatment of human immunodeficiency virus infection. N Engl J Med 326: 1037–1042

Hamilton J D, Hartigan P M, Simberkoff M S et al 1992 A controlled trial of early versus late treatment with zidovudine in symptomatic human immunodeficiency infection: results of the Veterans Affairs Cooperative Study. N Engl J Med 326: 437–443

Hughes W T 1991 Prevention and treatment of pneumocystis carinii pneumonia. Annu Rev Med 42: 287–295

Jacobson M A, Bacchetti P, Kolokathis A et al 1991 Surrogate markers for survival in patients with AIDS or AIDS related complex treated with zidovudine. Br Med J 302: 73–78

Lambert J S, Seidlin M, Reichman R C et al 1990 2′,3′-Dideoxyinosine (ddI) in patients with the acquired immunodeficiency syndrome or AIDS-related complex: a phase 1 trial. N Engl J Med 322: 1333–1340

Lane H C, Davey V, Kovacs J A et al 1990 Interferon-alpha in patients with asymptomatic human immunodeficiency virus (HIV) infection. A randomised, placebo-controlled trial. Ann Intern Med 112: 805–811

Larder B A, Darby G, Richman D D 1989 HIV with reduced sensitivity to zidovudine (AZT) isolated during prolonged therapy. Science 243: 1731–1734

Leoung G S, Feigl Jr D W, Montgomery A B et al 1990 Aerosolized pentamidine for prophylaxis against pneumocystis carinii pneumonitis – the San Francisco Community Prophylaxis Trial. N Engl J Med 323: 769–775

Levine A M 1992 AIDS-associated malignant lymphoma. Med Clin North Am 76: 253–268

McGowan Jr J E, Chesney P J, Crossley K B et al 1992 Guidelines for the use of systemic glucocorticosteroids in the management of selected infections. J Infect Dis 165: 1–13

Maiman M, Fruchter R G, Serur E et al 1990 Human immunodeficiency virus infection and cervical neoplasia. Gynecol Oncol 38: 377–382

Meng T C, Fischl M A, Boota A M et al 1992 Combination therapy with zidovudine and dideoxycytidine in patients with advanced human immunodeficiency virus infection. A phase I/II study. Ann Intern Med 116: 13–20

Miles S A, Mitsuyasu R T, Moreno J et al 1991 Combined therapy with recombinant G-CSF and erythropoietin decreases hematologic toxicity from zidovudine. Blood 77: 2109–2117

Mitsuyasu R T 1991 Use of recombinant interferons and hematopoietic growth factors in patients infected with human immunodeficiency virus. Rev Infect Dis 13: 979–984

Moss A R, Bacchetti P 1989 Natural history of HIV infection. AIDS 3: 55–61

Nordic Medical Research Councils' HIV Therapy Group 1992 Double blind dose–response study of zidovudine in AIDS and advanced HIV infection. Br Med J 304: 13–17

Pedersen C, Lindhart B O, Jensen B L et al 1989 Clinical course of primary HIV infection: consequences for subsequent course of infection. Br Med J 299: 154–157

Quinn T C, Strober W, Janoff E N et al 1992 Gastrointestinal infections in AIDS. Ann Intern Med 116: 63–77

Royce R A, Luckmann R S, Fusaro R E et al 1991 The natural history of HIV-1 infection: staging classifications of disease. AIDS 5: 355–364

Rutherford G W, Lifson A R, Hessol N A et al 1990 Course of HIV-1 infection in a cohort of homosexual and bisexual men: an 11 year follow up study. Br Med J 301: 1183–1188

Saag M S, Powderly W G, Cloud G A et al 1992 Comparison of amphotericin B with fluconazole in the treatment of acute AIDS-associated cryptococcal meningitis. N Engl J Med 326: 83–89

St Clair M H, Martin J L, Tudor-Williams G et al 1991 Resistance to ddI and sensitivity to AZT induced by a mutation in HIV-1 reverse transcriptase. Science 253: 1557–1559

Schmitt F, Bigley J, McKinnis R 1988 Neuropsychological outcome of zidovudine treatment of patients with AIDS and AIDS related complex. N Engl J Med 299: 819–821

Scoular A, French P, Miller R F 1991 Mycobacterium avium-intracellulare infection in the acquired immunodeficiency syndrome. Br J Hosp Med 46: 295–300

Smith D, Forbes A, Gazzard B 1992 A simple scoring system to diagnose pneumocystis carinii pneumonia in high-risk individuals. AIDS 6: 337–338

Snider Jr D E, Roper W L 1992 The new tuberculosis. N Engl J Med 326: 703–705

Sperling R S, Stratton P, O'Sullivan M J et al 1992 A survey of zidovudine use in pregnant women with human immunodeficiency virus infection. N Engl J Med 326: 857–861

Squire S B, Elford J, Tilsed G et al 1991 Open access clinic providing HIV-1 antibody results on day of testing: the first twelve months. Br Med J 302: 1383–1386

Studies of Ocular Complications of AIDS (SOCA) Research Group, in collaboration with the AIDS Clinical Trials Group 1992 Mortality in patients with the acquired immunodeficiency syndrome treated with either foscarnet or ganciclovir for cytomegalovirus retinitis. N Engl J Med 326: 213–220

Tudor-Williams G, St Clair M H, McKinney R E et al 1992 HIV-1 sensitivity to zidovudine and clinical outcome in children. Lancet 339: 15–19

Vella S, Giuliano M, Pezzotti P et al 1992 Survival of zidovudine-treated patients with AIDS compared with that of contemporary untreated patients. JAMA 267: 1232–1236

Volberding P A, Lagakos S W, Koch M A et al 1990 Zidovudine in asymptomatic human immunodeficiency virus infection: a controlled trial in persons with fewer than 500 CD4-positive cells per cubic millimeter. N Engl J Med 322: 941–949

Wachter R M, Luce J M, Hopewell P C 1992 Critical care of patients with AIDS. JAMA 267: 541–547

World Health Organization 1991 Current and future dimensions of the HIV/AIDS pandemic – a capsule summary. WHO, Geneva

Zwi A B, Cabral A J R 1991 Identifying 'high risk situations' for preventing AIDS. Br Med J 303: 1527–1529

10

Hepatitis C and the haematologist

G. Dusheiko   B. Wonke   S. M. Donohue

A viral agent responsible for most cases of post-transfusion hepatitis was recognized after serological tests for hepatitis A and hepatitis B viruses became available in 1974 (Feinstone et al 1975). The enigmatic name of non-A, non-B (NANB) hepatitis was given to classify this form of hepatitis. Although in the ensuing years many groups of investigators subsequently claimed to have identified the aetiological agent of NANB hepatitis or developed serological tests, none of the claims or tests could be validated (Dienstag 1983b). Despite this difficulty, however, a considerable body of information on NANB hepatitis in humans and chimpanzees was compiled. Finally, in 1989, Houghton and co-workers succeeded in isolating nucleic acid of the major NANB agent by recombinant DNA technology (Kuo et al 1989, Choo et al 1989, 1990). A viral protein (5-1-1) was expressed in bacteria from the open reading frame of the cDNA clone. Immunoblot analysis was performed on bacterial lysates using serum obtained from chimpanzees which had been experimentally infected with NANB hepatitis. This enabled detection of circulating antibody. A radioimmunoassay was then developed for detection of antibody in patients with chronic NANB hepatitis.

The timely identification of this agent, which has been given the name hepatitis C virus (HCV), and the development of specific serological tests for the diagnosis of HCV have rapidly enhanced our understanding of type C hepatitis, and have improved the treatment of this disease.

Preliminary epidemiological assessment suggests that most cases of NANB hepatitis in Europe, the Americas, and the Far East are caused by hepatitis C. There are approximately 100 million type C hepatitis carriers globally. About 175 000 new cases are said to occur annually in the USA and in Europe, and 350 000 cases per year in Japan. Because HCV is a parenterally transmitted virus, the agent is of particular interest to haematologists.

VIROLOGY OF HCV

The putative NANB virus was previously thought to possess a lipid envelope, and to be approximately 50–80 nm in diameter. HCV is now believed to be an enveloped virus, approximately 50 nm in size, and is known to possess an

RNA genome of 9379 nucleotides (Fig. 10.1). There are preliminary reports of viral particles which have been visualized by electron microscopy (Abe et al 1989). The genomic organization suggests some homology to flavi- or pestiviruses, but HCV may be sufficiently unique to be placed in its own genus (Takamizawa et al 1991). Genomic sequences have been published for the prototype strain isolated in the USA (HCV-1), and two strains isolated in Japan (HCV-J and HCV-JH). Partial sequences of other isolates are being reported from other geographical regions (Chen et al 1991). There are probably at least five major genotypes of hepatitis C.

The viral genomic RNA is a single stranded plus sense RNA, with a single long open reading frame. The gene product is a viral polyprotein precursor of 3011 amino acids, which undergoes proteolytic post-translational cleavage to yield structural (core, and envelope) and non-structural (proteases, helicases, RNA-dependent RNA polymerase) proteins. To some extent, knowledge of the nature of HCV proteins is based on predictions made from nucleotide sequences, but an increasing number of proteins are being recombinantly expressed.

The structural proteins are derived from the 5′ third of the genome (Okamoto et al 1990), and the non-structural proteins from the 3′ (NS1 to NS5) regions. The 5′ end begins with a non-coding region of at least 341 bases. This sequence of HCV appears to be highly conserved, with a high

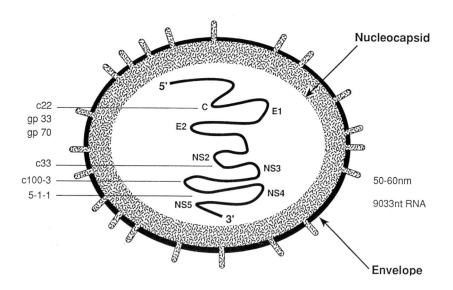

Fig. 10.1 A stylized depiction of the hepatitis C virus, showing an artistic representation of the viral particle, RNA genome, non-coding 5′ region, coding region, and proteins expressed from the viral genome and used in serological assays. C, nucleocapsid protein-coding region; E, envelope protein-coding region, NS, non-structural region.

degree of sequence homology amongst most isolates sequenced to date (Han et al 1991, Choo et al 1991). Two glycosylated proteins, gp35 and gp70, may be coded by the E1 and E2 regions of the genome, analogous to the NS1 region of flaviviruses, and could be envelope proteins of the HCV (Hijikata et al 1991b). Variable and hypervariable regions within the putative envelope glycoproteins have been described (Hijikata et al 1991a, Weiner et al 1991). These regions may code for important antigenic sites, and are probably involved in escape from host immunity, perhaps accounting for the fact that HCV infections are frequently persistent. This genomic diversity will have important implications in vaccine development and immunodiagnostic testing.

DIAGNOSIS OF HCV

HCV antibodies

The first commercially available diagnostic tests were based on antibodies to an expressed protein (c100-3) derived from the NS3/NS4 region. This antigen represents 363 amino acids of viral sequence from the NS4 region (4% of total viral protein), and includes a fusion protein (superoxide dismutase) for expression in yeast. To date, there are no serological tests for antigens of HCV in serum, as the virus circulates at a concentration below the level of detection of antigen by standard immunoassays. Most of the sero-epidemiological and diagnostic studies of hepatitis C were initially based on the prevalence of antibodies to the non-structural c100-3 protein. More recently, other antigens have been expressed, including a 22 kDa structural protein of HCV, whose coding region has been mapped to the amino terminal region of the HCV polyprotein, and which is ostensibly a nucleocapsid (core) antigen of HCV (Harada et al 1991). A second series of non-structural antigens, including c33 and c200, have been derived from the NS3 and NS4 regions and expressed in yeast or *Escherichia coli*. Together these antigens are the basis for second generation solid-phase enzyme-linked immunoassays (ELISA; Ortho Laboratories, New Jersey, and Abbott Laboratories, Chicago, USA) for antibodies to HCV, which considerably improve the sensitivity of diagnosis. NS5 epitopes have been incorporated in third generation ELISAS.

 An immunodominant epitope within the capsid antigen has been identified (Nasoff et al 1991) and antibodies to the core antigen, anti-c22, usually appear earlier than those to c100-3 (Fig. 10.2). Anti-c22 has been identified in blood donors who were previously involved in transmitting hepatitis C, but in whose serum anti-c100-3 was not detectable. Antibodies to core epitopes have also been detected in patients with chronic NANB hepatitis who were previously negative for anti-c100-3 (Fig. 10.3) (Brown et al 1992). The antibodies detected are probably not neutralizing as they are found in chronic carriers. In contrast, it is suspected, but unproven, that antibodies to the E (envelope) glycoproteins are neutralizing. Assays based on antibodies to synthetic

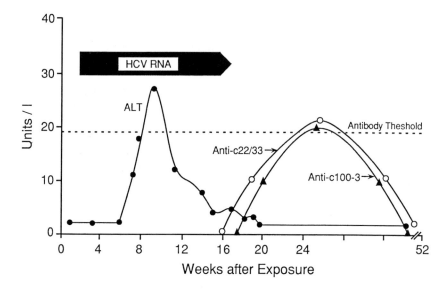

Fig. 10.2   Serological course in acute resolving HCV infection.

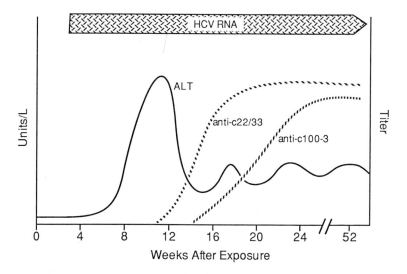

Fig. 10.3   Serological course in chronic hepatitis C infection.

peptides derived from immunodominant regions of both core and non-structural antigens have been developed, which minimize non-specific reactions (Hosein et al 1991). IgM antibody tests have also been developed. The clearance of IgM anti-HCV may distinguish between acute, resolving disease and chronic disease (Quiroga et al 1991).

Supplemental antibody tests

Initial surveys of antibody to hepatitis C in blood donors indicated a high rate of false positive tests. This has necessitated the development of 'supplemental' assays for confirmation of a positive anti-HCV result. The most widely used supplemental test is the recombinant immunoblot assay (RIBA) in which four HCV antigens are fixed to a nitrocellulose filter, along with control proteins. The four antigens comprise one structural (c22) and three non-structural antigens (c33, c100-3, 5-1-1). The strips are incubated with serum specimens; antibodies, if present, bind to the antigens and are detected by a colour reaction. Serum samples are scored as positive if antibodies to two antigens are present.

A close correlation has been found between 4-RIBA positive samples and viraemia, which enables discrimination between infective and non-infective donors (Van der Poel et al 1991). The proportion of RIBA positive donors varies from region to region. In Western Europe 20–40% of ELISA reactive donors are RIBA reactive, and about the same proportion have detectable HCV RNA by polymerase chain reaction (PCR). RIBAs are a valuable adjunct to donor testing. Unfortunately, the tests are ten times more expensive than ELISAs, are relatively insensitive, may give indeterminate results, and are not ideally configured for verification of a positive ELISA. A third generation of RIBA tests will incorporate NS5 epitopes. Several other assays for verification of a positive ELISA are available, including neutralization assays, and automated recombinant immunoblot assays ('matrix' assays).

HCV RNA testing

Since the antigens of HCV are present in very low quantities, direct tests for viraemia in HCV have relied on the detection of HCV RNA in serum. RNA detection necessitates an amplification of the circulating HCV RNA, and thus sensitive assays for HCV RNA have been developed, based on the PCR. In this test, HCV RNA is extracted from virus-infected serum or plasma, reversely transcribed to DNA, and amplified by appropriate primers homologous to HCV RNA by the enzyme TAQ polymerase in a programmable thermal cycler. RNA can then be detected by ethidium bromide staining of a gel, or by autoradiography. RNA is detected in the majority (60–80%) of anti-HCV positive patients, and is also detectable in a percentage of anti-HCV negative patients with chronic NANB hepatitis (Kato et al 1990).

The plasma concentration of virions has been estimated to range from 10^2 to 5×10^7/ml (Ulrich et al 1990). Sensitivity of the test is improved by using an internal (nested) set of primers, and by using primers derived from the 5' untranslated region of the genome, which is highly conserved. There is little standardization of the PCR assay at present (Cristiano et al 1991). Nonetheless, assays for HCV RNA are proving valuable in establishing the presence of HCV RNA in clinical samples, in the diagnosis of HCV in acute and chronic antibody negative patients, and in monitoring antiviral therapy (Farci et al 1991). Three basic temporal patterns of viraemia have been observed: transient viraemia in acute resolving NANB hepatitis; viraemia lasting for several years in chronic NANB hepatitis; and intermittent viraemia in chronic NANB hepatitis, with an initial transient phase followed by recurrence after many months (Garson et al 1990).

HCV RNA can also be detected in formalin-fixed, paraffin-embedded liver biopsies by PCR, and has been detected by insitu hybridization.

Serological diagnosis: acute hepatitis C

Anti-c100-3 appears in the circulation after a mean interval of 15 weeks from the acute illness and first elevations of alanine aminotransferase (ALT) (Lee et al 1991). Although roughly one-third of seroconversions take place early in the acute phase of the disease, sometimes as early as 2 weeks (Lim et al 1991), seroconversion can be delayed for a year or longer. The average time from transfusion to detectable seroconversion is of the order of 11–12 weeks with the first generation tests, and 7–8 weeks with the second generation tests. Anti-c33 or anti-c22 not infrequently appear a week or two earlier than anti-c100-3. Antibodies to HCV are found in a varying proportion of patients with acute sporadic NANB hepatitis depending upon the geographical location, mode of acquisition of hepatitis and severity of the disease. Seroconversion occurs much less frequently, and in lower titre, in acute self-limiting infections compared with those that progress to become chronic (Alter et al 1989, Alter & Sampliner 1989, Nishioka et al 1991). Thus tests for anti-HCV are of limited benefit in diagnosing acute hepatitis C. The presence of anti-HCV antibodies therefore seems to largely reflect active replication of HCV. A proportion of patients with sporadically acquired NANB hepatitis remain anti-HCV seronegative, however, and it will be important to define whether these patients represent HCV infection with poor serological response, or are infected with HCV variants or with other unclassified NANB agents.

During the early phase of primary HCV infection, serum HCV RNA is the only diagnostic marker of infection, and RNA testing therefore remains the only means of diagnosis in seronegative patients. Unfortunately, the test is only available in research laboratories. Serum HCV RNA has been detected within 1–3 weeks of transfusion in patients with hepatitis C, and usually lasts less than 4 months in patients with acute self-limited hepatitis C, but may persist for decades in patients with chronic disease (Farci et al 1991).

A suitable immunodiagnostic test for resolved infection and immunity is not available, but antibodies to the envelope region are being sought.

Serological diagnosis: chronic hepatitis C

Anti-HCV antibodies persist in the majority of patients with chronic post-transfusion NANB hepatitis. In studies in chimpanzees, anti-HCV (i.e.

anti-c100-3) was not neutralizing, because primates with high levels of this antibody were also shown to have high titres of circulating HCV (Bradley et al 1990). The development and maintenance of current diagnostic antibodies to HCV therefore appears to reflect concomitant virus replication, and consequently a high potential for infectivity.

A proportion of patients with chronic hepatitis C may improve spontaneously, but the number of patients who do so is unclear. These patients lose antibody after follow-up of at least 5 years, and usually develop normal serum aminotransferases (Tanaka et al 1991a). Other patients may have a decline in anti-HCV titre with time (Alter et al 1989).

HCV RNA usually persists in patients with abnormal serum aminotransferases and anti-HCV. However, HCV RNA, and hence viraemia, can also be found in patients with normal liver function tests. Isolates of HCV in individual patients may show nucleotide substitutions with time, suggesting that the HCV RNA mutates at a rate similar to those of other RNA viruses (Ogata et al 1991). Preliminary reports have suggested that the HCV antigens can be detected in liver biopsy preparations in chronic carriers (Krawczynski et al 1992).

EPIDEMIOLOGY AND TRANSMISSION OF HEPATITIS C

Transmission

Although the precise mode of acquisition of hepatitis C is often uncertain, hepatitis C is known to be transmitted by parenteral, or inapparent parenteral, contact routes. The virus circulates in relatively low titres in blood, but transmission by blood transfusion, and blood products including factor VII, factor IX, fibrinogen and cryoglobulin has been unequivocally documented. A number of studies in chimpanzees have documented serial passage of NANB hepatitis (now known to be HCV) using sera derived from blood donors implicated in cases of NANB post-transfusion hepatitis (Alter et al 1978). Similarly, transmission among intravenous drug abusers through shared needles accounts for the high prevalence of infection in this group. Transmission after needle-stick injury may also occur.

Community-acquired transmission

Surveillance data had suggested that sporadic NANB hepatitis represents between 20% and 42% of all diagnosed cases of hepatitis. The majority of cases of NANB hepatitis cannot be accounted for by past blood transfusion, or indeed an identifiable source of parenteral exposure to this virus. The disease is prevalent in many parts of the world where the transmission cannot be explained by blood transfusion or intravenous drug abuse. The precise mechanism of most cases of transmission of community-acquired disease is uncertain, but transmission by close person-to-person contact from carriers of

HCV is the most plausible method of explaining transmission in these societies. Transmission by insect vectors remains a speculative possibility.

It can be speculated that the disease may have been spread in the early postwar years in several countries through syringe transmission and intra-muscular injection without adequate sterilization or disposable equipment (Dull 1961). Sexual transmission seems certainly possible, albeit a relatively inefficient and infrequent means. Anti-HCV has been found in 11% of sexual partners of anti-HCV positive intravenous drug abusers, and may correlate with the presence of HIV (Tor et al 1990). The overall HCV infection rate is also higher in sexually promiscuous groups (prostitutes, 8.9%; clients of prostitutes, 16.3%; homosexual men, 5.4%) than in voluntary blood donors (0.4%)in Spain (Sanchez-Quijano et al 1990). Significantly more homosexual than heterosexual subjects attending a sexually transmitted disease clinic were positive for anti-HCV, and the prevalence of anti-HCV correlates with the lifetime number of sexually transmitted diseases (Tedder et al 1991). Other studies, however, have not found a high prevalence of sexual transmission in partners of anti-HCV positive haemophiliacs (Schulman & Grillner 1990).

Transmission by saliva (or saliva containing blood) and by a human bite has been reported (Abe & Inchauspe 1991, Wang et al 1991, Dusheiko et al 1990). Dental surgeons in New York have a higher prevalence of anti-HCV antibody compared to blood donors (Klein et al 1991). In the USA, the proportion of patients with type C hepatitis with a history of blood transfusion has declined in the past 7 years, whereas, in contrast, the proportion with a history of parenteral drug use has increased. By 1987, only 5% of cases of NANB in the USA were transfusion associated, whereas 42% were related to drug abuse. Approximately 40% were of unknown source (Alter 1991a,b). The advent of serological testing has shown that most community-acquired NANB hepatitis is also due to hepatitis C, and anti-HCV is detectable in 28–58% of community-acquired NANB hepatitis. The rate of positivity is higher in patients who progress to chronicity; for example, Bortolotti et al (1991) found a prevalence of 71% in patients who progressed to chronicity compared with 25% of those who recovered. It would appear that patients with no history of transfusion are just as likely to go on to chronic hepatitis. A substantial proportion of acute community-acquired cases remain unclassified, and studies using PCR to detect HCV RNA remain the only diagnostic means to exclude another virus.

Fulminant hepatitis is more common in sporadic compared with transfusion-acquired NANB hepatitis. Hepatitis C is a rare cause of fulminant hepatitis.

Intrafamilial transmission

The role of intrafamilial transmission requires clarification. Although house-hold transmission appears to be relatively infrequent, the true attack rate may be underestimated, since the prevalence of HCV infection in family members is based on the current diagnostic tests which usually reflect chronic infection rather than resolved disease. In Japan, up to 8% of family members of a patient with HCV have been found to be anti-HCV positive, but no specific relative could be linked to HCV positivity, making it difficult to identify the route of infection (Kiyosawa et al 1991).

Maternal–infant transmission

Mother–infant transmission has been observed, but appears to be relatively uncommon. The importance of this route remains controversial. Wejstal et al (1990) showed that children born to anti-HCV positive mothers acquired passively transferred antibodies that were present transiently in serum and disappeared within 7 months. Giovannini et al (1990) studied 49 children born to HIV positive mothers and found 25 mother–children pairs positive for anti-HCV. Although maternal anti-HCV antibodies fell to undetectable levels in all 25 infants by 2–4 months of age, in 11 active production of antibody was observed between 6 and 12 months. Six of these had abnormal serum enzymes (Giovannini et al 1990). A disturbing finding, however, has been the detection of persistent HCV RNA in serum in the absence of anti-HCV in newborn babies delivered by women who were anti-HCV positive, suggesting silent transmission of HCV (Thaler et al 1991). Thus the current evidence seems to suggest that perinatal transmission may occur, particularly in highly viraemic and anti-HIV positive mothers. It is not clear, however, how important this route is in perpetuating the reservoir of human infection, and the natural history of the carrier state in children is unknown.

Population studies

The prevalence of type C hepatitis in blood donors has now been ascertained in many countries. The positive immunoassay rate ranges from 0.18% to 1.4%. In most Western countries, the prevalence ranges from 0.2% to 0.7%; in Japan and Southern Europe, 0.9% to 1.2%. A higher prevalence has been found in Southern Italy and Eastern Europe than in Northern Europe (Rassam & Dusheiko 1991). The prevalence in commercial (paid) donors is higher (10–15%) (Dawson et al 1991). There remains considerable controversy regarding the specificity of the screening ELISA assay (Barbara & Contreras 1991) as the ELISAs are poorly specific in low-risk blood donors, and only 20–60% of donors have a positive supplemental test (RIBA II). Supplemental RIBA testing is highly predictive of infectivity, and correlates with the intensity of the ELISA result.

A higher prevalence has been found in Africans; for example, in South Africa up to 4.2% of Black men are anti-HCV positive (Coursaget et al 1990, Ellis et al 1990). False positive results can occur in stored serum, particularly if it is obtained from tropical areas.

Most anti-HCV positive donors give no history of blood transfusion, but a proportion admit to previous drug use. Clustering of HCV infections has been reported in Japan (Ito et al 1991).

Hepatitis C in recipients of blood or blood products

A high prevalence of anti-HCV is found in many risk groups exposed to blood or blood components, particularly where a single unit containing the virus contaminates the batch.

Post-transfusion hepatitis C

Prior to the introduction of HCV screening, the incidence of post-transfusion NANB hepatitis ranged from 2% to 19% (Dienstag 1983a). The incidence of NANB hepatitis has declined since 1985 to 2–4% due to the interdiction of high-risk blood donors, and, in some countries, screening for serum aminotransferases and antibody to hepatitis B core antigen. The recently introduced second generation tests based on structural (core) ELISAs have been shown to detect positivity in samples unreactive to the earlier 'first generation' tests using the c100 non-structural proteins alone.

Serological testing now indicates that seroconversion to anti-HCV occurs in 85–100% of patients with chronic post-transfusion NANB hepatitis (Esteban et al 1990). In studies of post-transfusion hepatitis (PTH) in Spain, seroconversion to anti-c100-3 occurred 6–8 weeks after transfusion in 38%, between 20 and 26 weeks after transfusion in 56%, and 38–52 weeks after transfusion in 6% (Esteban et al 1989). In some patients a very early appearance of anti-HCV may be due to passively acquired antibody from the donor blood.

Retrospective studies have shown a higher prevalence of anti-HCV at onset in those developing chronic disease (83%) than those who recover from post-transfusion hepatitis. Anti-HCV persists for years and even decades in chronic hepatitis C but may decline in titre or disappear with resolution.

Anti-HCV testing should effect at least a further 50% reduction in the incidence of post-transfusion hepatitis. In Spain, and Japan, the incidence has already been reduced from 9.6% and 4.6% to 1.6% and 1.9% respectively (Esteban et al 1990, Japanese Red Cross 1991).

The incidence of post-transfusion hepatitis C has decreased in the USA since the implementation of donor screening for surrogate markers and antibodies to HCV (Donahue et al 1992). This risk was 3.84% per patient (0.45% per unit transfused) for those transfused before the introduction of surrogate markers. For patients who received transfusions after October 1986 with blood screened for surrogate markers, the risk of seroconversion was 1.54% per patient (0.19% per unit). For patients receiving transfusions since the addition in May 1990 of screening for antibodies to HCV, the risk was 0.57% per patient (0.03% per unit). The current risk of PTH is about 3% per 10 000 units transfused (Widell et al 1991). Although the cost effectiveness of screening is unknown, screening is demanded by countries willing and able to pay for health care. Blood banks in the USA voluntarily began testing donations for anti-HCV in 1990, and there has been a decline in post-transfusion hepatitis C since then (Donahue et al 1992). In the UK, despite the demonstrable imprecision of donor screening, and the relatively low incidence of post-transfusion NANB hepatitis, the number of cases per year necessitates screening (Contreras et al 1991), and this was initiated in September 1991. Since May 1985, all plasma donations have been tested for antibody to HIV-1 by ELISA. In the USA, serum ALT is determined for each donation, which is considered safe if the ALT level is less than two times the established upper limit of normal. Although this test is required by the USA and several Western European countries it is not required in the UK.

Blood derivatives

Safe derivatives are those sterilized by heating (80°C for 10 hours) or other methods, such as by the fractionation method used (cold ethanol, Conn). The products generally considered safe are albumin, thrombin, fibrinolysin, normal immunoglobulin. Human immunoglobulin is generally regarded as a safe product, but there are occasional reports of transmission by inadequately prepared batches of intravenous immunoglobulin (Lever et al 1984). Solvent detergent inactivation and pasteurization have been shown to reduce the risk of transmitting HCV infection (Pistello et al 1991). Dry heating of factor VIII does not reduce the risk of transmission.

Haemophilia

It has been known for some time that many haemophilia patients have biochemical evidence of hepatitis. The advent of hepatitis C testing has shown that the highest prevalences worldwide are found in haemophilia patients, 50–90% of whom are anti-HCV positive, depending upon age, duration of infection, factor VIII requirement, and the source of factor VIII (Schramm et al 1989, Lee & Kernoff 1990, Brettler et al 1990). The high prevalence in haemophilia reflects the frequent use of factor VIII, which is derived from thousands of donors. In the USA, source plasma for these pools is still derived from paid donors.

Haemophilia patients may be HCV RNA positive without detectable anti-HCV, particularly if also infected with HIV (Simmonds et al 1990). These patients may also have evidence of infection with hepatitis B, hepatitis D or HIV which modulates the expression of the disease (Lee & Kernoff 1990). The prognosis may be worse for those haemophilia patients infected with HIV and HCV.

Recent evidence has confirmed that chronic hepatitis is not an insignificant disease in haemophilia patients; for example, a recent survey of the prevalence of HCV in this group suggested a rate of 3.2/100 000, which is ten times the expected prevalence. In this survey, all the notified patients had cirrhosis. Interestingly, coexistent alcoholism and HBV infection were cofactors in some (Colombo et al 1991). A form of NANB hepatitis with a short incubation period (4–19 days) earlier reported in haemophilia patients probably reflects a shortened incubation period due to infusion of a large inoculum of hepatitis C (Hruby & Schauf 1978).

The prevention of transmission of viral hepatitis to haemophilia patients will depend upon donor safety screening and HBsAg (hepatitis B surface antigen) and HCV screening as well as HIV screening. Zero infection is not attainable, but the risk of transmission of NANB virues has been improved by anti-HCV testing. All haemophilia patients should be vaccinated against hepatitis B and anti-HBs levels monitored yearly.

Virus inactivation procedures have also improved the safety of treatment. In particular, pasteurized factor VIII and factor IX concentrates (heated at 80°C for 72 hours) are currently the safest products. Solvent detergent inactivation, in which viral inactivation is achieved by addition of lipid solvents during purification procedures, inactivates lipid-coated viruses. Hot vapour treatment has also reduced the number of reported cases of HCV infection, but is not infallible (Mannucci et al 1990). The recent development of recombinant factor VIII concentrate should eliminate HCV, but the expense of the product is limiting at the present time.

There is a relatively low rate of sexual transmission in female sexual partners of haemophilia patients, of whom 2.7% were anti-HCV positive (Brettler et al 1992).

Thalassaemia major

The prevalence of anti-HCV is high in multiply transfused patients with thalassaemia major, but varies geographically according to the source of the blood administered to patients, and according to geographical region (Wonke et al 1990). The second commonest cause of death in thalassaemia major patients is liver disease due to blood-borne viral hepatitis. These patients are at risk of multiple viral infections, including HBV, cytomegalovirus, and HIV. Repeated transfusion resulting in iron overload may also aggravate the liver disease in these patients, and have immunological effects.

HCV in leukaemia and bone marrow transplantation

It is apparent that HCV infection is a hazard for patients with acute and chronic leukaemia in view of their requirements for blood and blood products during therapy. However, current serological tests may underestimate the prevalence of the disease, as immunosuppressed patients are less likely to have detectable anti-HCV. PCR for HCV RNA will sometimes be required to diagnose infection.

In one study, anti-HCV has been measured in 50 children with leukaemia who had chronic liver disease and were observed for 1–12.6 years after therapy was withdrawn (Locasciulli et al 1991b). Reactive sera were also tested by recombinant immunoblotting assay; 24% of children were persistently anti-HCV positive, 22% were transiently anti-HCV positive and 54% were negative. Mean ALT levels during follow-up were significantly higher in those positive for anti-HCV. Liver histology in 37 patients showed signs of chronic hepatitis in all patients with persistent anti-HCV. These results suggest that HCV plays a significant role in the aetiology of chronic hepatitis in leukaemia patients and that persistent anti-HCV activity correlates with a more severe chronic hepatitis, which could jeopardize the final outcome of children cured of leukaemia.

Antibody to HCV was investigated in sera of 128 Italian patients treated with allogeneic bone marrow transplantation (Locasciulli et al 1991a). The overall prevalence of anti-HCV positivity was 28.6%. The presence of pretransplant anti-HCV positivity did not seem to predict a more severe liver disease. Post-transplant liver disease (due to venocclusive disease or subacute hepatitis) and post-transplant elevations in ALT occurred regardless of anti-HCV serology. In patients tested for anti-HCV after bone marrow transplant, the number of patients in whom liver failure contributed to death was comparable in anti-HCV positive and anti-HCV negative patients. Approximately half of 17 patients with documented post-transplant seroconversion to anti-HCV had an exacerbation of hepatitis concomitant with the appearance of anti-HCV. Histological changes were generally more severe in anti-HCV positive patients: chronic hepatitis was diagnosed in 9/11 anti-HCV positives, compared with 1/7 anti-HCV negative cases. It would appear that hepatitis C may contribute to morbidity in these patients.

Complex hepatitis can be encountered in treated leukaemia patients. Kanamori et al (1992) described two Japanese patients with acute leukaemia who died of fulminant hepatitis caused by HCV after an allogeneic bone marrow transplant. Both had developed post-transfusion hepatitis during chemotherapy to induce remission; 6 months after blood transfusion, both were positive for anti-HCV and HCV RNA. In each case, there was a transient improvement in liver function after the transplant. However, within 5 months of receiving the transplant and coincident with the withdrawal of cyclosporine A, each patient developed an acute exacerbation of hepatitis. The fulminant hepatitis may, therefore, have been caused by the reactivation of HCV induced by the immunosuppressive therapy followed by reconstitution of the immune system (Krawczynski et al 1992).

Prolonged remissions in leukaemia have been reported in patients with acute myeloid or hairy cell leukaemia who developed hepatitis (Barton & Conrad 1979, Brody et al 1981).

Aplastic anaemia

Mild to moderate shortening of red cell survival may occur in viral hepatitis (Cawein et al 1960). In rare cases, agranulocytosis or aplastic anaemia develops during viral hepatitis, and acute NANB hepatitis complicated by fatal aplastic anaemia is a well-described entity (Perrillo et al 1981, Zeldis et al 1983, Tzakis et al 1988). Although hepatitis-associated aplastic anaemia is uncommon in the West, almost one-quarter of cases of aplastic anaemia in children in areas where hepatitis is endemic are attributable to viral hepatitis (Liang et al 1990). Hepatitis C has been sought as the possible aetiological agent inducing bone marrow suppression. However, most reports suggest that hepatitis C does not account for the majority of cases (Pol et al 1990).

In a French bone marrow transplant unit, anti-HCV prevalence among patients with hepatitis-associated aplastic anaemia was 16%, in aplastic anaemia of unknown cause it was 10%, and in aplastic anaemia of known cause it was 8%. It is likely that another NANB agent is responsible for most cases of hepatitis-associated aplastic anaemia (Pol et al 1990). There thus appears to be an interesting association between a non-A, non-B, non-C agent inducing aplastic anaemia and fulminant hepatitic failure (Van Dam et al 1990, Kawahara et al 1991). Hibbs et al (1992a) studied 28 patients with aplastic anaemia within 90 days of the onset of jaundice or hepatitis and three patients who developed aplastic anaemia following liver transplantation for NANB hepatitis. Hepatitis C was measured in serum, bone marrow, and liver samples by PCR and antibody testing; 36% were HCV RNA positive. However, hepatitis C viraemia was associated with transfusions received after the onset of aplasia: 58% of patients with hepatitis-associated aplasia who had received more than 20 units of blood products at the time were positive, compared with 19% who had received 20 units or less. HCV was not found in blood and bone marrow samples. None of three livers from NANB hepatitis patients who developed aplastic anaemia after liver transplantation contained HCV RNA.

To test the hypothesis that HCV viraemia is associated with aplastic anaemia among patients in Thailand, 53 non-transfused hospitalized aplastic anaemia patients and 39 non-transfused controls hospitalized for other conditions were studied (Hibbs et al 1992b). HCV viraemia was found in 5.7% non-transfused patients and 5.1% of non-transfused controls. Thus, although some cases of aplastic anaemia may be related to HCV infection, it appears that HCV does not account for most cases. These results implicate a novel non-A, non-B, non-C agent in both hepatitis-associated aplasia and fulminant hepatitis, rather than hepatitis C.

Radical treatment may be needed for such patients. A 6-year-old boy who received an orthotopic transplant for hepatic failure after NANB hepatitis and subsequently developed severe aplastic anaemia has been reported (Kawahara et al 1991). His aplastic anaemia was treated successfully with a marrow transplant from his sister. The patient remains alive without clinical chronic active hepatitis or need for blood product therapy.

Other groups

The prevalence of viral hepatitis C in intravenous drug users is extremely high (70–92%) because of repeated exposure to carriers of HCV through shared, contaminated needles. Community-based outbreaks of NANB hepatitis due to intravenous drug use have been identified (MMWR 1989). Several other groups have been shown to be at risk. These include haemodialysed patients, particularly in endemic areas such as the Middle East or Japan (Oguchi et al 1990). The disease has been transmitted by coagulum pyelolithotomy, in which the coagulum is prepared from a mixture of cryoprecipitate, thrombin and calcium chloride (McVary & O'Conor 1989). Anti-HCV is apparently also common in other transplant patients requiring frequent blood transfusions, including renal and liver transplant recipients (Baur et al 1991, Poterucha et al 1991, Ponz et al 1991). Liver transplantation is a relatively common therapeutic necessity for patients with cirrhosis due to hepatitis C, and recurrent hepatitis C disease is apparently common in these patients post transplant. In all these groups, previously positive patients may lose antibody after the procedure due to immunosuppression (Read et al 1991a). The role of immunosuppression in the expression of liver disease caused by HCV remains to be determined (Read et al 1991b). Hepatitis C has also been transmitted by organ transplantation, and may cause severe postorgan transplantation liver disease (Pereira et al 1991).

Nosocomial or occupational exposure is being evaluated. Health care workers appear to be at comparatively low risk (Polywka & Laufs 1991, Hofmann & Kunz 1990). However, there are well-documented instances of needlestick transmission of HCV, and of NANB hepatitis after surgery, or even hospitalization, without transfusion (Giusti et al 1987).

PREVALENCE OF ANTI-HCV IN CHRONIC LIVER DISEASE

Serological testing has shown a high prevalence of anti-HCV in patients with chronic active hepatitis and/or cirrhosis considered to be due to NANB hepatitis (Alter et al 1989). The majority (75–95%) of patients with post-transfusion chronic NANB hepatitis in the USA and Europe are positive for anti-HCV. The disease in many persons with chronic NANB hepatitis may or may not be associated with a history of blood transfusion. The prevalence varies according to the background endemicity of hepatitis C in the population (Pohjanpelto et al 1991). Tests for anti-HCV are now important in establishing a diagnosis of what was formerly considered cryptogenic cirrhosis.

Immunological disease

Autoimmune hepatitis

There are conflicting reports regarding the occurrence of hepatitis C antibodies in patients with autoimmune liver disease. Clearly the ELISA for anti-HCV is prone to false positive results in patients with high concentrations of immunoglobulins in serum (McFarlane et al 1990). These false reactive anti-HCV antibodies in patients with anti-smooth muscle antibody may actually disappear with immunosuppressive treatment, as globulin levels decrease (Schvarcz et al 1990). However, Italian patients with autoimmune chronic active hepatitis appear to have a high frequency of genuine exposure to HCV, whereas seropositivity in English patients usually represents a false positive result. It is therefore not certain whether anti-HCV in patients with chronic active hepatitis represents persistent anti-HCV from earlier disease, whether the autoimmune disease is induced by HCV (Lenzi et al 1991), or whether autoantibodies in autoimmune hepatitis patients cross-react with HCV-related antigens (Onji et al 1991). In Japan, 80% of patients with chronic NANB hepatitis have circulating antibodies to a pentadecapeptide (Gor), an epitope of normal hepatocytes; this phenomenon may represent an autoimmune response peculiar to type C hepatitis (Mishiro et al 1990).

Up to 50% of patients with type II autoimmune hepatitis (anti-liver kidney microsomal (LKM) antibody positive) are anti-HCV positive; and anti-HCV and anti-LKM in association may also represent another example of molecular mimicry. Anti-HCV positive patients with anti-LKM autoimmune chronic active hepatitis are usually male, older, and have lower titres of anti-LKM than patients without anti-HCV. The target antigen of antibodies to LKM is a portion of the cytochrome P450IID6 molecule; anti-LKM is not directed to a c100-3 epitope, but some sequence homology between HCV and cytochrome P450 may exist (Manns et al 1991). This association has some therapeutic implications, as the autoimmune disease is responsive to corticosteroids, and may be aggravated by α-interferon.

Cryoglobulinaemia

Cryoglobulinaemia has been associated with hepatitis C. The prevalence of antibodies to HCV was investigated in 52 unselected patients with mixed cryoglobulinaemia and in 84 patients with other systemic immunological diseases. Anti-HCV was detected by ELISA and the specificity was evaluated by a recombinant-based immunoblot assay.

Evidence of hepatitis C was found in 54% of mixed cryoglobulinaemia patients, and the finding was confirmed by recombinant-based immunoblot assay in all cases. Anti-HCV was more common in those with liver biopsy abnormalities and raised serum ALT. It would appear that HCV plays a role in the pathogenesis of this immunological disease (Ferri et al 1991), and indeed the disease improves with therapy of hepatitis C. Interferon treatment may alleviate the clinical manifestations of the disease (Waters & Cook 1992, Ferri et al 1991, Durand et al 1991).

Alcoholic liver disease

In several countries, a higher prevalence of anti-HCV has been found in patients with alcoholic liver disease. The prevalence of hepatitis C antibodies correlates with the severity of liver injury, and is higher in patients with cirrhosis than in those with only fatty change (Pares et al 1990). The relationship is a complex one (Mendenhall et al 1991), which apparently reflects in part the higher rate of transfusions in alcoholics with decompensated liver disease and a common environmental risk.

Hepatocellular carcinoma

Serological analysis of patients with hepatocellular carcinoma (HCC) has shown a high prevalence of anti-HCV in patients with HCC. Several case-control studies in Europe have suggested that up to 70% of male patients with HCC are anti-HCV positive (Tanaka et al 1991b, Bruix et al 1989). The highest prevalence of HCV in HCC is found in Italian, Japanese and Spanish patients; the prevalence is lower in Chinese and African patients, in whom the disease is more commonly associated with chronic hepatitis B. Since HCV is an RNA virus, it is believed that chronic HCV infection induces necroinflammatory change which progresses to cirrhosis and eventual malignant transformation (Levrero et al 1991). In Japan, at least, a history of transfusion has been documented in 42% of anti-HCV positive patients with HCC. The mean interval between the date of transfusion and the diagnosis of cirrhosis and HCC is usually long: 21 and 29 years, respectively (Kiyosawa et al 1990).

CLINICAL FEATURES

Acute hepatitis C

The mean incubation period of hepatitis C is 6–12 weeks. However, with a large inoculum, such as in cases following administration of factor VIII, the incubation period is reduced to 4 weeks or less (Bamber et al 1981, Lim et al 1991). The acute course of HCV infection is clinically mild, and the peak serum ALT elevations are less than those encountered in acute hepatitis A or B. Only 25% of cases are icteric. Subclinical disease is common; such patients may first present decades later with sequelae such as cirrhosis or HCC. During the early clinical phase the serum ALT levels may fluctuate, and may become normal or near normal, making the determination of true convalescence difficult. Severe or fulminant hepatitis C is rare, but may occur. The diagnosis of such cases requires confirmation by HCV RNA testing. Arthritis, rashes, glomerulonephritis, vasculitis, neurological syndromes have been reported. The histological features of acute hepatitis C are similar to those seen in hepatitis A or B, except sinusoidal cell activation is marked. The distinction from evolving chronic hepatitis C can be difficult.

Chronic hepatitis C

The clinical and epidemiological features of transfusion-associated and sporadic NANB hepatitis have been well documented, albeit that the disease previously required identification by prospective biochemical monitoring. The disease has a disturbing propensity to progress to chronic hepatitis; 50–75% of patients with type C post-transfusion hepatitis continue to have abnormal serum aminotransferase levels after 12 months, and chronic hepatitis histologically (Lee et al 1991). The risk of chronic infection after sporadic hepatitis C is probably similar.

Most patients with chronic hepatitis C are asymptomatic, or only mildly symptomatic. In symptomatic patients, fatigue is the most common complaint, and is variously described as lack of energy, increased need for sleep or fatiguability. Many patients do not give a history of acute hepatitis or jaundice. Physical findings are generally mild and variable, and there may be no abnormalities. With more severe disease, spider angiomata and hepatosplenomegaly may be found. Serum aminotransferases decline from the peak values encountered in the acute phase of the disease, but remain 2–8 times normal.

The serum ALT concentrations may fluctuate over time, and may even intermittently be normal. Many patients have a sustained elevation of the serum aminotransferases. The relationship between HCV RNA in serum and serum aminotransferases is complex, and although most patients with raised serum ALT are HCV RNA positive, the converse is not always true.

The spectrum of chronic disease varies. Most patients appear to have an indolent, only slowly progressive course with little increase in mortality after 20 years. However, cirrhosis develops in approximately 20% of patients with chronic disease within 10 years, albeit that the cirrhosis remains indolent and only slowly progressive for a prolonged period (Patel et al 1991, Berman et al 1979, Koretz et al 1980, Mattsson 1989). The disease is not necessarily benign, however, and rapidly progressive cirrhosis can occur. Older age of infection, concomitant alcohol abuse, concurrent HBV or HIV infection or other illness may be important aggravating co-factors. With the development of cirrhosis, weakness, wasting, oedema, and ascites become progressive problems. Older patients may present with complications of cirrhosis, or even HCC. With progressive disease, the laboratory values become progressively more abnormal. The finding of AST (aspartate aminotransferase) greater than ALT, low albumin and prolonged prothrombin time suggest cirrhosis. Low levels of autoantibodies may also become detectable.

Two main pathological forms of chronic hepatitis – chronic active hepatitis and chronic persistent hepatitis – occur in hepatitis C; these terms require reassessment in the light of new information on the evolution of the hepatitis. Chronic persistent hepatitis is generally referred to as chronic viral hepatitis with minor histological changes, a benign course and a good prognosis. The disease may persist for many years without evidence of progression to chronic active hepatitis. The patient's health remains good (Wejstal et al 1987, Vucelic et al 1988).

However, in some patients the lesion can be progressive, and it is not easy to project the prognosis for patients seen at one point in time (Lai et al 1991). A characteristic histological pattern of mild chronic hepatitis with portal lymphoid follicles and varying degrees of lobular activity is found in many patients (Scheuer et al 1992). Chronic active hepatitis refers to chronic inflammatory and sometimes fibrotic liver lesion with varied histological features. Episodes of hepatic necrosis may progress at variable rates to cirrhosis; the lesion may revert in some patients to inactive hepatitis.

Interestingly, routine screening of blood donors for anti-HCV indicates that a significant proportion of asymptomatic anti-HCV positive blood donors indeed have progressive liver disease. Several histological studies in asymptomatic anti-HCV positive donors have shown that 45–62% had chronic active hepatitis, and 7–15% had active cirrhosis (Alberti et al 1991). Progression to hepatocellular carcinoma is also well documented, and, despite the indolent and slowly progressive nature of the disease in many, it is apparent from serological testing for anti-HCV that HCV is a leading cause of morbidity from liver disease in the Western world.

MANAGEMENT

Acute hepatitis C

The management of acute sporadic or transfusion-related hepatitis C is along conventional lines, and is largely non-specific and supportive. The diagnosis remains one of exclusion in most, although, if the patient is seen early enough, HCV RNA in serum may be detectable at the time that the serum aminotransferases are elevated. Anti-HCV may be detectable particularly in severe, icteric cases, and in most of those patients destined to go on to chronic disease. Many patients will not be jaundiced. The serum aminotransferases should be measured at weekly intervals; during the recovery phase, these levels should be measured periodically (monthly to three monthly), as the determination of true convalescence in this illness can be difficult.

Approximately 50% of patients will still have elevated serum aminotransferases 6 months after diagnosis. Patients should be encouraged to rest during the acute, severe phase of the illness. Most patients can be effectively cared for at home. A gradual return to normal activity is encouraged. The diet should be as palatable as possible. Potentially hepatotoxic medications may aggravate the hepatic injury. Oral contraceptives can probably be continued. Exhausting exercise should be discouraged until the serum aminotransferases are normal. Hospitalization is indicated for patients with more severe symptoms, a serum bilirubin level greater than 200 mEq/l, or a prothrombin time that is prolonged for more than 3 seconds, neuropsychiatric symptoms, spontaneous bleeding or persistent vomiting.

Therapeutic trials of α-interferon have been undertaken. Most have not reduced the rate of chronic disease, but might indicate an amelioration of the severity of the chronic hepatitis lesion. A trial of β-interferon in Japan, given intravenously for 1–3 months, did significantly reduce the risk of chronic hepatitis (Omata et al 1991). Until these findings can be reproduced, however, the advisability of routine administration of interferon for acute hepatitis C is uncertain. Liver transplantation is necessary for the treatment of fulminant hepatitis C in cases where indices indicate a high probability of a fatal outcome.

Chronic hepatitis C

Asymptomatic patients detected through blood screening will require a supplemental test to verify their HCV status, as the rate of false positive anti-HCV tests in low-risk donors is high. Ideally HCV RNA should be measured in all patients to confirm viraemia, but the test is not generally available for routine diagnosis. If the test is reproducibly positive, then serum aminotransferases, bilirubin, alkaline phosphatase, and prothrombin time should be measured. In patients whose lifestyle or geographical origin suggest that they are at risk of other forms of viral hepatitis, HBsAg and HIV infection need also to be considered. In equivocal cases, the diagnosis of chronic hepatitis C may still require confirmation, and careful exclusion of all other forms of chronic hepatitis, including alcoholism, inborn errors of metabolism, hepatoxicity, and disease of the biliary tract. Because autoimmune hepatitis is treated differently, it is particularly advisable to exclude this diagnosis by measuring the titres of anti-smooth muscle and anti-LKM antibodies even in those with a positive anti-HCV test, and to measure HCV RNA in anti-HCV positive patients in whom interferon is contemplated.

In patients with more than two-fold elevations in serum aminotransferases, a liver biopsy to ascertain the degree of inflammatory activity and fibrosis in the liver should be considered. The patient should be monitored for 1–3 months to assess the trend in serum aminotransferases.

Relapses and remissions can occur. Prospective studies have suggested that 10–20% of patients with chronic NANB hepatitis develop cirrhosis within a 10-year period. However, in many patients the disease is silently and insidiously progressive, even after cirrhosis is present. Nonetheless, morbidity from cirrhosis and hepatocellular carcinoma is well established, and individuals with chronic hepatitis C with elevated ALT and chronic hepatitis histologically should be considered for antiviral therapy.

Major restrictions need not be placed on the lifestyle of the patient with compensated hepatitis C. The drinking of excess spirituous liquor is discouraged, as there is evidence that the combination of type C hepatitis and alcohol abuse may be detrimental. Small quantities of beer and wine are permissable. The patient should be counselled and advised not to donate blood. It is not yet clear how efficiently hepatitis C may be transmitted by sexual contact. This can apparently occur, however, in highly viraemic individuals after prolonged contact. It is prudent, therefore, to test regular sexual partners for anti-HCV.

α-Interferon

Preliminary therapeutic trials of α-interferon indicated that a proportion of patients may respond to treatment with this agent. Larger, placebo-controlled studies have indicated that approximately 50% of patients will have normal serum aminotransferases after treatment courses of α-interferon of approximately 3 million units three times a week for 6 months compared with 5–10% of untreated controls (Davis et al 1989, Di Bisceglie et al 1989).

Both anti-c100-3 positive and negative patients respond, presumably reflecting the insensitivity of the anti-c100-3 test (Ohnishi et al 1991, Marcellin et al 1990). Serum HCV RNA may become undetectable in patients after 4–8 weeks of α-interferon treatment in patients who respond, but an undetectable HCV RNA at the end of treatment does not preclude relapse in patients.

However, after stopping treatment for 6 months, one-half of the responsive patients will promptly relapse. Serum aminotransferases usually increase in patients who are HCV RNA positive at the end of therapy (Chayama et al 1991). Our studies at the Royal Free Hospital indicate that 20% of patients have a prolonged response to therapy and do not develop elevated serum aminotransferases (Varagona et al 1992). These patients also become negative for HCV RNA. Other regimens are being evaluated (Kakumu et al 1990). Initiating therapy with a somewhat higher dose of 15–20 million units per week and prolonging therapy for a year may result in lower relapse rates. However, relapses still occur after higher doses, and patients have more side-effects at higher doses.

Interferon is of benefit in haemophiliacs. In a UK study 18 patients were randomized to treatment with α2b-interferon, or no treatment for 12 months; four of the 10 treated patients had normal serum ALT, compared to none of the eight controls. After all had been treated, 9/16 had responded. When first and second biopsies (performed under factor VIII control) were compared, the treated group showed improvement (Makris et al 1991). Interferon is generally well tolerated in this group and bleeding does not occur at injection sites. Alternatively, interferon can be given intravenously thrice weekly in this group.

Similarly, the response of thalassaemia patients is not different to those of other groups. We have determined the response to therapy in 12 patients with thalassaemia and chronic hepatitis C. Recombinant α2b (3–6 mu thrice weekly) was given for 6 months (Fig. 10.4). Seven (58%) patients had normal ALT during treatment; 57% of these relapsed when treatment was stopped, however. Responders had high NK (natural killer) cell activity measured within 16–24 hours of commencing treatment. HCV RNA was negative in serum in five of seven responders at the end of treatment (Donohue et al 1993). Response (and relapse) rates are therefore similar in this group. The cost of 6 months of treatment is at least $3000.00. Treatment should not be continued beyond 3 months in patients who do not have reduced levels of serum ALT. Responsive patients usually exhibit histological improvement, and may have a decrease in collagen III propeptide concentrations (Schvarcz et al 1991).

Unfortunately responsiveness to α-interferon remains somewhat unpredictable; patients with cirrhosis respond less well, however. Most patients will tolerate the treatment quite well; many develop flu-like symptoms, some develop severe psychological side-effects, and patients with cirrhosis are at risk of developing significant thrombocytopenia and leukopenia, and therefore infections (Renault & Hoofnagle 1989). Response rates are lower in patients with cirrhosis. Responders seem to show less diversity in the hypervariable region (E2/NS1), perhaps because they are infected with a uniform population of virus, or because of a differential sensitivity of particular genotypes (Okada et al 1992). Thyroid abnormalities occur in

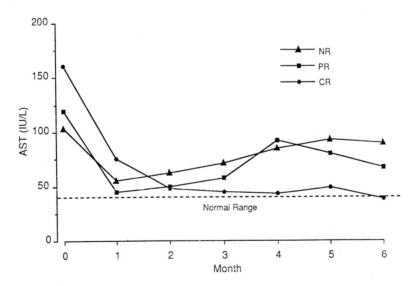

Fig. 10.4 Mean serum AST levels of interferon in a group of 12 thalassaemia patients treated with α2b-interferon for 6 months. NR, non-responders; PR, partial responders; CR, complete responder.

approximately 3% of treated patients. When can treatment be considered successful? It is reasonable to infer that patients with normal serum ALT for more than a year after stopping interferon treatment, negative HCV RNA for more than a year, with histologically improved disease activity, and a normal serum procollagen III peptide have had a good response.

Some patients may actually worsen on treatment with interferon, and develop increased serum aminotransferases. A positive anti-HCV antibody in patients with autoimmune disease remains a pitfall in diagnosis, which has implications for treatment (Davis 1991). Such patients require confirmation by immunoblot assay, or HCV RNA, as they may require corticosteroid therapy rather than α-interferon (Czaja et al 1991).

It is possible that such patients have an underlying autoimmune abnormality associated with hepatitis C and exacerbated by interferon treatment. For such patients, and for patients who do not respond to treatment, ribavirin may be an alternative (Reichard et al 1991, Di Bisceglie et al 1992). This nucleoside analogue has been shown to suppress HCV replication, but is weakly efficacious, and doses above 1.2 g per day are associated with mild haemolytic anaemia. Several trials of ribavirin for hepatitis C are now in progress.

SUMMARY

In 1989, taking advantage of new recombinant DNA technology, the major agent of NANB hepatitis was isolated, and serological tests were developed. Preliminary epidemiological assessment indicates that hepatitis C is an important cause of chronic liver disease, cirrhosis and hepatocellular carcinoma worldwide. Molecular virology of HCV has identified differences between the prototype strain and other isolates. Serological assays have been developed which enable the diagnosis of chronic hepatitis C. Assays for HCV RNA are being used to study viraemia. The availability of markers of hepatitis C has facilitated the study of the epidemiology and natural history of the disease, and has improved its treatment.

KEY POINTS FOR CLINICAL PRACTICE

- The prevalence of anti-HCV in several haematological diseases is high, due to blood and blood product administration.
- At least 50% of patients with hepatitis C virus infection develop chronic hepatitis.
- Approximately 20% of persons with chronic hepatitis C may develop cirrhosis within 10 years.
- α-Interferon treatment should be considered in patients with two-fold elevated aminotransferases, HCV RNA in serum and a liver biopsy showing chronic hepatitis.

- Response rates on treatment are 50%; 20–30% may have a prolonged response to treatment.
- Severe thrombocytopenia, leucopenia, decompensated cirrhosis or thyroid disease are contraindications to interferon treatment. Patients with cirrhosis respond poorly.

REFERENCES

Abe K, Inchauspe G 1991 Transmission of hepatitis C by saliva. Lancet 337: 248
Abe K, Kurata T, Shikata T 1989 Non-A, non-B hepatitis: visualization of virus-like particles from chimpanzee and human sera. Arch Virol 104: 351–355
Alberti A, Chemello L, Cavalletto D et al 1991 Antibody to hepatitis C virus and liver disease in volunteer blood donors. Ann Intern Med 114: 1010–1012
Alter M J 1991a Inapparent transmission of hepatitis C: footprints in the sand. Hepatology 14: 389–391
Alter M J 1991b Hepatitis C: a sleeping giant. Am J Med 91 (Suppl 3B): 112S–115S
Alter M J, Sampliner R E 1989 Hepatitis C: and miles to go before we sleep. N Engl J Med 321: 1538–1540 (Editorial)
Alter H J, Purcell R H, Holland P V et al 1978 Transmissible agent in non-A, non-B hepatitis. Lancet 1: 459–463
Alter H J, Purcell R H, Shih J W et al 1989 Detection of antibody to hepatitis C virus in prospectively followed transfusion recipients with acute and chronic non-A, non-B hepatitis. N Engl J Med 321: 1494–1500
Bamber M, Murray A, Arborgh B A M et al 1981 Short incubation non-A, non-B hepatitis transmitted by factor VIII concentrates in patients with congenital coagulation disorders. Gut 22: 854–859
Barbara J A, Contreras M 1991 Non-A, non-B hepatitis and the anti-HCV assay. Vox Sang 60: 1–7
Barton J C, Conrad M E 1979 Beneficial effects of hepatitis in patients with acute myelogenous leukaemia. Ann Intern Med 90: 188–190
Baur P, Daniel V, Pomer S et al 1991 Hepatitis C-virus (HCV) antibodies in patients after kidney transplantation. Ann Hematol 62: 68–73
Berman M, Alter H J, Ishak K G et al 1979 The chronic sequelae of non-A, non-B hepatitis. Ann Intern Med 91: 1–6
Bortolotti F, Tagger A, Cadrobbi P et al 1991 Antibodies to hepatitis C virus in community-acquired acute non-A, non-B hepatitis. J Hepatol 12: 176–180
Bradley D W, Krawczynski K, Ebert J W et al 1990 Parenterally transmitted non-A, non-B hepatitis: virus-specific antibody response patterns in hepatitis C virus-infected chimpanzees. Gastroenterology 99: 1054–1060
Brettler D B, Alter H J, Dienstag J L et al 1990 Prevalence of hepatitis C virus antibody in a cohort of hemophilia patients. Blood 76: 254–256
Brettler D B, Mannucci P M, Gringeri A et al 1992 The low risk of hepatitis C virus transmission among sexual partners of hepatitis C-infected hemophilic males: an international, multicenter study. Blood 80: 540–543
Brody S A, Russel W G, Krantz S B et al 1981 Beneficial effect of hepatitis in leukemic reticuloendotheliosis. Arch Intern Med 141: 1080–1081
Brown D, Powell L, Morris A et al 1992 Improved diagnosis of chronic hepatitis C infection by detection of antibody to multiple epitopes: confirmation by antibody to synthetic oligopeptides. J Med Virol 38: 167–171
Bruix J, Barrera J M, Calvet X et al 1989 Prevalence of antibodies to hepatitis C virus in Spanish patients with hepatocellular carcinoma and hepatic cirrhosis. Lancet 2: 1004–1006
Cawein M J, Hagedorn A B, Owen C A 1960 Anemia of hepatic disease studied with radiochromium. Gastroenterology 38: 324–331
Chayama K, Saitoh S, Arase Y et al 1991 Effect of interferon administration on serum hepatitis C virus RNA in patients with chronic hepatitis C. Hepatology 13: 1040–1043
Chen P-J, Lin M-H, Tu S-J et al 1991 Isolation of a complementary DNA fragment of hepatitis C virus in Taiwan revealed significant sequence variations compared with other

isolates. Hepatology 14: 73–78

Choo Q L, Kuo G, Weiner A J et al 1989 Isolation of a cDNA clone derived from a blood-borne non-A, non-B viral hepatitis genome. Science 244: 359–362

Choo Q L, Weiner A J, Overby L R et al 1990 Hepatitis C virus: the major causative agent of viral non-A, non-B hepatitis. Br Med Bull 46: 423–441

Choo Q L, Richman K H, Han J H et al 1991 Genetic organization and diversity of the hepatitis C virus. Proc Natl Acad Sci USA 88: 2451–2455

Colombo M, Mannucci P M, Brettler D B et al 1991 Hepatocellular carcinoma in hemophilia. Am J Hematol 37: 243–246

Contreras M, Barbara J A, Anderson C C et al 1991 Low incidence of non-A, non-B post-transfusion hepatitis in London confirmed by hepatitis C virus serology. Lancet 337: 753–757

Coursaget P, Bourdil C, Kastally R et al 1990 Prevalence of hepatitis C virus infection in Africa: anti-HCV antibodies in the general population and in patients suffering from cirrhosis or primary liver cancer. Res Virol 141: 449–454

Cristiano K, Di Bisceglie A M, Hoofnagle J H et al 1991 Hepatitis C viral RNA in serum of patients with chronic non-A, non-B hepatitis: detection by the polymerase chain reaction using multiple primer sets. Hepatology 14: 51–55

Czaja A J, Taswell H F, Rakela J et al 1991 Frequency and significance of antibody to hepatitis C virus in severe corticosteroid-treated autoimmune chronic active hepatitis. Mayo Clin Proc 66: 572–582 (see Comments)

Davis G L 1991 Hepatitis C virus antibody in patients with chronic autoimmune hepatitis: pitfalls in diagnosis and implications for treatment. Mayo Clin Proc 66: 647–650 (Editorial; Comment)

Davis G L, Balart L A, Schiff E R et al 1989 Treatment of chronic hepatitis C with recombinant interferon alfa. A multicenter randomized, controlled trial. Hepatitis Interventional Therapy Group. N Engl J Med 321: 1501–1506

Dawson G J, Lesniewski R R, Stewart J L et al 1991 Detection of antibodies to hepatitis C virus in US blood donors. J Clin Microbiol 29: 551–556

Di Bisceglie A M, Martin P, Kassianides C et al 1989 Recombinant inteferon alfa therapy for chronic hepatitis C. A randomized, double-blind, placebo-controlled trial. N Engl J Med 321: 1506–1510

Di Bisceglie A M, Shindo M, Fong T-L et al 1992 A pilot study of ribavirin therapy for chronic hepatitis C. Hepatology 16: 649–654

Dienstag J L 1983a Non-A, non-B hepatitis. I. Recognition, epidemiology, and clinical features. Gastroenterology 85: 439–462

Dienstag J L 1983b Non-A, non-B hepatitis. II. Experimental transmission, putative virus agents and markers, and prevention. Gastroenterology 85: 743–768

Donahue J G, Muñoz A, Ness P M et al 1993 The declining risk of post-transfusion hepatitis C virus infection. N Engl J Med 327: 369–373

Donohue S M, Wonke B, Hoffbrand A V et al 1993 Alpha interferon in the treatment of chronic hepatitis C infection in thalassaemia major. Br J Haematol 83: 491–497

Dull H B 1961 Syringe transmitted hepatitis: a recent epidemic in historic perspective. JAMA 176: 413–418

Durand J M, Lefevre P, Harle J R et al 1991 Cutaneous vasculitis and cryoglobulinaemia type II associated with hepatitis C virus infection. Lancet 337: 499–500

Dusheiko G M, Smith M, Scheuer P J 1990 Hepatitis C transmitted by a human bite. Lancet 336: 503–504

Ellis L A, Brown D, Conradie J D et al 1990 Prevalence of hepatitis C in South Africa: detection of anti-HCV in recent and stored serum. J Med Virol 32: 249–251

Esteban J I, Esteban R, Viladomiu L et al 1989 Hepatitis C virus antibodies among risk groups in Spain. Lancet 2: 294–297

Esteban J I, Gonzalez A, Hernandez J M et al 1990 Evaluation of antibodies to hepatitis C virus in a study of transfusion-associated hepatitis. N Engl J Med 323: 1107–1112

Farci P, Alter H J, Wong D et al 1991 A long-term study of hepatitis C virus replication in non-A, non-B hepatitis. N Engl J Med 325: 98–104

Feinstone S M, Kapikian A Z, Purcell R H et al 1975 Transfusion associated hepatitis not due to viral hepatitis type A or B. N Engl J Med 292: 767–770

Ferri C, Greco F, Longombardo G et al 1991 Antibodies to hepatitis C virus in patients with mixed cryoglobulinemia. Arthritis Rheum 34: 1606–1610

Garson J A, Ring C, Tuke P et al 1990 Enhanced detection by PCR of hepatitis C virus RNA. Lancet 336: 878–879

Giovannini M, Tagger A, Ribero M L et al 1990 Maternal-infant transmission of hepatitis C virus and HIV infections: a possible interaction. Lancet 335: 1166 (Letter)

Giusti G, Galanti B, Gaeta G B et al 1987 Etiological, clinical and laboratory data of post-transfusion hepatitis: a retrospective study of 379 cases from 53 Italian hospitals. Infection 15: 111–114

Han J H, Shyamala V, Richman K H et al 1991 Characterization of the terminal regions of hepatitis C viral RNA: identification of conserved sequences in the 5' untranslated region and poly(A) tails at the 3' end. Proc Natl Acad Sci USA 88: 1711–1715

Harada S, Watanabe Y, Takeuchi K et al 1991 Expression of processed core protein of hepatitis C virus in mammalian cells. J Virol 65: 3015–3021

Hibbs J R, Frickhofen N, Rosenfeld S J et al 1992a Aplastic anemia and viral hepatitis: non-A, non-B, non-C. JAMA 267: 2051–2054

Hibbs J R, Issaragrisil S, Young N S 1992b High prevalence of hepatitis C viremia among aplastic anemia patients and controls from Thailand. Am J Trop Med Hyg 46: 564–570

Hijikata M, Kato N, Ootsuyama Y et al 1991a Hypervariable regions in the putative glycoprotein of hepatitis C virus. Biochem Biophys Res Commun 175: 220–228

Hijikata M, Kato N, Ootsuyama Y et al 1991b Gene mapping of the putative structural region of the hepatitis C virus genome by in vitro processing analysis. Proc Natl Acad Sci USA 88: 5547–5551

Hofmann H, Kunz C 1990 Low risk of health care workers for infection with hepatitis C virus. Infection 18: 286–288

Hosein B, Fang C T, Popovsky M A et al 1991 Improved serodiagnosis of hepatitis C virus infection with synthetic peptide antigen from capsid protein. Proc Natl Acad Sci USA 88: 3647–3651

Hruby M A, Schauf V 1978 Transfusion related short incubation hepatitis in hemophiliac patients. JAMA 240: 1355–1357

Ito S, Ito M, Cho M J et al 1991 Massive sero-epidemiological survey of hepatitis C virus: clustering of carriers on the southwest coast of Tsushima, Japan. Jpn J Cancer Res 82: 1–3

Japanese Red Cross Non-A Non-B Hepatitis Research Group 1991 Effect of screening for hepatitis C virus antibody and hepatitis B virus core antibody on incidence of post-transfusion hepatitis. Lancet 338: 1040–1041

Kakumu S, Arao M, Yoshioka K et al 1990 Recombinant human alpha-interferon therapy for chronic non-A, non-B hepatitis: second report. Am J Gastroenterol 85: 655–659

Kanamori H, Fukawa H, Maruta A et al 1992 Case report: fulminant hepatitis C viral infection after allogeneic bone marrow transplantation. Am J Med Sci 303: 109–111

Kato N, Yokosuka O, Omata M et al 1990 Detection of hepatitis C virus ribonucleic acid in the serum by amplification with polymerase chain reaction. J Clin Invest 86: 1764–1767

Kawahara K, Storb R, Sanders J et al 1991 Successful allogeneic bone marrow transplantation in a 6.5-year-old male for severe aplastic anemia complicating orthotopic liver transplantation for fulminant non-A-non-B hepatitis. Blood 78: 1140–1143

Kiyosawa K, Sodeyama T, Tanaka E et al 1990 Interrelationship of blood transfusion, non-A, non-B hepatitis and hepatocellular carcinoma: analysis by detection of antibody to hepatitis C virus. Hepatology 12: 671–675

Kiyosawa K, Sodeyama T, Tanaka E et al 1991 Intrafamilial transmission of hepatitis C virus in Japan. J Med Virol 33: 114–116

Klein R S, Freeman K, Taylor P E et al 1991 Occupational risk for hepatitis C virus infection among New York City dentists. Lancet 338: 1539–1542

Koretz R L, Stone O, Gitnick G L 1980 The long term course of non-A, non-B post-transfusion hepatitis. Gastroenterology 79: 893–898

Krawczynski K, Beach M J, Bradley D W et al 1992 Hepatitis C virus antigen in hepatocytes: immunomorphologic detection and identification. Gastroenterology 103: 622–629

Kuo G, Choo Q L, Alter H J et al 1989 An assay for circulating antibodies to a major etiologic virus of human non-A, non-B hepatitis. Science 244: 362–364

Lai E C S, Ng I O L, You K T et al 1991 Hepatic resection for small hepatocellular carcinoma: the Queen Mary Hospital experience. World J Surg 15: 654–659

Lee C A, Kernoff P B 1990 Viral hepatitis and haemophilia. Br Med Bull 46: 408–422

Lee S-D, Hwang S-J, Lu R-H et al 1991 Antibodies to hepatitis C virus in prospectively followed patients with posttransfusion hepatitis. J Infect Dis 163: 1354–1357

Lenzi M, Johnson P J, McFarlane I G et al 1991 Antibodies to hepatitis C virus in autoimmune liver disease: evidence for geographical heterogeneity. Lancet 338: 277–280

Lever A M L, Webster A D B, Brown D et al 1984 Non-A, non-B hepatitis occurring in agammaglobulinaemic patients after intravenous immunoglobulin. Lancet 2: 1062–1064

Levrero M, Tagger A, Balsano C et al 1991 Antibodies to hepatitis C virus in patients with hepatocellular carcinoma. J Hepatol 12: 60–63

Liang D C, Lin K H, Lin D T et al 1990 Post hepatitic aplastic anaemia in children in Taiwan, a hepatitis prevalent area. Br J Haematol 74: 487–491

Lim S G, Lee C A, Charman H et al 1991 Hepatitis C antibody assay in a longitudinal study of haemophiliacs. Br J Haematol 78: 398–402

Locasciulli A, Bacigalupo A, Vanlint M T et al 1991a Hepatitis C virus infection in patients undergoing allogeneic bone marrow transplantation. Transplantation 52: 315–318

Locasciulli A, Gornati G, Tagger A et al 1991b Hepatitis C virus infection and chronic liver disease in children with leukemia in long-term remission. Blood 78: 1619–1622

McFarlane I G, Smith H M, Johnson P J et al 1990 Hepatitis C virus antibodies in chronic active hepatitis: pathogenetic factor or false-positive result? Lancet 335: 754–757

McVary K T, O'Conor V J 1989 Transmission of nonA/nonB hepatitis during coagulation pyelolithotomy. J Urol 141: 923–925

Makris M, Preston F E, Triger D R et al 1991 A randomized controlled trial of recombinant interferon-α in chronic hepatitis C in hemophiliacs. Blood 78: 1672–1677

Manns M P, Griffin K J, Sullivan K F et al 1991 LKM-1 autoantibodies recognize a short linear sequence in P450IID6, a cytochrome P-450 monooxygenase. J Clin Invest 88: 1370–1378

Mannucci P M, Zanetti A R, Colombo M et al 1990 Antibody to hepatitis C virus after a vapour-heated factor VIII concentrate. The Study Group of the Fondazione dell'Emofilia. Thromb Haemost 64: 232–234

Marcellin P, Giostra E, Boyer N et al 1990 Is the response to recombinant alpha interferon related to the presence of antibodies to hepatitis C virus in patients with chronic non-A, non-B hepatitis? J Hepatol 11: 77–79

Mattsson L 1989 Chronic non-A, non-B hepatitis with special reference to the transfusion-associated form. Scand J Infect Dis Suppl 59: 1–55

Mendenhall C L, Seeff L, Diehl A M et al 1991 Antibodies to hepatitis B virus and hepatitis C virus in alcoholic hepatitis and cirrhosis: their prevalence and clinical relevance. Hepatology 14: 581–589

Mishiro S, Hoshi Y, Takeda K et al 1990 Non-A, non-B hepatitis specific antibodies directed at host-derived epitope: implication for an autoimmune process. Lancet 336: 1400–1403

MMWR 1989 Non-A, non-B hepatitis-Illinois. MMWR 38: 529–531

Nasoff M S, Zebedee S L, Inchauspé G et al 1991 Identification of an immunodominant epitope within the capsid protein of hepatitis C virus. Proc Natl Acad Sci USA 88: 5462–5466

Nishioka K, Watanabe J, Furuta S et al 1991 Antibody to the hepatitis C virus in acute hepatitis and chronic liver diseases in Japan. Liver 11: 65–70

Ogata N, Alter H J, Miller R H et al 1991 Nucleotide sequence and mutation rate of the H strain of hepatitis C virus. Proc Natl Acad Sci USA 88: 3392–3396

Oguchi H, Terashima M, Tokunaga S et al 1990 Prevalence of anti-HCV in patients on long-term hemodialysis. Nippon Jinzo Gakkai Shi 32: 313–317

Ohnishi K, Nomura F, Nakano M 1991 Interferon therapy for acute posttransfusion non-A, non-B hepatitis: response with respect to anti-hepatitis C virus antibody status. Am J Gastroenterol 86: 1041–1049

Okada S, Akahane Y, Suzuki H et al 1992 The degree of variability in the amino terminal region of the E2/NS1 protein of hepatitis C virus correlates with responsiveness to interferon therapy in viremic patients. Hepatology 16: 619–624

Okamoto H, Okada S, Sugiyama Y et al 1990 The 5'-terminal sequence of the hepatitis C virus genome. Jpn J Exp Med 60: 167–177

Omata M, Yokosuka O, Takano S et al 1991 Resolution of acute hepatitis C after therapy with natural beta interferon. Lancet 338: 914–915

Onji M, Kikuchi T, Michitaka K et al 1991 Detection of hepatitis C virus antibody in patients with autoimmune hepatitis and other chronic liver diseases. Gastroenterol Jpn 26: 182–186

Pares A, Barrera J M, Caballeria J et al 1990 Hepatitis C virus antibodies in chronic alcoholic patients: association with severity of liver injury. Hepatology 12: 1295–1299

Patel A, Sherlock S, Dusheiko G et al 1991 Clinical course and histological correlations in post-transfusion hepatitis C: the Royal Free Hospital experience. Eur J Gastroenterol Hepatol 3: 491–495

Pereira B J G, Milford E L, Kirkman R L et al 1991 Transmission of hepatitis C virus by organ transplantation. N Engl J Med 325: 454–460

Perrillo R P, Pohl D A, Roodman S T et al 1981 Acute non-A, non-B hepatitis with serum sickness-like syndrome and aplastic anaemia. JAMA 245: 494–496

Pistello M, Ceccherini-Nelli L, Cecconi N et al 1991 Hepatitis C virus seroprevalence in Italian haemophiliacs injected with virus-inactivated concentrates: five year follow-up and correlation with antibodies to other viruses. J Med Virol 33: 43–46

Pohjanpelto P, Tallgren M, Farkkila M et al 1991 Low prevalence of hepatitis C antibodies in chronic liver disease in Finland. Scand J Infect Dis 23: 139–142

Pol S, Driss F, Devergie A et al 1990 Is hepatitis C virus involved in hepatitis-associated aplastic anemia? Ann Intern Med 113: 435–437

Polywka S, Laufs R 1991 Hepatitis C virus antibodies among different groups at risk and patients with suspected non-A, non-B hepatitis. Infection 19: 81–84

Ponz E, Campistol J M, Barrera J M et al 1991 Hepatitis C virus antibodies in patients on hemodialysis and after kidney transplantation. Transplant Proc 23: 1371–1372

Poterucha J J, Rakela J, Ludwig J et al 1991 Hepatitis C antibodies in patients with chronic hepatitis of unknown etiology after orthotopic liver transplantation. Transplant Proc 23: 1495–1497

Quiroga J A, Campillo M L, Catillo I et al 1991 IgM antibody to hepatitis C virus in acute and chronic hepatitis C. Hepatology 14: 38–43

Rassam S W, Dusheiko G M 1991 Epidemiology and transmission of hepatitis C infection. Eur J Gastroenterol 3: 585–591

Read A E, Donegan E, Lake J et al 1991a Hepatitis C in patients undergoing liver transplantation. Ann Intern Med 114: 282–284

Read A E, Donegan E, Lake J et al 1991b Hepatitis C in liver transplant recipients. Transplant Proc 23: 1504–1505

Reichard O, Andersson J, Schvarcz R et al 1991 Ribavirin treatment for chronic hepatitis C. Lancet 337: 1058–1061

Renault P F, Hoofnagle J H 1989 Side effects of alpha interferon. Semin Liver Dis 9: 273–277

Sanchez-Quijano A, Rey C, Aguado I et al 1990 Hepatitis C virus infection in sexually promiscuous groups. Eur J Clin Microbiol Infect Dis 9: 610–612

Scheuer P J, Ashrafzadeh P, Sherlock S et al 1992 The pathology of hepatitis C. Hepatology 15: 567–571

Schramm W, Roggendorf M, Rommel F et al 1989 Prevalence of antibodies to hepatitis C virus (HCV) in haemophiliacs. Blut 59: 390–392

Schulman S, Grillner L 1990 Antibodies against hepatitis C in a population of Swedish haemophiliacs and heterosexual partners. Scand J Infect Dis 22: 393–397

Schvarcz R, von-Sydow M, Weiland O 1990 Autoimmune chronic active hepatitis: changing reactivity for antibodies to hepatitis C virus after immunosuppressive treatment. Scand J Gastroenterol 25: 1175–1180

Schvarcz R, Glaumann H, Weiland O et al 1991 Histological outcome in interferon alpha-2b treated patients with chronic posttransfusion non-A, non-B hepatitis. Liver 11: 30–38

Simmonds P, Zhang L Q, Watson H G et al 1990 Hepatitis C quantification and sequencing in blood products, haemophiliacs, and drug users. Lancet 336: 1469–1472

Takamizawa A, Mori C, Fuke I et al 1991 Structure and organization of the hepatitis C virus genome isolated from human carriers. J Virol 65: 1105–1113

Tanaka E, Kiyosawa K, Sodeyama T et al 1991a Significance of antibody to hepatitis C virus in Japanese patients with viral hepatitis: relationship between anti-HCV antibody and the prognosis of non-A, non-B post-transfusion hepatitis. J Med Virol 33: 117–122

Tanaka K, Hirohata T, Koga S et al 1991b Hepatitis C and hepatitis B in the etiology of hepatocellular carcinoma in the Japanese population. Cancer Res 51: 2842–2847

Tedder R S, Gilson R J, Briggs M et al 1991 Hepatitis C virus: evidence for sexual transmission. Br Med J 302: 1299–1302

Thaler M M, Park C-K, Landers D V et al 1991 Vertical transmission of hepatitis C virus. Lancet 338: 17–18

Tor J, Llibre J M, Carbonell M et al 1990 Sexual transmission of hepatitis C virus and its relation with hepatitis B virus and HIV. Br Med J 301: 1130–1133

Tzakis A G, Arditi M, Whitington P F et al 1988 Aplastic anemia complicating orthotopic liver transplantation for non-A, non-B hepatitis. N Engl J Med 319: 393–396

Ulrich P P, Romeo J M, Lane P K et al 1990 Detection, semiquantitation, and genetic variation in hepatitis C virus sequences amplified from the plasma of blood donors with elevated alanine aminotransferase. J Clin Invest 86: 1609–1614

Van der Poel C L, Cuypers H T M, Reesink H W et al 1991 Confirmation of hepatitis C virus infection by new four-antigen recombinant immunoblot assay. Lancet 337: 317–319

Van Dam J, Farraye F A, Gale R P et al 1990 Fulminant hepatic failure following bone marrow transplantation for hepatitis-associated aplastic anemia. Bone Marrow Transplant 5: 57–60

Varagona G, Brown D, Kibbler H et al 1992 Response, relapse and retreatment rates and viraemia in chronic hepatitis C treated with α2b interferon. A phase III study. Eur J Gastroenterol Hepatol 4: 707–712

Vucelic B, Hadzic N, Dubravcic D 1988 Chronic persistent hepatitis. Long term prospective study on the natural course of the disease. Scand J Gastroenterol 23: 551–554

Wang J-T, Wang T-H, Lin J-T et al 1991 Hepatitis C virus RNA in saliva of patients with post-transfusion hepatitis C infection. Lancet 337: 48

Waters V V, Cook L 1992 Prevalence of hepatitis B in pregnant women. JAMA 267: 1919

Weiner A J, Brauer M J, Rosenblatt J et al 1991 Variable and hypervariable domains are found in the regions of HCV corresponding to the flavivirus envelope and NS1 proteins and the pestivirus envelope glycoproteins. Virology 180: 842–848

Wejstal R, Lindberg J, Lundin P et al 1987 Chronic non-A, non-B hepatitis. A long-term follow-up study in 49 patients. Scand J Gastroenterol 22: 1115–1122

Wejstal R, Hermodsson S, Iwarson S et al 1990 Mother to infant transmission of hepatitis C virus infection. J Med Virol 30: 178–180

Widell A, Sundstrom G, Hansson B G et al 1991 Antibody to hepatitis-C-virus-related proteins in sera from alanine-aminotransferase-screened blood donors and prospectively studied recipients. Vox Sang 60: 28–33

Wonke B, Hoffbrand A V, Brown D et al 1990 Antibody to hepatitis C virus in multiply transfused patients with thalassaemia major. J Clin Pathol 43: 638–640

Zeldis J B, Dienstag J L, Gale R P 1983 Aplastic anemia and hepatitis. Am J Med 74: 64–68

11

Oral iron chelation therapy

F. N. Al-Refaie   A. V. Hoffbrand

Since 1988 when the topic of iron chelation with orally active drugs was reviewed in *Recent Advances in Haematology* (Kontoghiorghes & Hoffbrand 1988), clinical trials have been carried out worldwide with the compound 1,2-dimethyl-3-hydroxypyrid-4-one (L_1, CP20). Shorter term trials have also been undertaken with other compounds including 1,2-diethyl-3-hydroxypyrid-4-one (CP94, Table 11.1), N, N'-bis(o-hydroxybenzyl) ethylenediamine-N, N'-diacetic acid (HBED), desferrithiocin (DFT) and pyridoxal isonicotinoyl hydrazone (PIH). Nevertheless, no single compound has yet emerged as a widely available pharmaceutical preparation. The purpose of the present review is mainly to summarize current results in patients and in experimental animals and tissue culture with the orally active chelator L_1. Other recent reviews of the field of iron chelation include those of Hershko (1989), Grady & Hershko (1990a,b), Kontoghiorghes (1992) and Brittenham (1992).

Table 11.1   The hydroxypyrid-4-ones

R_1 (see Fig. 11.1)	R_2 (see Fig. 11.1)	CP nomenclature	L_1 nomenclature
CH_3	CH_3	20	L_1
CH_3	CH_2CH_3	21	L_1NEt
CH_3	$CH_2CH_2CH_3$	22	
CH_3	$CH(CH_3)_2$	23	
CH_3	$CH_2CH_2CH_2CH_3$	24	
CH_3	$CH_2CH_2CH_2CH_2CH_3$	25	
CH_3	$CH_2CH_2CO_2H$	38	
CH_3	CH_2CH_2OH	40	
CH_3	$CH_2CH_2CH_2OH$	41	
CH_3	$CH_2CH_2CH_2CH_2OH$	42	
CH_3	$CH_2CH_2OCH_3$	51	$L_1NMeOEt$
CH_3	$CH_2CH_2CH_2OCH_2CH_3$	52	
CH_3	$(CH_2)_2COOCH_2CH_3$	55	
CH_3	$CH_2CH=CH_2$		L_1NAll
CH_3	$CH(CH_2)_2$		L_1NCPr
CH_2CH_3	CH_3	93	EL_1
CH_2CH_3	CH_2CH_3	94	EL_1NEt
CH_2CH_3	$CH_2CH_2OCH_3$	96	$EL_1NMeOEt$

Et = ethyl, MeO = methoxy, All = allyl, CPr = cyclopropyl.

ANIMAL STUDIES

Despite the widespread clinical trials with L_1, carefully controlled studies in both normal and iron-loaded animals are still needed for L_1 and other potential orally active chelators. The studies that have been performed with the hydroxypyridine group of compounds are summarized below.

Mice

Kontoghiorghes (1987) reported that L_1 and L_1NEt (CP21) given intragastrically (i.g.) caused ^{59}Fe excretion in iron overloaded or normal mice comparable to that with intraperitoneal (i.p.) desferrioxamine (DFX). The excretion caused by CP21, CP22 and CP23 was significantly more than that caused by L_1; the most hydrophobic compounds, CP24 and CP25, caused increased toxicity (Gyparaki et al 1987).

Porter et al (1990) subsequently studied the oral efficacy and acute toxicity of several hydroxypyridine compounds in iron loaded mice. With all compounds studied the majority of ^{59}Fe excretion at lower doses was faecal. As the dose increased the proportion excreted in urine increased. The dose–response curves were linear for most of the chelators including L_1 over the range 0–750 mg/kg. Iron excretion was equivalent after i.p. or i.g. administration. The most effective compounds orally were CP22, CP51 and CP94. The increase in excretion of ^{59}Fe for each mg/kg administered orally ranged from 0.15% for CP55 to 3.67% for CP22. L_1 was associated with a 0.85% increase. The LD_{50} for these compounds in iron overloaded mice ranged between 99 mg/kg for CP24 and 2783 mg/kg for CP55. The LD_{50} for L_1, given i.p., was 983 mg/kg. At lethal doses of each chelator, death occurred by convulsions. The interval between i.p. administration of compound and death was shorter with the lipophilic compounds (e.g. within 5 minutes for CP22) compared with the more hydrophillic compounds (2–8 hours for L_1). The LD_{50} for iron overloaded animals was higher than for non-iron overloaded animals showing a protective effect for iron loading against acute toxicity. Those compounds with higher lipid solubility (K_{part}, defined as the ratio of the concentrations of the compound between an organic phase usually n-octanol and water buffered to pH 7.4) were associated with lower LD_{50}.

There was a significant correlation between lipid solubility and efficacy of the chelator ($r = 0.6$) and between efficacy and acute toxicity (LD_{50}) ($r = 0.84$), i.e. chelators with higher lipid solubility were more effective but more toxic. The ratio of LD_{50} to the dose required to cause 200% increase in iron excretion was calculated and it was suggested that compounds with the highest ratio possess the best balance between these two parameters and, therefore, between toxicity and efficacy. CP94 and CP51 were found to have the highest ratio (10.5 and 8.4 respectively) while the ratio for L_1 was 4.2 (Porter et al 1990).

In order to assess the chronic toxicity of hydroxypyridine compounds and their effect on iron loading, several of these chelators and DFX were administered i.p. to iron overloaded mice (with i.p. iron–dextran) at a dose of 200 mg/kg/day for up to 60 days (Porter et al 1991). At the end of the study all oral compounds and DFX caused a highly significant reduction in diffuse Perls positive material in the liver while no change was observed in granular deposits. Liver iron removal after 60 days ranged from 37% with L_1 to 63% with CP51 compared with 46% with DFX given as an i.p. injection at a similar dose. No significant reduction in splenic or cardiac iron was observed with any chelator.

There were no deaths in iron overloaded animals receiving the chelators, while significant mortality occurred in the non-iron overloaded animals. L_1 also caused a significant fall of white cell count (leukopenia rather than selective neutropenia) and of haemoglobin in both iron overloaded and non-overloaded animals and a significant rise in MCV (mean corpuscular volume) only in non-overloaded animals (Table 11.2).

No histological abnormalities of brain, kidney, spleen, bone marrow, lung, eye, heart or joints were observed. In the liver, however, intracytoplasmic eosinophilic inclusion bodies were noted in the centrilobular hepatocytes with all the chelators but not with DFX in both iron overloaded and non-overloaded animals. These changes were most marked with CP51 and CP21 and least marked with L_1 and CP94. At the end of the study no adrenal enlargement was noted and no biochemical changes were observed apart from a rise in serum albumin which accompanied the use of CP21 and CP51.

Nortey et al (1992) studied the efficacy of L_1 and related compounds in iron overloaded, ^{59}Fe-labelled mice. Chelators were given i.g. at a dose of 200 mg/kg. L_1NAll was the most effective of the compounds studied causing a $639 \pm 82\%$ increase in ^{59}Fe excretion whereas EL_1NMeOEt (CP96) was the least effective ($260 \pm 28\%$). L_1 and L_1NEt (CP21) were less effective than L_1NAll but more effective than other chelators studied. L_1 and L_1NCPr had similar efficacy at increasing ^{59}Fe excretion, predominantly (>90%) in the faeces.

Rats

In the first of the studies in rats Kontoghiorghes et al (1987a) compared L_1 with DFX for their ability to remove iron and for their site of action. Intraperitoneal administration of the chelators (200 mg/kg) to iron overloaded and non-overloaded rats labelled with ^{59}Fe induced comparable ^{59}Fe mobilization. However, most of the ^{59}Fe remained in the rats even after prolonged chelation. Specific labelling of the iron pool in hepatocytes was achieved by using ^{59}Fe-ferritin. This iron pool was shown to be equally accessible to both chelators given i.p. and also to oral L_1. All rats were alive after 7 months of daily therapy. L_1 induced hypersalivation within minutes of administration and this continued for 1–2 hours.

In a later study L_1 was given orally to normal rats at a dose of 200 mg/kg for 90 days and at 200 mg b.d. for a further 60 days (Kontoghiorghes et al

Table 11.2   Animal toxicity of hydroxypyrid-4-one (CP) iron chelators

Toxicity	Animal species (iron status)	Chelator	Dose (mg/kg)/ route	Study
Leukopenia	Mice (normal & iron loaded)	CP20	200/i.p.	Porter et al (1991)
	Rats (normal)	CP20	200/i.g.	Kontoghiorghes et al (1989)
	Rats (normal)	CP20	300/i.p., i.g.	Grady et al (1992)
Anaemia	Mice (normal & iron loaded)	CP20	200/i.p.	Porter et al (1991)
	Rats (normal)	CP20	300/i.p.	Grady et al (1992)
	Rats (normal)	CP20	200/i.g.	Kontoghiorghes et al (1989)
Low RBC	Rats (normal)	CP20	300/i.p.	Grady et al (1992)
	Mice (normal & iron loaded)	CP20	200/i.p.	Porter et al (1991)
Low PCV	Rats (normal)	CP20	300/i.p.	Grady et al (1992)
High MCV	Mice (normal)	CP20	200/i.p.	Porter et al (1991)
	Rats (normal)	CP20	300/i.p.	Grady et al (1992)
High serum cholesterol	Rats (normal)	CP20	DR/i.g., i.p.	Grady et al (1992)
Hyper-salivation	Rats (normal & iron loaded)	CP20	200/i.g., i.p.	Kontoghiorghes et al (1987a)
	Rats (normal)	CP20	75–300/i.g.	Grady et al (1992)
	Rats (normal)*	CP20	42–63/i.g.	Bergeron et al (1992)
	Rats (normal)†	CP94	50-75/i.g.	Bergeron et al (1992)
Adrenal enlargement	Rats (normal)	CP20	DR/i.g., i.p.	Grady et al (1992)
Inclusion body (liver)	Mice (normal)	CP20, CP21, CP51, CP93, CP94	200/i.p.	Porter et al (1991)
Atrophy of Sp., Th.	Rats (normal)	CP20	DR/i.g., i.p.	Grady et al (1992)
Atrophy of testes	Rats (normal)	CP20	DR/i.p.	Grady et al (1992)
Reduced weight gain	Rats (normal)	CP20	300/i.p.	Grady et al (1992)
Death	Mice (normal)‡	CP20, CP51 CP93, CP94	200/i.p.	Porter et al (1991)
	Rats (normal)¶	CP94	300/i.g.	Grady et al (1991)
	Rats (normal)**	CP94, CP51	200/i.g.	Kontoghiorghes (1990)
	Monkeys (iron loaded)††	CP94	75/p.o.	Bergeron et al (1992)

Sp. = spleen, Th. = thymus, DR = dose-related, i.p. = intraperitoneal, i.g. = intragastric, p.o. = oral, RBC = red blood cells, PCV = packed cell volume, MCV = mean corpuscular volume.
*40% of animals. †60% of animals. ‡At 60 days: 3/9 of animals on CP20; 2/6 of animals on CP51; 1/5 of animals on CP93; 1/8 of animals on CP94. ¶8/10 of animals at 4 weeks. **6/6 of animals at 5 months. ††1/4 of animals at 19 hours.

1989). A fall in white blood cell count was observed at 30 and 150 days. No change in haematological indices was seen with a 60 mg/kg dose for 36 days.

Venkataram & Rahman (1990) gave L_1 at a dose of 200 mg/kg/day to iron overloaded rats. The chelation efficiency (ratio of iron excreted to the capacity of the dose of L_1 to chelate iron in forming 3:1 complexes) for L_1 was found to be 1.3%, similar to that observed in normal rats by Bergeron et al (1992) (see p. 190). There was no difference in the amount of iron excreted in faeces before and after L_1 administration by any route.

Chronic toxicity studies of L_1 in normal rats were carried out by Grady et al (1992). Three groups of normal rats were given L_1 daily at doses of 75, 150 and 300 mg/kg i.p. A fourth group was given 300 mg/kg/day orally. Animals given L_1 i.p. at 300 mg/day failed to gain weight normally. When the same dose was given i.g. no inhibition of growth was observed. At all doses, marked hypersalivation was noted 10 minutes after drug administration. L_1 caused a dose-related increase in the size of the adrenals and a decrease in the size of the thymus, spleen and testes. No biochemical changes were observed during the study apart from a dose-related increase in serum cholesterol. No significant changes were seen in haematological indices when L_1 was given at a dose of 75–150 mg/kg i.p. At 300 mg/kg i.p. L_1 caused a fall in red cell and white cell counts, haemoglobin and haematocrit by about 50% and a rise in MCV. When L_1 was given i.g. the effect on red cell indices was markedly reduced while suppression of the white cell count remained significant (Table 11.2).

In another study, CP94 was found to be significantly more toxic than L_1 in normal rats (Grady et al 1991). Four weeks of oral administration of CP94 at a dose of 300 mg/kg/day caused the death or premature sacrifice of eight of ten animals, while no animals succumbed to a similar dose of L_1. CP94 caused similar organ changes to those caused by L_1, but they were more pronounced at doses one third less. Similar findings were reported by Kontoghiorghes (1990) and Nortey et al (1992). EL_1NEt (CP94) and $L_1NMeOEt$ (CP51) caused the death of all rats ($n = 6$) within 2–5 months of i.g. administration of the drug at a dose of 200 mg/kg, 5 days a week. In contrast L_1 was not associated with a single death when given i.g. at a similar dose for up to 8 months.

In order to determine the selectivity of the oral iron chelator for iron in different body compartments, Zevin et al (1992) employed selective radio-iron probes to introduce tracer iron into the two major iron storage pools: hepatic parenchyma and reticuloendothelial system. These studies were performed in hypertransfused rats and showed that the oral chelators (CP94 and CP20 (L_1)) are able to mobilize iron from both hepatocellular and reticuloendothelial stores with an efficiency comparable to that of DFX. Iron mobilized from the liver was excreted in bile while up to half of the iron removed from reticuloendothelial stores was cleared by the kidneys. The rest was excreted in the bile.

Florence et al (1992) utilized a new animal model of iron overload in order to determine the site of chelation by various iron chelators at a subcellular level. Rats were iron overloaded by being fed on ferrocene (Longueville & Crichton 1986). This was shown to produce stable hepatic iron stores which did not decrease 2 weeks after the cessation of iron loading. When oral L_1 or

CP94 or i.p. DFX was administered there were significant decreases in total hepatic and ferritin iron, while there were no consistent changes in ferritin protein. Analysis of the iron content of the subcellular organelles showed a significant decrease in both cytosolic and lysosomal fractions. It was concluded, therefore, that both L_1 and CP94 when given orally are capable of removing iron from hepatic ferritin and haemosiderin. L_1 also caused a significant reduction in ferritin iron and protein content of spleen. Neither brain nor heart showed any significant fall in iron content after chelation. There was no alteration in haematological indices during the 2-week period of the study.

The chelation efficiencies of L_1, CP94 and DFX were compared in a more recent animal study (Bergeron et al 1992). When non-iron overloaded rats were given L_1 or CP94 orally or subcutaneous (s.c.) DFX, the chelation efficiencies were found to be 1.2%, 7.1% and 2.8% respectively. These figures are comparable with those observed in iron overloaded monkeys (see below). Most of the excreted iron was found in bile (86%, 69% and 75% respectively). Hypersalivation was noted in 40% of rats treated with L_1 and in 60% of those treated with CP94 after a dose of 450 µmol/kg.

Rabbits

Kontoghiorghes & Hoffbrand (1986) showed that when L_1 or L_1NEt was given to iron overloaded (with i.m. iron–dextran) ^{59}Fe-labelled rabbits at a dose of 200 mg/kg, they caused iron excretion comparable to that promoted by a similar dose of DFX. The ^{59}Fe excretion by these drugs was predominantly faecal. However, when L_1 and L_1NCPr were given by Nortey et al (1992) to iron overloaded ^{59}Fe-labelled rabbits at a similar dose, the contribution of faecal ^{59}Fe excretion was less than 50% of the total. The drugs caused significant and comparable increases in 24-hour urine iron and ^{59}Fe excretion.

Monkeys

Bergeron et al (1992) also studied the effects of L_1, CP94 and DFX in iron overloaded monkeys. The chelation efficiencies of the three chelators were 2.1%, 7.4% and 5.5% respectively, while the percentages of iron excreted in urine were 70%, 38% and 55% respectively, the rest of the iron being excreted in the faeces. There were no significant changes in blood counts or in kidney and liver function profiles. Only CP94 was associated with toxicity. When four monkeys were given this drug at a dose of 450 µmol/kg (75 mg/kg), one of the animals died after about 19 hours and tested positive for blood in urine and faeces. No definite cause of death was found on postmortem examination.

In summary, the animal studies have shown the oral effectiveness of the hydroxypyridine chelators at inducing iron excretion and shown that the more lipid-soluble compounds tend to be more effective but more toxic. In contrast to humans, substantial iron excretion occurs by the faecal route. The major side-effects noted with L_1 have been leukopenia, macrocytosis of red cells and hypersalivation (see Table 11.2).

CELL CULTURE STUDIES

Several in vitro experiments have studied the physicochemical properties of the different compounds in the hydroxypyridine group of oral chelators and the relation between these properties and the efficacy and toxicity of the compounds.

Porter et al (1988) investigated the efficiency of various iron chelators in mobilizing iron from ^{59}Fe-labelled hepatocytes in culture. Following the addition of chelators to the culture medium the rate of ^{59}Fe release was increased above that of the control. There was a significant correlation between the percentage of iron release and the lipid solubility of the compound with a maximum mobilization by compounds with a K_{part} close to 1. Compounds with a K_{part} higher than 1 were less effective although the difference was not significant.

Compounds with higher iron-binding constants, i.e. 4-one compounds (Fig. 11.1A) (log $\beta = 36$), were more effective than those with lower iron-binding constants, i.e. 2-one compounds (Fig. 11.1B) (log $\beta = 32$), over a wide range of concentrations but particularly at low concentrations of chelator. At higher concentrations of chelator and with more prolonged incubation times, more lipophilic compounds were associated with lower cell viability as determined by higher lactate dehydrogenase levels in the culture supernatant.

Culture of myocardial cells was utilized by Hershko et al (1991a) to assess the efficiency of several hydroxypyridine compounds and of DFX in mobilizing ^{59}Fe and in inhibiting lipid peroxidation induced by iron as indicated by cellular malonaldehyde (MDA) content. At a low molar concentration of chelators (0.1 mmol/l), DFX was more effective than the hydroxypyridines in reducing the iron content of the iron loaded heart cell (52% versus 9–16%). At a higher concentration (1 mmol/l) all hydroxypyridine compounds were as effective or more effective than DFX (87–89% versus 83%).

When DFX and CP94 were used at a concentration of 1 mmol/l, rapid mobilization of cellular iron was observed, reaching a plateau after 6 hours. Iron mobilization by both compounds was associated with a reduction in cellular MDA content. However, there was no correlation between the MDA level and the amount of iron removed; DFX reduced MDA more than CP94 did despite the greater efficiency of CP94 for iron chelation.

The effect of chelator (CP94 and DFX) concentration on chelating efficiency was also evaluated. At concentrations of 0.1 and 0.25 mmol/l, DFX was more effective than CP94, while at concentrations of 0.75 and 1.0 mmol/l the opposite was true. It was concluded, therefore, that effective mobilization

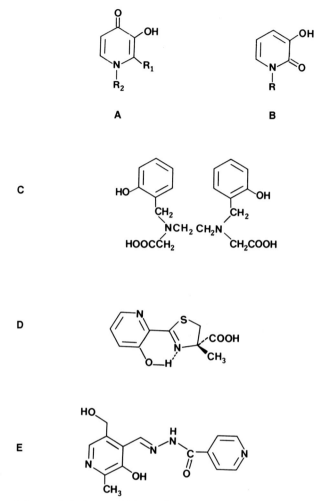

Fig. 11.1 Iron chelators: **A.** hydroxypyrid-4-one; **B.** hydroxypyrid-2-one; **C.** HBED [*N, N'*-bis(*o*-hydroxybenzyl)ethylenediamine-*N, N'*-diacetic acid]; **D.** DFT (deferrithiocin); **E.** PIH (pyridoxal isonicotinoyl hydrazone).

of iron by CP94 and probably by other hydroxypyridines requires a drug/iron ratio exceeding 3:1 permitting the formation of a hexadentate complex.

Pattanapanyasat et al (1992) studied the effect of hydroxypyridine (CP) compounds and DFX on human lymphocytes. CP compounds and DFX caused a dose-dependent inhibition of the proliferative response after 4 hours of exposure. At a concentration of 100 µmol both DFX and CP compounds caused 70% inhibition and at 200 µmol 100% inhibition. These concentrations were not associated with a change in cell viability, but higher concentration of chelators or more prolonged exposure (72 hours) resulted in reduced cell viability. The inhibitory effect of CP compounds was higher than that of DFX. Greater inhibition was observed among CP compounds with increasing K_{part}. Presaturation of CP and DFX with ferric ion diminished their inhibitory effect on DNA synthesis. It was suggested, therefore, that both DFX and CP compounds exert their effect by chelating iron with subsequent inhibition of DNA synthesis. DFX has previously been shown to inhibit lymphocyte ribonucleotide reductase which is a rate-limiting enzyme in DNA synthesis (Hoffbrand et al 1976). All chelators studied at these concentrations had no effect, in short-term cultures, on protein synthesis, assessed by [^{3}H]leucine incorporation or on T-cell activation markers (transferrin and interleukin-2 receptors).

Ganeshaguru et al (1992) showed that L_1 at the higher concentration of 1 mmol/l caused substantial inhibition of DNA, RNA and protein synthesis and cell viability in phytohaemagglutinin-stimulated lymphocytes. Similar inhibition was observed with DFX at this high concentration. Their actions were, however, different. Whereas L_1 increased both dATP and dTTP concentrations in the cells, DFX, like hydroxyurea (a known ribonucleotide reductase inhibitor), decreased dATP and increased dTTP concentration suggesting DFX inhibits DNA synthesis by chelating iron from ribonucleotide reductase. Both L_1 and DFX decreased the cell concentration of dsDNA. However, there was increased recovery of dsDNA with time on removal of L_1 while removal of DFX did not allow substantial recovery. These findings indicate different mechanisms of iron removal and cytotoxicity for L_1 and DFX which remain to be defined.

CLINICAL STUDIES WITH L_1

PHARMACOKINETICS

Several reports are now available on the pharmacokinetics of L_1 in humans (Kontoghiorghes et al 1990a,b, Olivieri et al 1990, Matsui et al 1991).

Absorption

L_1 is rapidly absorbed since it appears in the blood within 5–10 minutes of ingestion with a half-life ($T_{1/2}$) of absorption of 0.7–32.4 minutes (Kontoghiorghes et al 1990b). The peak serum concentration (C_{max}) in one study of five patients was 132 ± 44 µmol/l at an L_1 dose of 3 g with peak levels observed 12–120 minutes after L_1 ingestion (Kontoghiorghes et al 1990a,b). In another study of 14 patients C_{max} was 125.8 ± 15.0 µmol/l at an L_1 dose of 25 mg/kg and occurred 45–60 minutes after L_1 ingestion. A second peak at 240 minutes was observed in one patient (Matsui et al 1991).

Clearance

More than 90% of the drug is eliminated from plasma in most patients within 5–6 hours of ingestion. The $T_{1/2}$ for elimination from plasma ranged from 46.6 to 134.2 minutes (74.3 ± 28.7) in one study (Kontoghiorghes et al 1990b) with a mean $T_{1/2}$ in another study of 159.6 ± 20.5 minutes (Matsui et al 1991). Most of the drug (79–99%) is recovered from urine mainly as L_1 glucuronide but also as free L_1 and L_1–iron complex (Kontoghiorghes et al 1990b). Urinary iron excretion (UIE) was found to be significantly and independently related to L_1 trough concentrations (before morning dose) and to serum ferritin levels (Matsui et al 1991).

Increased faecal iron excretion was observed in two studies from one centre (Olivieri et al 1990, Collins et al 1992). This accounted for 15% (0–28%) of the total iron excretion in the first study of six patients and 1–30% of iron excretion in the second study of four patients. No similar increase in faecal iron was found in two patients studied in another trial and no L_1 was found in their faecal extracts (Kontoghiorghes et al 1990a, Sheppard & Kontoghiorghes 1991).

Metabolism

The major route of L_1 metabolism is glucuronidation (Goddard & Kontoghiorghes 1989). When urine samples from patients taking L_1 are treated with glucuronidase the L_1–glucuronide complex peak disappears from the chromatogram with a proportional increase in the L_1 peak. This peak accounts for most of the L_1 administered to the patient. L_1 glucuronide reaches a peak concentration in plasma in 2–3 hours after L_1 ingestion (Kontoghiorghes et al 1990b). Since L_1 glucuronide is not capable of binding iron, it is possible that the speed of L_1 glucuronidation may correlate inversely with the efficacy of L_1 to chelate iron but this remains to be established.

Factors which may influence L_1 pharmacokinetics and efficacy

Simultaneous ingestion of food with L_1 significantly reduced the peak serum concentration of L_1 from 125.8 ± 15.0 to 95.0 ± 11.4 (P<0.05). There was, however, no change in the total area under the curve of L_1 concentration in plasma or an effect on UIE (Matsui et al 1991). The effect of the frequency of L_1 administration on UIE was evaluated in one study (Al-Refaie et al 1992a). When the same daily dose of L_1 was administered in four divided doses instead of two, substantially more iron excretion was induced in three of the eight patients studied. More frequent administration had no effect or an opposite effect in the other patients. Larger studies are therefore required to evaluate the effect of dose size and frequency on iron excretion and also to establish whether more frequent administration of smaller doses of L_1 compared with less frequent larger doses will affect the incidence and severity of side-effects.

Vitamin C was found to have no effect on UIE in two trials (Töndury et al 1990, Al-Refaie et al 1992a). However, neither trial was large enough to determine the exact effect of vitamin C therapy, both in vitamin C deficient and replete patients. Al-Refaie et al (1992a) observed a fall in leukocyte ascorbate levels 3–5 months from the commencement of L_1 treatment in seven of ten patients during L_1 therapy. None of these patients became symptomatic.

The possible contribution of dietary iron to L_1-induced UIE was assessed by Olivieri et al (1990). No increase in UIE in two normal volunteers was observed when L_1 complexed to iron was administered orally.

Finally, there has been some evidence that long-term use of L_1 may be associated with a fall in serum L_1 trough concentrations (Matsui et al 1991). This was presumed to be due to reduced absorption or increased metabolism. The latter possibility is supported by the results of an in vitro study which has shown that L_1 induces its own metabolism by human hepatocytes in culture (Neuman et al 1991). As there was significant correlation between UIE and L_1 trough concentrations, it was suggested that it may be necessary to increase the dose of L_1 if negative iron balance is to be maintained in the long term (Matsui et al 1991). However, in none of the long-term clinical trials has a decline in efficacy of L_1 been documented.

SHORT-TERM TRIALS

Initial short-term (less than 1 month) studies showed that L_1 is effective in promoting UIE comparable to that with s.c. DFX. DFX (MW 657) forms a 1:1 iron–chelator complex whereas L_1 (MW 139) forms a 1:3 iron–chelator complex. L_1 and DFX are therefore approximately equivalent iron chelators on a weight basis. Initial phase I studies in patients with myelodysplasia (MDS) and thalassaemia major (TM) showed that single doses of L_1 up to 3 g were well tolerated with nausea in some patients as the only side-effect. UIE was related to the size of the dose and to the iron load of the patient (Kontoghiorghes et al 1987b,c, Kontoghiorghes & Hoffbrand 1989). UIE related more closely to the number of units of blood transfused than to serum ferritin. UIE was also increased by increasing the frequency of L_1 ingestion to two, three or more times daily. It was not clear, and still remains to be established, whether UIE is greater if the same total daily dose is given singly or divided into smaller doses, although variation in the pattern of response from patient to patient is apparent. No constant effect of vitamin C was established in contrast to the findings with DFX where vitamin C usually increases UIE.

Olivieri et al (1990) gave L_1 to 26 patients with TM. At 50 mg/kg/day, L_1 induced UIE of 12.3 ± 6.7 (mean $\pm$ SD) mg/24 h and DFX 18.2 ± 15.3 mg/24 h. When the L_1 dose was increased in five patients to 75 mg/kg/day divided into three doses UIE rose from a mean of 13.8 to a mean of 26.7 mg/24 h. This was comparable to the UIE induced by 50 mg/kg/day of DFX in these five patients. In six patients faecal iron excretion rose from 8.5 ± 0.9 to 12.2 ± 0.9 mg/day at an L_1 dose of 75mg/kg/day. This accounted for a mean of 15% (0–28%) of the total iron excretion in these patients.

More recently, this group compared L_1 with DFX in four regularly transfused patients with sickle cell anaemia (Collins et al 1992). Their mean serum ferritin was 2853 ug/l. In three patients L_1 at 75 or 100 mg/kg/day induced 1.5–2 times more UIE than DFX at 50 mg/kg/day and achieved a net mean iron excretion of 0.68 mg/kg/day. The average intake of iron from blood transfusions in regularly transfused TM patients is approximately 0.50 mg/kg/day. Faecal iron excretion accounted for 1–30% of total iron excretion, the patient with the lowest serum ferritin and least UIE excreting the greatest proportion of iron in the faeces.

LONG-TERM CLINICAL TRIALS

Seven groups have so far reported results of long-term (>4 weeks) L_1 therapy (Table 11.3) and other such trials are in progress. These have largely been in patients with TM but patients with other transfusion-dependent congenital or acquired refractory anaemias have been included. The aims have been to observe the effect of L_1 on iron stores and organ function and to determine possible adverse effects. In some studies, control groups have been treated in parallel with DFX. An exact comparison between the results from these different studies is difficult because of variation in dose of L_1 used, differences in expression of iron excretion (mg/24 h or mg/kg/24 h) and of changes in serum ferritin. Nevertheless, an overall picture is emerging that L_1 therapy is capable of stabilizing or reducing iron overload in patients receiving regular blood transfusions, the largest falls occurring in the patients starting with the highest iron stores assessed either by serum ferritin or by number of previous transfusions. Because of better compliance and because patients are capable of taking L_1 7 days a week, for some patients it has proved more effective than DFX, although with comparable doses daily UIE is about 50% greater with s.c. DFX than with L_1. Faecal iron excretion is probably also greater in response to DFX than to L_1.

The first long-term trial, from the Royal Free Hospital, London, was reported by Bartlett et al (1990) and Kontoghiorghes et al (1990a). Thirteen patients were given L_1 for 1–15 months. UIE correlated with L_1 dose and number of blood units transfused but not with serum ferritin which showed no overall change. In contrast to the results of Olivieri et al (1990, 1992a) faecal iron excretion was not found to be increased by L_1. Subsequently, the same group gave L_1 long term to ten TM patients (Al-Refaie et al 1992a). In this study mean serum ferritin did fall significantly over the 7–13-month trial period (Table 11.3).

Töndury et al (1990, 1992) gave 12 TM patients L_1 (51–93 mg/kg/day) for 9–27 months. UIE was similar to that with DFX 50 mg/kg/day. Serum ferritin fell progressively in nine patients and rose in the others (Table 11.3).

Olivieri and colleagues have performed several long-term studies and it is likely that the same patients after more prolonged follow-up are included in the more recent reports. L_1 was given to 11 patients with TM (Olivieri et al 1991a). Serum ferritin fell significantly over the trial period (16.4 ± 3.6 months). Eight of the 11 patients could be age- and serum ferritin-matched

Table 11.3 Long-term clinical trials with L_1

Trial	No. of patients	Diagnosis	Duration of treatment (months) (range, $X \pm SD$)	L_1 dose (mg/kg/day)	Serum ferritin (µg/l) (range, $X \pm SD$) Initial	Final	UIE (mg/day) (range, $X \pm SD$)
Bartlett et al (1990), Kontoghiorghes et al (1990a)	13	TM × 9, MDS × 2, RCA × 2	1–15 (6.5 ± 5.2)	86–150	3000–14000 (9060 ± 3340)	3000–16000 (8860 ± 3580)*	18.2–126 (47.4 ± 28.4)
Al-Refaie et al (1992a)	11	TM	7–13 (11.4 ± 1.9)	85–119	1000–9580 (5549 ± 3333)	738–7435 (4126 ± 2278)♦	9.6–41.1 (23.0 ± 11.2)
Töndury et al (1990, 1992)	12	TM	9–27 (19.9 ± 7.1)	51–93	1380–11500 (5503 ± 3537)	231–10000 (3891 ± 2966)*	11.4–59.1 (30.2 ± 14.2)
Olivieri et al (1991a)	11	TM	(16.4 ± 3.6)	75	3636 ± 4185	2564 ± 2115♦	22.9 ± 12.0
Olivieri et al (1992a)	15	TM	12–30 (21.5 ± 7.3)	75–100	4325 ± 4028	2608 ± 2153♦	0.2–1.5 mg/kg (0.6 ± 0.3)mg/kg
Olivieri et al (1992b)	1	TI	9	75	2174	251	11–109♦ (53.0 ± 30.0) 13–40♦♦
Agarwal et al (1992a,b)	52	TM × 51, HbE/Thal × 1	3–21 (14.2 ± 6.8)	75–100	1048–18600 (6926 ± 3335)	870–12300♦ (4703 ± 2885)♦	24.0 ± 14.0♦♦ 18.4–110.4♦♦ (42.3 ± 37.1)
Goudsmit (1991), Goudsmit & Kersten (1992)	6	MDS × 4, AA × 1, HbE/Thal × 1	4–16 (11.3 ± 5.0)	31–63	2220–4800 (3497 ± 1167)	144–4320* (2882 ± 1737)	12.1–45.7 (24.6 ± 12.1)
Jaeger et al (1992)	3	MDS	0.7–5.4	2.5 (g/day)	2913–4802	NA	15.7–22.6 (19.1 ± 3.5)
Carnelli et al (1992)	22	TM	1–16 (3.9 ± 3.5)	50	NA	NA	2.8–21.0 (13.2 ± 4.7)

NA = not available, UIE = urinary iron excretion, TM = thalassaemia major, MDS = myelodysplastic syndrome, AA = aplastic anaemia, RCA = red cell aplasia, TI = thalassaemia intermedia.
*P>0.05. ♦P<0.05. ♦♦P<0.005. ♦♦UIE in the first 6 months. ♦♦UIE in the final 6 months. ♦UIE in the first 3 months. ♦Mean fall in serum ferritin: 3641 (20 months, $n = 11$); 2373 (15 months, $n = 14$); 1799 (9 months, $n = 19$); 1465 (5 months, $n = 8$). ♦♦UIE at L_1 dose of 100 mg/kg/day ($n = 47$).

with eight DFX-treated patients. Final serum ferritin was significantly (P<0.05) lower in the L_1-treated patients than in the DFX-treated patients.

In a more recent report 15 patients were given L_1 for 12–30 months (Olivieri et al 1992a). Serum ferritin fell from a mean of 4325 µg/l to a mean of 2608 µg/l. UIE was highly variable (range 0.226–1.45 mg/kg/day) and related to initial serum ferritin. Age-matched and serum ferritin-matched controls treated with s.c. DFX over the same period showed no significant change in serum ferritin. Stainable iron in the liver was reduced in ten patients and unchanged in five.

Further evidence that L_1 can decrease body iron stores has been recently obtained by the same group (Olivieri et al 1992b). L_1 was given to a 29-year-old man with thalassaemia intermedia. After 9 months the serum ferritin had fallen progressively from 2174 µg/l initially to 251 µg/l and liver iron from 14.6 mg/g dry weight to 1.9 mg/g with a corresponding fall in UIE.

The largest group of patients studied so far is in Bombay where Agarwal et al (1992a,b) gave L_1 to 52 patients at a dose of 75–100 mg/kg/day. UIE in five patients averaged 17.4 mg/24 h compared to 21.5 mg/24 h induced by 50 mg/kg/day of s.c. DFX. After 3–21 months 46 patients (88.5%) showed an absolute fall in serum ferritin ranging between 1465 and 3641 µg/l. There were significant correlations between UIE and L_1 dose, initial serum ferritin and patient age but no relation was found between UIE and units of blood transfused. More recently Agarwal et al (1993) have shown that 40 of 40 patients excreting >0.5 g/kg/day of iron but only 16 of 30 excreting <0.5 g/kg/day showed a fall in serum ferritin.

Other long-term trials have been reported by Goudsmit (1991), Goudsmit & Kersten (1992), Jaeger et al (1992) and Carnelli et al (1992). These have confirmed the efficacy of L_1 at increasing iron excretion and have shown variable effects on serum ferritin (Table 11.3).

Changes in non-transferrin-bound iron (NTBI) levels

NTBI is present in the plasma of inadequately chelated patients with transfusional iron overload and is thought to be particularly toxic to the heart and other organs (Gutteridge et al 1985). Al-Refaie et al (1992a,b) monitored the level of NTBI, measured by a modification of the method described by Singh et al (1990), in the sera of the patients they gave L_1. There was a significant fall in the mean level of NTBI after 6 months of L_1 therapy which was not accompanied by a similar change in serum ferritin during the same period. The authors suggested therefore that NTBI levels may prove to be valuable in monitoring the efficacy of iron chelation. Moreover, they found that NTBI was more closely related than serum ferritin to clinical complications of severe iron overload.

Other changes

Both Al-Refaie et al (1992a) and Agarwal et al (1992a) observed lightening of skin colour in patients initially heavily pigmented within 1–3 months of commencement of L_1 therapy. Al-Refaie et al (1992a) also observed a significant decline in serum aspartate aminotransferase (AST) levels in three of ten patients followed for 11–12 months. More recently Olivieri et al (1992a) reported improvement in cardiac function (assessed by radionuclide angiography) associated with decreased cardiac iron (assessed by magnetic resonance imaging) in one patient with iron-related cardiac disease at the start of L_1 therapy.

ADVERSE EFFECTS

In general L_1 has been well tolerated and compliance has been good. However, a number of possible adverse effects have now been reported not all of which could have been predicted from animal studies (Table 11.4).

Musculoskeletal symptoms (MSS)

Bartlett et al (1990) first reported the onset of joint pains and muscle stiffness and pain in four of 13 patients receiving long-term L_1 therapy. These symptoms occurred as early as 3 weeks after commencing treatment. In two patients, the symptoms disappeared despite continuation of the drug, but in a third patient the ankle swelling gradually resolved only after stopping L_1 therapy. In the fourth patient, symptoms remained intermittent both on and off the drug. Al-Refaie et al (1992a) reported similar problems in three of 11 TM patients. In two, the symptoms resolved spontaneously despite continuing L_1 therapy while in the third the pain disappeared 48 hours after stopping L_1 but reappeared (although to a lesser degree) after re-starting L_1. There was no significant correlation between these symptoms and the patients' autoantibody status (see pp 202–205).

Agarwal et al (1992a,b) reported similar symptoms in 20 (38.5%) of their 52 patients. Sixteen had pain and four also developed joint swelling. Two patients had myalgia and one fever. Symptoms disappeared in nine cases after temporary discontinuation of L_1 therapy for 7–45 days. L_1 could be re-started at full dose without reappearance of the symptoms in three patients and at a reduced dose (50 mg/kg) in six cases. In the remaining 11 patients the symptoms disappeared after reducing the dose of L_1. The incidence of MSS in Bombay has been 20 of 52, four of 40 and three of 30 at L_1 doses of 100, 75 and 50 mg/kg/day respectively. Arthroscopy in seven patients showed excess of iron in synovium, cartilage and joint fluid but no L_1 (Agarwal et al 1993).

Berkovitch et al (1992) noted bilateral knee joint pain, stiffness and swelling in three of 15 patients treated long term but in none was it necessary to discontinue the drug. L_1 concentration was estimated in synovial fluid aspirate and was found to be similar to that in serum. No L_1–iron complexes were detectable in the synovial fluid.

Table 11.4 Incidence of adverse effects during L_1 therapy

Trial centre	No. of patients	MSS	Autoantibodies				ZD	GIS	AST changes	AGC	Reference(s)
			RhF		ANA						
			Initial	Final	Initial	Final					
London	24	7	4	4	4	6	4	3	6	3	Bartlett et al (1990), Hoffbrand et al (1989), Al-Refaie et al (1992a, 1993), Veys et al (1993)
Bern	12	0	NA	NA	NA	NA	0	0	0	0	Töndury et al (1990, 1992), Berkovitch et al (1992), Olivieri et al (1991a, 1992b)
Toronto	15	3	5	4	4	2	0	0	0	0	
Bombay	52(104)*	20	4	6	6	10	1*	7	2	1*	Agarwal et al (1992a,b, 1993), Goudsmit (1991), Goudsmit & Kersten (1992), Kersten (personal communication, 1993)
Amsterdam	25	1	NA	NA	0	1	2	4	0	1	
Dusseldorf	6	0	NA	NA	NA	NA	1	1	0	0	Jaeger et al (1992), Jaeger (personal communication, 1993)
Milan	22	2	NA	NA	0	0	0	0	5	0	Carnelli et al (1992), Carnelli (personal communication, 1993)
Total Incidence	156(208)*	33 (21%)	13 (14.3%)	14 (15.4%)	14 (10.2%)	19 (13.8%)	8 (3.9%)	15 (9.6%)	13 (8.3%)	5 (2.4%)	

MSS = musculoskeletal symptoms, ZD = zinc deficiency, GIS = gastrointestinal symptoms, AST = aspartate transaminase, AGC = agranulocytosis
RhF = rheumatoid factor, ANA = antinuclear antibodies.
*A case of agranulocytosis and a case of zinc deficiency have subsequently occurred in Bombay among 104 patients receiving L_1 (Agarwal et al 1993).

Haematological changes

The most serious of the reported L_1-associated adverse reactions are five cases of agranulocytosis three of which have occurred in London (Table 11.5). The

Table 11.5 L_1-induced agranulocytosis

Case	Age(y)/Sex	Diagnosis	Duration on continuous L_1	L_1 dose/day	Time to recovery	Associated features
1	28/F	BDA	6 weeks	105 mg/kg	3 weeks	LW red cell antibody
2	20/F	TM	6 weeks	105 mg/kg	7 weeks	Multiple red cell antibodies
3	63/M	MDS	6 weeks	79 mg/kg	8 days	
4	40/F	MDS	1 year	50 mg/kg	10 days	
5	10/F	TM	10 months	75 mg/kg	7 days	

BDA = Blackfan–Diamond anaemia, TM = thalassaemia major, MDS = myelodysplastic syndrome.

first was a 28-year-old woman with Blackfan–Diamond anaemia who developed agranulocytosis and thrombocytopenia 6 weeks after receiving L_1 at a dose of 105 mg/kg/day (Hoffbrand et al 1989). She had previously received L_1 for 4 months at a lower dose of 50 mg/kg/day and for 3 weeks at 105 mg/kg/day when she developed an LW red cell antibody. Thrombocytopenia recovered 10 days after discontinuing L_1 therapy and agranulocytosis after 3 weeks.

The second case was a 20-year-old woman with TM who developed agranulocytosis 11 weeks after starting L_1 therapy and 6 weeks after being on a full dose (105 mg/kg) (Al-Refaie et al 1993). The patient had pre-existing red cell alloantibodies (anti-D, C, Kell and Kpa). The neutrophil count recovered 7 weeks after discontinuing L_1. The third case, a man of 63 with myelodysplasia and red cell aplasia developed agranulocytosis after receiving L_1 (79 mg/kg/day) for 6 weeks. The agranulocytosis recovered after 8 days. This patient was given G-CSF from the onset of agranulocytosis (unpublished). All three patients suffered severe infections at the time of agranulocytosis and required parenteral antibiotic therapy.

Several experiments have been performed to elucidate the role of L_1 in the pathogenesis of agranulocytosis. When compared with normal individuals, no increased sensitivity of the second patient's bone marrow myeloid progenitors (CFU-GM) to L_1 was found (Cunningham et al 1993). The drug was cleared from plasma and converted to a glucuronide in this patient at the same rate as in other patients and no abnormal metabolite could be detected in plasma or urine by high-performance liquid chromatographic analysis. No evidence for a drug-dependent antimyeloid antibody has been found in plasma obtained during the period of agranulocytosis in either the second or third patients (Al-Refaie et al 1993, Veys et al 1993).

A fourth less severe case of agranulocytosis has been reported in a patient of 40 with myelodysplasia who had received L_1 at a dose of 50 mg/kg/day for a year (Goudsmit 1991, Goudsmit & Kersten 1992). Agranulocytosis recovered within 10 days of discontinuing all drugs including L_1. However re-treatment with L_1 induced no change in white cell count for over one year when agranulocytosis recurred, reversible within five days of stopping L_1. A fifth case of agranulocytosis, lasting one week on G-CSF treatment, occurred in a female TM patient aged 10 years in Bombay 28 months after starting L_1 and 10 months after continuous therapy with L_1 at 75 mg/kg/day (Agarwal et al 1993).

It is not clear why three of the five cases of L_1-associated agranulocytosis have been encountered in London. The drug, which was synthesized at the Royal Free Hospital, has been checked by mass spectroscopy, thin-layer chromatography and elemental analysis and its purity appears to be equivalent to that synthesized at other centres. On balance, it seems most probable that agranulocytosis is due to a toxic mechanism to marrow progenitors occurring in patients with pre-existing fragile white cell production and with individual sensitivity to the drug. A similar mechanism of agranulocytosis has been described for chlorpromazine and other drugs (Pisciotta & Santos 1965, Pisciotta 1965). As mentioned earlier neutropenia is one of the side-effects of L_1 given in high doses long term to experimental animals.

Zinc deficiency

Previous experimental work and animal studies have showed L_1 to be a specific iron chelator with high binding constant for iron (Log β = 36) and lower affinity for other heavy metals such as zinc and copper (Kontoghiorghes 1987). None of the earlier short- and long-term trials reported a change in serum zinc levels or increased urinary zinc excretion. Recently, however, Al-Refaie et al (1992a) reported a decrease of serum zinc levels to subnormal values (<11.5 µmol/l) in four of ten patients after 7–13 months of L_1 therapy. This fall was accompanied by increased 24-hour urinary zinc excretion in eight patients (mean 15.2 ± 5.0 µmol/24 h, range 4.7–23.4 µmol/24 h, normal <9 µmol/24 h). The amount of zinc excreted could not be related to the dose of L_1 or to the iron load of the patients. Two patients became symptomatic with dermatological changes of dry, itchy, scaling patches on the limbs. These disappeared with zinc supplementation (220 mg/day). Several other studies have recently reported zinc deficiency in patients receiving L_1 therapy (Table 11.4). It is known that patients with diabetes mellitus excrete more zinc in the urine than normal individuals (Honnorat et al 1992). As many severely iron overloaded patients have diabetes, increased urinary zinc excretion may therefore be partly attributed to diabetes in these patients. Among the patients studied by Al-Refaie et al (1992a), zinc deficiency was indeed more marked in those with diabetes mellitus. More recently, Fielding et al (1993) have shown that zinc excretion in response to L_1 is most marked in patients with overt diabetes, less so in patients with only biochemical evidence of diabetes and least in patients with normal glucose tolerance.

In view of the infrequency of zinc deficiency in patients receiving L_1, it seems likely that dietary intake of zinc is usually sufficient to prevent the deficiency, despite increased zinc excretion during L_1 therapy, even in diabetic patients. In any event, zinc deficiency with L_1 is a minor problem since it can easily be corrected by oral zinc therapy. Zinc excretion is certainly not of the magnitude encountered in patients receiving the parenteral iron chelator diethyltriamine penta-acetic acid (Pippard et al 1986).

Gastrointestinal symptoms

In all the trials L_1 has generally been well tolerated. However, 15 patients have been reported to have gastrointestinal complaints. Three patients in London developed nausea on starting the treatment or on increasing the dose of L_1. The symptoms lasted for a few days and required no treatment (Al-Refaie et al 1992a). Seven of 52 patients in India complained of minor gastrointestinal symptoms (Agarwal et al 1992a). These included anorexia, nausea (3), altered taste (3), vomiting (2) and epigastric disturbances (2). The symptoms subsided within 15 days with or without antacids and metoclopramide. Two patients, however, required temporary discontinuation of the drug. Other reports of gastrointestinal symptoms in patients receiving L_1 therapy are summarized in Table 11.4.

Liver function

Al-Refaie et al (1992a) reported a transient fluctuating rise of the plasma level of liver AST shortly after the commencement of L_1 therapy in five patients, three of whom were anti-hepatitis C virus (HCV) positive. The AST levels eventually settled in all the patients despite continuation of L_1 therapy. Agarwal et al (1992a) reported fluctuation of the liver enzymes AST and ALT (alanine aminotransferase) in two of their patients. This was attributed in both cases to post-transfusion hepatitis. One patient was positive for hepatitis B surface antigen and HCV antibody while the other patient was persistently negative for both tests. A transient increase in plasma transaminase levels was also reported by Carnelli et al (1992) in five of 22 patients receiving L_1 therapy. These five patients were also found to be anti-HCV positive. Bartlett et al (1990) had previously reported a transient increase in plasma AST in one patient. However, this was considered to be secondary to excessive alcohol consumption and settled on abstinence.

Autoantibodies

In view of the musculoskeletal symptoms in some patients, it is important to exclude drug-induced immune mechanisms. Bartlett et al (1990) reported no change in the incidence of positive antinuclear antibody (ANA) tests in 13 patients (Table 11.4). Two were weakly positive initially (titres 1/40, 1/20), and remained so during the trial. For rheumatoid factor (RhF) there was a rise in the titre (1/80 to 1/160 and 1/80 to 1/640) in two patients with no change in the incidence of positive tests during the trial period. In the second trial in London, Al-Refaie et al (1992a) found minor changes in the incidence and titre of ANA. Initially one patient was positive (titre of 1/160) and another patient weakly positive (titre of 1/40). After 11 months of L_1 three patients were weakly positive (1/40) and one patient was positive at a titre of 1/320. If only those patients with clearly positive ANA (titre >1/80) are considered, there was a change in the titre in only one patient and no increase in incidence of positive tests. In order to assess the significance of these results an unselected group of patients with TM ($n = 51$) were tested for the presence of ANA and RhF. Nine (17.6%) were positive for RhF and none was positive for ANA (Al-Refaie et al 1992a).

Agarwal et al (1992a,b) found a rise in the incidence of positive ANA tests (>1/80) among their 52 patients from 11.5% (six patients) initially to 19.2% (ten patients). There was also a slight rise in the incidence of positive RhF tests (>1/80) from initially 7.7% (four patients) to 11.5% (six patients). Anti-dsDNA antibody was invariably negative while antihistone antibody (AHA) was not tested.

On the other hand, Mehta et al (1991a,b) reported a case they suggested had L_1-induced systemic lupus erythematosus (SLE). An 18-year-old patient with TM taking L_1 had a positive ANA and AHA but was negative for anti-dsDNA antibody. These tests had not been performed before L_1 therapy. The patient's symptoms (low-grade fever, anorexia, nausea, muscle and joint pain and abdominal pain) persisted despite discontinuation of L_1. His ANA titre also increased from 1/80 to 1/160. Subsequently he developed symptoms of a urinary tract infection with anaemia, leukocytosis, haematuria and bacteriuria with urine cultures growing *Klebsiella*. These symptoms improved after starting parenteral antibiotic therapy. He was later given high-dose methylprednisolone but died on the second day of this therapy after developing tachypnoea, cyanosis, bilateral basal crepitations, tachycardia and hypertension. Permission for necropsy was denied.

An association between the fatal outcome of this case and the postulated L_1-induced SLE remains unsubstantiated, however. High doses of corticosteroids have previously been reported to cause sudden cardiac decompensation. This is more likely to occur in a patient with pre-existing heart disease secondary to iron overload. It is also possible that this patient died of septicaemia aggravating cardiac disease.

Mehta et al (1993) reported the presence of the same triad (positive ANA, positive AHA and negative anti-dsDNA) in five of 26 patients receiving L_1. Two of 51 thalassaemic patients not receiving L_1 were found to be positive for ANA and negative for AHA.

In none of the 12 patients studied by Olivieri et al (1991b) who received L_1 for up to 12 months could the development of positive ANA or RhF tests be demonstrated. Prior to the commencement of L_1 three were ANA positive, three were RhF positive and two were positive for both. None of these patients developed ANA or anti-dsDNA antibody during the trial. In a recent report of 15 patients with TM from the same group (Berkovitch et al 1992), ANA converted from negative to positive in three patients who also developed knee joint pain during L_1 therapy but only one patient remained positive despite continuation of L_1, RhF remained negative in all patients. Initially four of the 12 asymptomatic patients on L_1 had positive ANA and one has remained positive. RhF was initially positive in five of the 12 patients and remained positive in four patients. Anti-dsDNA antibody and AHA were negative in the 15 patients throughout the trial. Fifty-three DFX-treated patients with TM were also studied; 17 (32%) were found to have joint symptoms. Autoantibody results were obtainable on 14 of the 17 patients. Three had positive ANA (21%) and one had positive RhF (7%).

In summary, positive ANA and RhF tests are not infrequent findings in patients with TM whether receiving L_1 or DFX. In some studies there has been a slight increase in the incidence and titre of these antibodies among patients receiving L_1 but no consistent pattern of change has been found and no overall association with musculoskeletal pains or with other symptoms suggestive of SLE and the presence of autoantibodies been shown. It is important that careful monitoring for these antibodies and clinical features should be carried out in more patients receiving L_1 long term. Like Berdoukas (1991), we consider that the existence of an L_1-induced SLE syndrome remains unproven.

Deaths

Two patients died during the period of the first trial in London (Bartlett et al 1990). One patient with TM died from congestive heart failure and infection. She had not had L_1 for 5 weeks prior to death. The second patient, with MDS (refractory anaemia with excess of blasts), died from recurrent episodes of infection associated with profound neutropenia (present before commencing L_1) and progression of disease.

In Bombay four patients died during an L_1: one from refractory congestive heart failure and arrhythmia and three from infection (disseminated varicella and fungal infection, pyogenic meningitis, gastroenteritis and possible encephalitis) (Agarwal et al 1992a, b). All four patients were poor compliers with DFX and had high initial serum ferritin levels (8300–12 800 μg/l) and they were all splenectomized. None of them developed neutropenia during the episode of the illness which led to the death. One MDS patient (Kersten M J. Personal communication, 1993) died of infection without agranulocytosis after four months of L_1 therapy.

In summary, no individual appears to have died as a consequence of L_1 therapy. The main adverse effect is agranulocytosis with an incidence so far in long-term trials (> 4 weeks) of about 2%. Preliminary data suggests that G-CSF can be used to shorten the period of agranulocytosis. Whether the advantages of L_1 outweigh the risks depends on further trials but also on the prognosis for the patient when, for one reason or another (hypersensitivity, cost, compliance), DFX is not available.

OTHER POTENTIAL CLINICAL APPLICATIONS OF ORAL IRON CHELATORS

Malaria

The emergence of drug-resistant strains of malaria has resulted in a continuous search for new antimalarial compounds. As malarial parasites require iron for growth (Pollack 1989), several iron chelators have been assessed both in vitro and in vivo for their antimalarial activity. Recently the activity of DFX against human infection with *Plasmodium falciparum* was determined. When DFX was given to adults with asymptomatic parasitaemia, it was associated with a ten-fold enhancement of the rate of parasite clearance compared to placebo (Gordeuk et al 1992a). More recently, Gordeuk et al (1992b) have shown that addition of DFX to conventional antimalarial therapy reduces the duration of parasitaemia and of unconsciousness in patients with cerebral malaria.

CP compounds, like DFX, are known to inhibit the growth in vitro of malarial parasites (Heppner et al 1988). Hershko et al (1991b) studied the antimalarial activity of several CP compounds. The addition of any iron chelator at a concentration of a 5 μmol/l or higher to *P. falciparum* cultures was associated with a dose-related suppression of *P. falciparum*, with a maximal effect observed at a concentration of 20–45 μmol/l at 3 days of culture.

The subcutaneous administration of CP compounds in rats infected with *P. berghei* was associated with segregation of these compounds into two groups: L_1, CP38 and CP40 failed to suppress the malaria, whereas CP51, CP94 and CP96 had strong antimalarial effects, similar to, or better than, DFX. The lipophilic compounds were the most effective in suppressing malaria. However, animals treated with CP94 and CP96 failed to gain weight and with CP51 lost weight in contrast to the animals treated with L_1, CP38, CP40 and DFX where a weight gain was observed. Reduced toxicity, evident as a gain in weight, was achieved when lower doses (40 or 150 mg/kg/day) of the most effective compound (CP51) were used. This, however, was associated with a marked reduction in antimalarial activity. The oral use of CP94 at a dose of 300 mg/kg/day was associated with similar antimalarial activity and toxicity to the parenteral use of the same dose.

The discrepancies between these in vivo and in vitro results were explained by the fact that in vitro exposure to CP compounds was continuous and for 3 days. Therefore there was enough time for all chelators, regardless of their lipid solubility, to achieve a critical intracellular concentration. With in vivo administration, lipid solubility and other factors may become the dominant factors in determining the intracellular concentration of chelator and hence its antimalarial activity.

Anaemia of chronic disorders

The anaemia of chronic disorders is characterized by a low serum iron and total iron-binding capacity and increased iron stores with reduced iron incorporation into erythroblasts. The pathogenesis of this anaemia is thought to be related to cytokine release which results in decreased iron absorption, decreased iron release from macrophages (Beamish et al 1971), reduced red cell life span and inadequate erythropoietin response to anaemia (Vreugdenhil et al 1990a). Iron chelator drugs have been used in an attempt to increase iron transfer from endothelial cells to erythroblasts.

Giordano et al (1984) observed a significant increase in haemoglobin 24 hours after a single intramuscular injection of 1 g of DFX to patients with rheumatoid arthritis. This was sustained for the 2-week period of the study.

When L_1 was used at a dose of 2 g twice daily in six anaemic patients with rheumatoid arthritis for 3 weeks, a slight rise in haemoglobin was also observed with a significant increase in serum iron (Vreugdenhil et al 1989). In order to establish the mechanism of this L_1-associated antianaemic effect, Vreugdenhil et al (1990b) studied iron exchange between L_1 and transferrin and found that L_1 is able to remove a substantial amount of iron from transferrin, confirming earlier results by Hewitt et al (1989). However, it was also found that apotransferrin can remove iron from L_1. The direction of iron movement between L_1 and transferrin depended on their relative concentrations. It was therefore suggested that L_1 may mediate iron exchange between ferritin and transferrin resulting in more iron being available to erythroblasts. Alternatively L_1 may directly incorporate iron into erythroblasts.

Similar observations have been made by Evans et al (1992) when they studied time-dependent changes in the iron saturation of transferrin in serum samples taken from an iron overloaded patient and a normal volunteer who had taken L_1 orally. A decrease in transferrin saturation was observed within 1–3 hours in the patient's serum, whereas the reverse was observed in the normal volunteer 4–7 hours after L_1 administration.

In a later study, Vreugdenhil et al (1991) compared the iron-mobilizing and antianaemic effects of L_1 with those of erythropoietin. L_1 was given to six anaemic patients with rheumatoid arthritis at a dose of 2 g b.d. for 3 weeks; erythropoietin was given to ten similar patients at a dose of 240 U/kg s.c. three times per week for 3 weeks. In the erythropoietin group serum iron decreased from 5 to 2 µmol/l, transferrin increased from 43 to 50 µmol/l and ferritin fell from 180 to 118 µg/l (34%). In the L_1 group serum iron increased from 6 to 12 µmol/l and transferrin from 50 to 52 µmol/l, while serum ferritin fell from 118 to 78 µg/l. The increase in haemoglobin in the erythropoietin group was more pronounced than in the L_1 group (15% versus 7%). The authors concluded that L_1 has an iron-mobilizing effect comparable to that of erythropoietin although the underlying mechanism is different. They suggested that L_1 might enhance the effect of erythropoietin in the treatment of the anaemia of chronic disorders.

Free radical formation and related diseases

Iron is known to be effective in catalysing the formation of potentially toxic oxygen derivatives (Halliwell & Gutteridge 1986) which in turn have been implicated in the pathogenesis of several diseases such as rheumatoid arthritis (Blake et al 1984) and postischaemic perfusion injury (McCord 1987). DFX has been shown to suppress both acute and chronic inflammation in animal models (Yoshino et al 1984). However, a therapeutic trial of DFX in patients with rheumatoid arthritis had to be discontinued because of ocular and cerebral toxicity (Blake et al 1985). Giordano et al (1986) found a moderate improvement in several physical indices with improvement in joint function which lasted up to 6 weeks after DFX administration to patients with rheumatoid arthritis.

CP compounds have also been examined for their anti-inflammatory properties. Using a rat model of inflammation with acute pleurisy induced by carrageenin, Hewitt et al (1989) found that the most hydrophillic compounds were associated with the best anti-inflammatory effects. This effect was dose dependent. L_1 possessed the highest anti-inflammatory activity when administered by any route (i.p., i.g., s.c.) whereas other CP compounds were less effective especially after oral administration.

L_1 has also been shown to cause a slight improvement in serological and clinical indices in rheumatoid arthritis (Vreugdenhil et al 1991). Bartlett et al (1990) also noted a partial improvement with L_1 therapy in joint swelling and pain in a patient with MDS and arthritis. Further studies are clearly needed to establish whether there is a role for L_1 and other CP compounds in the treatment of rheumatoid arthritis and other diseases associated with iron-induced free radical formation.

Chelation of aluminium and other metals

DFX is effective in mobilizing aluminium in chronic renal failure patients with aluminium overload secondary to chronic dialysis (Brown et al 1982). However, the use of DFX in these patients was associated with increased visual and auditory toxicity (Cases et al 1988). The hydroxypyridines are as effective as DFX in binding aluminium (Sheppard & Kontoghiorghes 1989). In a preliminary study (Kontoghiorghes & Barr 1989) the effect of L_1 on aluminium mobilization was examined in 11 renal dialysis patients with aluminium overload (0.7–9.8 μmol/l) using a single oral dose of L_1 (1.5–3 g). In most patients plasma aluminium increased by 20–100% within the first few hours after L_1 administration but it then reached basal levels or decreased

24 hours later. In one patient an increase of aluminium in the peritoneal dialysis fluid was found.

Elorriaga et al (1991) found that L_1 given at a single dose of 200 mg/kg was able to remove a great amount of aluminium in aluminium-intoxicated rats with or without renal failure and there was a great increase in aluminium clearance (P<0.05). This single dose of L_1 was able to remove about 5% of the total aluminium body burden when the drug was given i.p. and about 4% when it was given orally. With more prolonged L_1 administration (6 weeks), L_1 was able to reduce aluminium in bone from values higher than 2.3 µmol/g to 1.1 µmol/g.

L_1 is therefore an effective aluminium chelator and if its long-term safety in these patients is established it has the potential to replace DFX in the treatment of aluminium overload in patients with chronic renal failure.

L_1 has also been shown to be effective in chelating other metals including plutonium (Taylor et al 1989), indium (Eybl et al 1989) and gallium (Eybl et al 1992).

OTHER ORAL IRON CHELATORS

HBED

HBED [N, N'-bis(o-hydroxybenzyl)ethylenediamine-N, N'-diacetic acid] (Fig. 11.1C) is a synthetic hexadentate ligand with high affinity to ferric ion (stability constant: Log β = 40). Affinity for other metals is lower than for iron but still appreciable, e.g. copper (10^{21}) and zinc (10^{18}) (l'Eplattenier et al 1967). Oral activity of HBED in animals is low but its dimethyl ester (dmHBED) possesses greater oral potency (Hershko et al 1984, Pitt et al 1986). The results of the animal studies in rats, mice and dogs were reviewed by Grady & Hershko (1990a,b). Orally administered HBED is about 70% as active in iron overloaded rats as an equivalent dose of DFX given parenterally whereas a similar oral dose of dmHBED is associated with four times greater iron excretion. The pattern of iron excretion in response to both compounds is similar to that with DFX, with the bulk of the iron appearing in the faeces.

The LD_{50} of both compounds exceeds 800 mg/kg when given orally or parenterally to normal mice. The oral or parenteral administration of HBED to normal mice at a dose of 200 mg/kg/day for 10 weeks was associated with growth reduction compared to that of control animals. No other evidence of toxicity was found. In rats the administration of HBED i.p. at doses up to 200 mg/kg/day for 12 weeks was not associated with toxicity whereas the oral administration of HBED at doses of 0.2% and 0.4% of the diet was associated with a significant decrease in growth rate and also in red cell count, haemoglobin, haematocrit and MCV. These changes were considered to reflect HBED-mediated iron deficiency. Abnormalities in serum biochemical measurements were also observed. Finally, there was no evidence of toxicity when HBED was administered at a dose of 100 mg/kg/day to beagle dogs for 6 weeks.

HBED appears to be a reasonably safe chelator, therefore, with a somewhat low oral efficacy compared to DFX. The dimethyl ester derivative is much more potent but is expensive to prepare and its chronic toxicity in animals has not yet been evaluated.

Desferrithiocin (DFT)

This is a naturally occurring siderophore isolated from *Streptomyces antibioticus* (Fig. 11.1D). Its tridentate molecule forms a 2:1 complex with ferric ion. It has high affinity and selectivity for iron (Log β = 30) (Wolfe 1990). The oral efficacy of DFT in iron overloaded rats was shown to be three times more than that of DFX given parenterally (Longueville & Crichton 1986). The chelation efficiency of DFT was estimated at 32.5% in iron overloaded monkeys (Bergeron et al 1990) compared to 6–28% in iron overloaded rats (Longueville & Crichton 1986).

Despite excellent oral efficacy this compound has shown significant toxicity in hepatocyte cultures (Baker et al 1985) and animal studies (Porter et al 1989). It has an LD_{50} of 300 mg/kg when given i.g. or s.c. to normal mice, whereas in normal rats the LD_{50} is lower at 227 mg/kg s.c. and 112 mg/kg i.p. (Porter et al 1989). Furthermore, long-term studies in rats and dogs showed significant toxicity including decreased body weight, renal dysfunction and neurological symptoms (Wolfe 1990).

In a recent study (Baker et al 1992a) the efficacy of DFT was further confirmed, but more evidence of toxicity was revealed. When ^{59}Fe-labelled ferrithiocin (DFT–iron chelate) was incubated with hepatocytes in culture, it was found to be a more effective donor of iron to hepatocytes than ^{59}Fe–transferrin and ^{59}Fe–DFX chelate (3.5 and 11.7 times respectively). In contrast to transferrin–iron and DFX–iron chelate, most of the iron donated from ferrithiocin was found in the membrane fraction of the cell. This was associated with increased cytotoxicity as evidenced by membrane disruption and increase in AST release. As a result of this apparent toxicity both in vitro and in vivo, DFT has been considered inappropriate for clinical application (Porter et al 1989, Baker et al 1992a).

PIH

PIH (pyridoxal isonicotinoyl hydrazone) (Fig. 11.1E), a tridentate ligand, is one of a family of aromatic hydrazones. It has high selectivity for binding to ferric ion with which it forms 2:1 complex with a stability constant (log β) of 28. The iron–PIH_2 complex breaks down as the pH of the solution reaches a value of about 2 (Brittenham 1990). PIH has been shown to be effective in vitro in mobilizing iron from macrophages, reticulocytes and hepatocytes (Ponka et al 1988, Baker et al 1992b). PIH has also been assessed in animal studies (Cikrt et al 1980, Hershko et al 1981, Williams et al 1982, Brittenham 1990, Gale et al 1991, Sookvanichsilp et al 1991). Studies in rats have shown that PIH (i.p. or i.g.) takes up iron from hepatocytes and enters bile as an iron–PIH_2 complex. Maximum biliary excretion was achieved at a dose of 2×125 mg/kg i.p. This was comparable to that induced by an equivalent dose of DFX (Cikrt et al 1980). However, no reduction in hepatic iron stores was observed when the drug was given orally to iron overloaded rats at a dose of 100 mg/kg/day for 10 weeks (Williams et al 1982). Recently, the oral efficacy of PIH in iron overloaded mice was compared with that of oral L_1 and i.p. DFX, each chelator being given at a dose of 300 mg/kg/day for 4 days. Total iron excreted over the 4-day period, expressed as µg/mouse, was: controls, 26; PIH, 31; DFX, 162; L_1, 208 (Gale et al 1991). The LD_{50} values of PIH in mice and rats were 5 and 1 g/kg given orally and i.p. respectively (Sookvanichsilp et al 1991). PIH was not associated with significant acute and chronic toxicity when administered to normal rats at a dose of 100 mg/kg/day for 2 weeks (Brittenham 1990).

Recently, PIH has been evaluated in phase I clinical trial in five normal and ten iron overloaded volunteers (Brittenham 1990). At an oral dose of up to 30 mg/kg/day for 2 weeks, PIH was associated with minimal side-effects. No haematological, biochemical, ophthalmological or audiological abnormalities developed. When administered to iron overloaded volunteers at a dose of 600 mg 8 hourly for 6 days, it was associated with a mean UIE of 0.12 ± 0.07 mg/kg/day. This disappointingly low chelation efficiency of PIH in man is insufficient to produce negative iron balance in patients with transfusional siderosis. It is probably due to reduced bioavailability of the drug (Brittenham 1990). Therefore, the search continues for other analogues of the drug which possess greater oral efficacy, although PIH may have some clinical value in iron overloaded patients not requiring regular transfusions, e.g. with thalassaemia intermedia.

KEY POINTS FOR CLINICAL PRACTICE

- A safe, cheap, orally active iron chelator is needed for patients who because of hypersensitivity, cost or lack of compliance cannot use desferrioxamine.
- Short- and long-term clinical trials have shown that iron chelation can now be carried out effectively with orally active drugs.
- L_1 (1,2-dimethyl-3-hydroxypyrid-4-one; CP20) is the most widely studied compound. It causes daily urine iron excretion equivalent to that of subcutaneous desferrioxamine given at the same or a 50% smaller daily dose.
- Iron excretion induced by L_1 is probably entirely via the urine.
- Long-term trials in patients with thalassaemia major, myelodysplasia, red cell aplasia, sickle cell anaemia and other conditions have shown that L_1 can reduce body iron stores despite continuing blood transfusions.

- The main adverse effects encountered have been agranulocytosis, musculoskeletal symptoms, gastrointestinal intolerance and zinc deficiency.
- It seems likely that L_1 or another orally active iron chelating agent will become commercially available. However, these compounds remain experimental and should only be administered to patients in the context of Ethical Committee approved trials.

REFERENCES

Agarwal M B, Gupte S S, Viswanathan C et al 1992a Long-term assessment of efficacy and safety of L_1, an oral iron chelator, in transfusion dependent thalassaemia: Indian trial. Br J Haematol 82: 460–466

Agarwal M B, Gupte S S, Viswanathan C et al 1992b Long-term assessment of efficacy and toxicity of L_1 (1,2-dimethyl-3-hydroxypyrid-4-one) in transfusion dependent thalassaemia: Indian trials. Drugs of Today 28 (Suppl A): 107–114

Agarwal M B, Gupte S S, Viswanathan C et al 1993 Long-term efficacy and toxicity of L_1-oral iron chelator in transfusion dependent thalassaemics over the last three years. Abstracts of the 5th International Conference of Thalassaemias and the Haemoglobinopathies, Nicosia, Cyprus, p 192

Al-Refaie F N, Wonke B, Hoffbrand A V et al 1992a Efficacy and possible adverse effects of the oral iron chelator 1,2-dimethyl-3-hydroxypyrid-4-one (L_1) in thalassaemia major. Blood 80: 593–599

Al-Refaie F N, Wickens D G, Wonke B et al 1992b Serum non-transferrin-bound iron in beta-thalassaemia major patients treated with desferrioxamine and L_1. Br J Haematol 82: 431–436

Al-Refaie F N, Veys P A, Wilkes S et al 1993 Agranulocytosis in a patient with thalassaemia major during treatment with oral iron chelator 1,2-dimethyl-3-hydroxypyrid-4-one. Acta Haematol (in press)

Baker E, Vitolo M L, Webb J 1985 Iron chelation by pyridoxal isonocotinol hydrazone and analogoues in hepatocytes in culture. Biochem Pharmacol 34: 3011–3017

Baker E, Wong A, Peter H et al 1992a Desferrithiocin is an effective iron chelator in vivo and in vitro but ferrithiocin is toxic. Br J Haematol 81: 424–431

Baker E, Richardson D, Gross S et al 1992b Evaluation of the iron chelation potential of hydrazones of pyridoxal, salicylaldehyde and 2-hydroxyl-1-naphthylaldehyde using the hepatocyte in culture. Hepatology 15: 492–501

Bartlett A N, Hoffbrand A V, Kontoghiorghes G J 1990 Long-term trial with the oral iron chelator 1,2-dimethyl-3-hydroxypyrid-4-one (L_1) II. Clinical observations. Br J Haematol 76: 301–304

Beamish M R, Davis A G, Eakins J D et al 1971 The measurement of reticuloendothelial iron release using iron–dextran. Br J Haematol 21: 617–622

Berdoukas V 1991 Antinuclear antibodies in patients taking L_1. Lancet 337: 672

Bergeron R J, Streiff R R, Wiegand J et al 1990 A comparative evaluation of iron clearance models. Ann NY Acad Sci 612: 378–393

Bergeron R J, Streiff R R, Wiegand J et al 1992 A comparison of the iron-chelating properties of 1,2-dimethyl-3-hydroxypyrid-4-one and deferoxamine. Blood 79: 1882–1890

Berkovitch M, Laxer R M, Matsui D et al 1992 Analysis of adverse rheumatologic effects of iron chelators in patients with homozygous beta thalassaemia (HBT). Blood 80 (Suppl 1): 7a

Blake D R, Gallagher P J, Potter A R et al 1984 The effect of synovial iron on the progression of rheumatoid disease. Arthritis Rheum 27: 495–501

Blake D R, Winyard P, Lunec J et al 1985 Cerebral and ocular toxicity induced by desferrioxamine. Q J Med 219: 345–355

Brittenham G M 1990 Pyridoxal isonicotinoyl hydrazone: an effective iron-chelator after oral administration. Semin Hematol 27: 112–116

Brittenham G M 1992 Development of iron-chelating agents for clinical use. Blood 80: 569–574

Brown D J, Ham K N, Dawborn J K et al 1982 Treatment of dialysis osteomalacia with desferrioxamine. Lancet ii: 343–345

Carnelli V, Spadaro C, Stefano V et al 1992 L_1 efficacy and toxicity in poorly compliant and/or refractory to desferrioxamine thalassaemia patients: interim report. Drugs of Today 28 (Suppl A): 119–121

Cases A, Kelly J, Sabater J et al 1988 Acute visual and auditory neurotoxicity in patients with end-stage renal disease receiving desferrioxamine. Clin Nephrol 29: 176–178

Cikrt M, Ponka P, Necas E et al 1980 Biliary iron excretion in rats following pyridoxal isonicotinoyl hydrazone. Br J Haematol 45: 275–283

Collins A F, Fassos F, Stobie S et al 1992 Iron balance and dose response studies of the oral iron chelator 1,2-dimethyl-3-hydroxypyrid-4-one (L_1) in iron-loaded patients with sickle cell disease (SCD). Blood 80 (Suppl 1): 80a

Cunningham J M, Hunter A B, Hoffbrand A V et al 1993 Differential toxicity of α-ketohydroxypyridine iron chelators and desferrioxamine to human hemopoietic precursors in vitro. (manuscript in preparation)

Elorriaga R, Alonso M, Olaizola I et al 1991 Effect of L_1 in aluminium removal: short and long-term experimental studies. Abstracts of the 3rd International Conference on Oral Chelators, Nice, France, p 8

Evans R W, Sharma M, Ogwang W et al 1992 The effect of alpha-ketohydroxypyridine chelators on transferrin saturation in vitro and in vivo. Drugs of Today 28 (Suppl A): 19–23

Eybl V, Koutenska M, Koutensky J et al 1989 Interaction of the 1,2-dialkyl-3-hydroxypyridin-4-one chelators with indium in vivo. Abstracts of the 1st International Symposium on Oral Chelation in the Treatment of Thalassaemia and Other Diseases, London, p 16

Eybl V, Svihovcova P, Koutensky J et al 1992 Interaction of L_1, L_1NAll and deferoxamine with gallium in vivo. Drugs of Today 28 (Suppl A): 173–175

Fielding A, Wonke B, Wickens D G et al 1993 Zinc excretion in thalassaemia major patients receiving the oral chelator 1,2-dimethyl-3-hydroxypyrid-4-one correlates with diabetic status. Br J Haematol 84 (Suppl 1): 65

Florence A, Ward R J, Peters T J et al 1992 Studies of in vivo iron mobilization by chelators in the ferrocene-loaded rat. Biochem Pharmacol 44: 1023–1027

Gale G R, Litchenberg W H, Smith A B et al 1991 Comparative iron mobilizing actions of deferoxamine, 1,2-dimethyl-3-hydroxypyrid-4-one and pyridoxal isonicotinoyl hydrazone in iron hydroxamate-loaded mice. Res Commun Chem Pathol Pharmacol 73: 299–313

Ganeshaguru K, Lally J M, Piga A et al 1992 Cytotoxic mechanisms of iron chelators. Drugs of Today 28 (Suppl A): 29–34

Giordano N, Fioravanti A, Sancasciani S et al 1984 Increased storage of iron and anaemia in rheumatoid arthritis: usefulness of desferrioxamine. Br Med J 289: 961–962

Giordano N, Sancasciani S, Borghi C et al 1986 Antianaemic and potential anti-inflammatory activity of desferrioxamine: possible usefulness in rheumatoid arthritis. Clin Exp Rheumatol 4: 25–29

Goddard J G, Kontoghiorghes G J 1989 Pharmacological studies of the orally active iron chelator 1,2-dimethyl-3-hydroxypyrid-4-one (L_1) in man. Abstracts of the 1st International Symposium on Oral Chelation in the Treatment of Thalassaemia and Other Diseases, London, p 38

Gordeuk V R, Thuma P E, Brittenham G M et al 1992a Iron chelation with desferrioxamine B in adults with asymptomatic *Plasmodium falciparum* parasitemia. Blood 79: 308–312

Gordeuk V, Thuma P, Brittenham G et al 1992b Effect of iron chelation therapy on recovery from deep coma in children with cerebral malaria. N Engl J Med 327: 1473–1477

Goudsmit R 1991 The oral iron chelator 1,2-dimethyl-3-hydroxypyrid-4-one (L_1), in the treatment of transfusion haemosiderosis. Ned Tijdschr Geneeskd 135 (45): 2133–2136

Goudsmit R, Kersten M J 1992 Long-term treatment of transfusion hemosiderosis with the oral iron chelator L_1. Drugs of Today 28 (Suppl A): 133–135

Grady R W, Hershko C 1990a An evaluation of the potential of HBED as an orally effective iron-chelating drug. Semin Hematol 27: 105–111

Grady R W, Hershko C 1990b HBED: a potential oral iron chelator. Ann NY Acad Sci 612: 361–368

Grady R W, Srinivasan R, Lemert R F et al 1991 DMHP (L_1) and DEHP (CP94): evidence of toxicity in rats. Abstracts of the 3rd International Conference on Oral Chelators, Nice, France, p 11

Grady R W, Srinivasan R, Dunn J B et al 1992 Evidence of toxicity due to 1, 2-dimethyl-3-hydroxypyrid-4-one (L_1) in normal rats. Drugs of Today 28 (Suppl A): 73–79

Gutteridge J M C, Rowley D A, Griffiths E et al 1985 Low-molecular weight iron complexes and oxygen radical reactions in idiopathic haemochromatosis. Clin Sci 68: 463–467

Gyparaki M, Porter J B, Hirani S et al 1987 In vivo evaluation of hydroxypyridone iron chelators in a mouse model. Acta Haematol 78: 217–221

Halliwell B, Gutteridge J M C 1986 Oxygen, free radicals and iron in relation to biology and medicine: some problems and concepts. Arch Biochem Biophys 246: 501–514

Heppner D G, Hallaway P E, Kontoghiorghes G J et al 1988 Antimalarial properties of orally active iron chelators. Blood 72: 358–361

Hershko C (ed) 1989 Iron chelating therapy. Clin Haematol 2: 195–501

Hershko C, Avramovici-Grisaru S, Link G et al 1981 Mechanism of in vivo iron chelation by pyridoxal isonicotinoyl hydrazone and other imino derivatives of pyridoxal. J Lab Clin Med 98: 99–108

Hershko C, Grady R W, Link G 1984 Phenolic ethyldiamine derivatives: a study of orally effective iron chelators. J Lab Clin Med 103: 337–346

Hershko C, Link G, Pinson A et al 1991a Iron mobilization from myocardial cells by 3-hydroxypyridin-4-one chelators: studies in rat heart cells in culture. Blood 77: 2049–2053

Hershko C, Theanacho E N, Spira D T et al 1991b The effect of N-alkyl modification on the antimalarial activity of 3-hydroxypyridin-4-one oral iron chelators. Blood 77: 637–643

Hewitt S D, Hider R C, Sarpong P et al 1989 Investigation of the anti-inflammatory properties of hydroxypyridinones. Ann Rheum Dis 48: 382–388

Hoffbrand A V, Ganeshaguru K, Hooton J W L et al 1976 Effect of iron deficiency and desferrioxamine on DNA synthesis in human cells. Br J Haematol 33: 517–526

Hoffbrand A V, Bartlett A N, Veys P A et al 1989 Agranulocytosis and thrombocytopenia in patient with Blackfan-Diamond anaemia during oral chelator trial. Lancet ii: 457

Honnorat J, Accominoti M, Broussolle C et al 1992 Effect of diabetes type and treatment on zinc status in diabetes mellitus. Biol Trace Elem Res 32: 311–316

Jaeger M, Aul C, Sohngen D et al 1991 Iron overload in polytransfused patients with MDS: use of L_1 for oral iron chelation. Abstracts of the 3rd International Conference on Oral Chelators, Nice, France, p 22

Kontoghiorghes G J 1987 Orally active alpha-ketohydroxypyridine iron chelators: effect on iron and other metal mobilisations. Acta Haematol 78: 212–216

Kontoghiorghes G J 1990 Design, properties and effective use of the oral chelator L_1 and other α-ketohydroxypyridines in the treatment of transfusional iron overload in thalassaemia. Ann NY Acad Sci 612: 339–350

Kontoghiorghes G J 1992 Advances in oral iron chelation in man. Int J Hematol 55: 27–38

Kontoghiorghes G J, Barr J 1989 Preliminary studies of aluminum removal in haemodialysis and peritoneal dialysis patients using 1,2-dimethyl-3-hydroxypyrid-4-one (L_1). Abstracts of the 1st International Symposium on Oral Chelation in the Treatment of Thalassaemia and Other Diseases, London, p 19

Kontoghiorghes G J, Hoffbrand A V 1986 Orally active α-ketohydroxypyridine iron chelators intended for clinical use: in vivo studies in rabbits. Br J Haematol 62: 607–613

Kontoghiorghes G J, Hoffbrand A V 1988 Prospects for effective and oral chelation in transfusional iron overload. Rec Adv Haematol 5: 75–98

Kontoghiorghes G J, Hoffbrand A V 1989 Clinical trials with oral iron chelator L_1. Lancet ii: 1398–1399

Kontoghiorghes G J, Sheppard L, Hoffbrand A V et al 1987a Iron chelation studies using desferrioxamine and the potential oral chelator, 1,2-dimethyl-3-hydroxypyridine-4-one, in normal and iron overloaded rats. J Clin Pathol 40: 404–408

Kontoghiorghes G J, Aldouri M A, Hoffbrand A V et al 1987b Effective chelation of iron in thalassaemia with the oral chelator 1,2-dimethyl-3-hydroxypyrid-4-one. Br Med J 295: 1509–1512

Kontoghiorghes G J, Aldouri M A, Sheppard L et al 1987c 1,2-Dimethyl-3-

hydroxypyrid-4-one an orally active chelator for the treatment of transfusional iron overload. Lancet i: 1294–1295

Kontoghiorghes G J, Nasseri-Sina P, Goddard G J et al 1989 Safety of oral iron chelator L$_1$. Lancet ii: 457–458

Kontoghiorghes G J, Bartlett A N, Hoffbrand A V et al 1990a Long-term trial with the oral iron chelator 1,2-dimethyl-3-hydroxypyrid-4-one (L$_1$). I. Iron chelation and metabolic studies. Br J Haematol 75: 295–300

Kontoghiorghes G J, Goddard G, Bartlett A N et al 1990b Pharmacokinetic studies in humans with the oral iron chelator 1,2-dimethyl-3-hydroxypyrid-4-one. Clin Pharmacol Ther 48: 255–261

l'Eplattenier F, Murase I, Martell A E 1967 New multidentate ligands. VI. Chelating tendencies of N,N'-di(2-hydroxybenzyl)ethylenediamine-N,N'-diacetic acid. J Am Chem Soci 89: 837–843

Longueville A, Crichton R R 1986 An animal model of iron overload and its application to study hepatic ferritin iron mobilization by chelators. Biochem Pharmacol 35: 3669–3678

McCord J M 1987 Oxygen-derived radicals: a link between reperfusion injury and inflammation. Fed Proc 46: 2402–2406

Matsui D, Klein J, Hermann C et al 1991 Relationship between the pharmacokinetics and iron excretion pharmacodynamics of the new oral iron chelator 1,2-dimethyl-3-hydroxypyrid-4-one in patients with thalassaemia. Clin Pharmacol Ther 50: 294–298

Mehta J, Singhal S, Revankar R et al 1991a Fatal systemic lupus erythematosus in patient taking oral iron chelator L$_1$. Lancet 337: 298

Mehta J, Singhal S, Chablani A et al 1991b L$_1$-induced systemic lupus erythematosus. Indian J Hematol Blood Transfus 9: 33–37

Mehta J, Singhal S, Mehta B C 1993 Oral iron chelator L$_1$ and autoimmunity. Blood 81: 1970–1971

Neuman M G, Klein J, Koren G et al 1991 Oral iron chelator L$_1$ induces its metabolism in vitro in human hepatocyte lines. Proceedings of the Sixteenth World Congress of Anatomic and Clinical Pathology, Vancouver, p 15

Nortey P, Barr J, Matsakis M et al 1992 Effect on iron excretion and animal toxicology of L$_1$ and other alpha-ketohydroxypyridine chelators. Drugs of Today 28 (Suppl A): 81–88

Olivieri N F, Koren G, Hermann C et al 1990 Comparison of oral iron chelator L$_1$ and desferrioxamine in iron-loaded patients. Lancet 336: 1275–1279

Olivieri N F, Koren G, Matsui D et al 1991a Oral iron chelation with 1,2-dimethyl-3-hydroxypyrid-4-one (L$_1$) in thalassaemia major: one year comparison with subcutaneous desferrioxamine. Blood 78 (Suppl 1): 369a

Olivieri N F, Koren G, Freedman M H et al 1991b Rarity of systemic lupus erythematosus after oral iron chelator L$_1$. Lancet 337: 924

Olivieri N F, Matsui D, Berkovitch M et al 1992a Superior effectiveness of the oral iron chelator L$_1$ vs. subcutaneous deferoxamine in patients with homozygous beta-thalassaemia (HBT): the impact of patient compliance during two years of therapy. Blood 80 (Suppl 1): 344a

Olivieri N F, Koren G, Maltsui D et al 1992b Reduction of tissue iron stores and normalization of serum ferritin during treatment with the oral iron chelator L$_1$ in thalassaemia intermedia. Blood 79: 2741–2748

Pattanapanyasat K, Webster H K, Tongtawe P et al 1992 Effect of orally active hydroxypyridinone iron chelators on human lymphocyte function. Br J Haematol 82: 13–19

Pippard M J, Jackson M J, Hoffman K et al 1986 Iron chelation using subcutaneous infusions of diethylene triamine penta-acetic acid (DTPA). Scand J Haematol 36: 466–472

Pisciotta A V 1965 Studies on agranulocytosis. VII. Limited proliferative potential of CPZ-sensitive patients. J Lab Clin Med 65: 241–247

Pisciotta A V, Santos A S 1965 Studies on agranulocytosis. VI. The effect of clinical treatment with chlorpromazine on nucleic-acid synthesis of granulocyte precursors in normal persons. J Lab Clin Med 65: 228–240

Pitt C G, Bao Y, Thompson J et al 1986 Esters and lactones of phenolic amino carboxylic acids: prodrugs for iron chelation. J Med Chem 29: 1231–1237

Pollack S 1989 P. falciparum iron metabolism. Malaria and the red cell: 2. Proceedings of the Second Workshop on Malaria and the Red Cell, pp 151–161

Ponka P, Richardson D, Baker E et al 1988 Effect of pyridoxal isonicotinoyl hydrazone and other hydrazones on iron release from macrophages, reticulocytes and hepatocytes. Biochim Biophys Acta 967: 122–129

Porter J B, Gyparaki M, Burke L C et al 1988 Iron mobilization from hepatocyte monolayer cultures by chelators: the importance of membrane permeability and the iron binding constant. Blood 72: 1497–1503

Porter J, Huens E, Hider R 1989 The development of iron chelating drugs. Baillières Clin Haematol 2: 257–292

Porter J B, Morgan J, Hoyes K P et al 1990 Relative oral efficacy and acute toxicity of hydroxypyridin-4-one iron chelators in mice. Blood 76: 2389–2396

Porter J B, Hoyes K P, Abeysinghe R D et al 1991 Comparison of the subacute toxicity and efficacy of 3-hydroxypyridin-4-one iron chelators in overloaded and nonoverloaded mice. Blood 78: 2727–2734

Sheppard L N, Kontoghiorghes G J 1989 New generation of α-ketohydroxypyridine iron chelators intended for clinical use and their metal binding properties. Abstracts of the 1st International Symposium on Oral Chelation in the Treatment of Thalassaemia and Other Diseases, London, p 2

Sheppard L N, Kontoghiorghes G J 1992 Synthesis and metabolism of L_1 and other novel α-ketohydroxypyridine iron chelators and their metal complexes. Drugs of Today 28 (Suppl A): 3–10

Singh S, Hider R C, Porter J B 1990 A direct method for quantification of non-transferrin-bound iron. Anal Biochem 186: 320–323

Sookvanichsilp N, Nakornchai S, Weerapradist W 1991 Toxicological study of pyridoxal isonicotinoyl hydrazone: acute and subchronic toxicity. Drug Chem Toxicol 14: 395–403

Taylor D M, Volf V, Kontoghiorghes G J 1989 Investigation of some hydroxypyridone derivatives as oral chelators for the treatment of plutonium poisoning. Abstracts of the 1st International Symposium on Oral Chelation in the Treatment of Thalassaemia and Other Diseases, London, p 17

Töndury P, Kontoghiorghes G J, Ridolfi-Lüthy A et al 1990 L_1 (1,2-dimethyl-3-hydroxypyrid-4-one) for oral iron chelation in patients with beta-thalassaemia major. Br J Haematol 76: 550–553

Töndury P, Wagner H P, Kontoghiorghes G J 1992 Update of long-term clinical trials with L_1 in Beta-thalassaemia major patients in Bern, Switzerland. Drugs of Today 28 (Suppl A): 115–117

Venkataram S, Rahman Y E 1990 Studies of an oral iron chelator: 1,2-dimethyl-3-hydroxypyrid-4-one. Br J Haematol 75: 274–277

Veys P A, Wilkes S, Al-Refaie F N et al 1993 The mechanism of agranulocytosis mediated by the oral iron chelator L_1. Br J Haematol 84 (Suppl 1): 64

Vreugdenhil G, Swaak A J G, Kontoghiorghes G J et al 1989 Efficacy and safety of oral iron chelator L_1 in anaemic rheumatoid arthritis patients. Lancet ii: 1398–1399

Vreugdenhil G, Wognum A W, van Eijk H G et al 1990a Anaemia in rheumatoid arthritis: the role of iron, vitamin B12, and folic acid deficiency, and erythropoietin responsiveness. Ann Rheum Dis 49: 93–98

Vreugdenhil G, Swaak A J G, De Jeu-Jaspars C et al 1990b Correlation of iron exchange between the oral iron chelator 1,2-dimethyl-3-hydroxypyrid-4-one (L_1) and transferrin and possible antianaemic effects of L_1 in rheumatoid arthritis. Ann Rheum Dis 49: 956–957

Vreugdenhil G, Nieuwenhuizen C, Swaak A J G 1991 EPO and L_1 have comparable iron mobilizing effects in rheumatoid arthritis. Abstracts of the 3rd International Conference on Oral Chelators, Nice, France, p 17

Williams A, Hoy T, Pugh A et al 1982 Pyridoxal complexes as potential chelating agents for oral therapy in transfusional overload. J Pharmacol 24: 730–733

Wolfe L C 1990 Desferrithiocin. Semin Hematol 27: 117–120

Yoshino S, Blake D R, Bacon P A 1984 The effect of desferrioxamine on antigen induced inflammation in the rat air pouch. J Pharm Pharmacol 36: 543–545

Zevin S, Link G, Grady R W et al 1992 Origin and fate of iron mobilized by the 3-hydroxypyridin-4-one oral chelators: studies in hypertransfused rats by selective radioiron probes of reticuloendothelial and hepatocellular iron stores. Blood 79: 248–253

12

Familial thrombophilia

F. E. Preston   E. Briët

The coagulation system is essentially a series of linked reactions involving zymogens, their respective serine proteases and cofactors. The system is controlled through a series of feedback mechanisms and by the action of inhibitors. The functions of the coagulation system are closely linked to those of the fibrinolytic system with fibrin being the natural substrate for the fibrinolytic enzyme, plasmin.

It is only within recent years that the physiological and clinical importance of blood coagulation inhibitors has become appreciated. Although antithrombin deficiency was first described in 1965, it was not until the 1980s, following the first reports of familial deficiencies of protein C and protein S, that coagulation inhibitors became generally recognized as being at least as important as procoagulants in the pathogenesis of venous thromboembolism.

Although a number of groups have provided estimates of the prevalence of familial thrombophilia, these have varied widely and the true figure remains unknown (Gladson et al 1988, Ben Tal et al 1989, Heijboer et al 1990). The reason for the discrepancy relates largely to the method of patient selection by the various groups. To date, there have been relatively few studies to determine the number of affected families within a particular population and most researchers have concentrated on the prevalence of the various types of familial thrombotic disorder in highly selected patient groups. Some workers have attempted to determine the prevalence of familial thrombophilia by determining plasma coagulation inhibitor concentrations in a large population of normal individuals and then calculating the figure from the number of results that are more than two standard deviations below the lower limit of the normal range. Unless additional family studies are also included this is clearly unsatisfactory since it is not possible to distinguish between individuals with the genetic defect and those whose level is at the lower limit of the normal range.

Although a positive family history might be considered a useful predictor of familial thrombophilia, this was not confirmed by Heijboer et al (1990). In this study, a positive family history was obtained in 67 of 277 unselected, consecutive patients with deep vein thrombosis. However, a specific abnormality was detected in only 11 of the 67 subjects. Consequently, although an inherited risk factor was present in approximately 25% of the 277 affected subjects this was identifiable in only 4%. This clearly indicates that a family history is not predictive of familial thrombophilia or, more likely, that we are currently unable to detect all abnormalities which predispose to thrombophilia.

There are different views as to what constitutes a positive family history of venous thromboembolism. Heijboer et al (1990) considered a positive family history to be present when, in addition to the affected proband, there was also a history of undoubted deep vein thrombosis or pulmonary embolus in a first or second degree relative. In our view, even this approach is somewhat imprecise since with an annual incidence of venous thrombosis in the general population of approximately 1 per 1000 per year, we can expect 25% of all patients with thrombosis to have a positive family history.

It is clear that in studies designed to determine the prevalence of familial thrombophilia stringent criteria should be applied to the definition of a positive family history. From our understanding of the coagulation system familial thrombophilia could be caused by any genetically determined defect of the coagulation or fibrinolytic systems that produces accelerated thrombin formation or delayed fibrin dissolution. The former could theoretically result from increased procoagulant activity or reduced coagulation activation inhibition. Impaired fibrinolysis, due either to reduced levels of profibrinolytic components or increased levels of fibrinolytic inhibitors, could have the same effect. Abnormal fibrin due to genetically determined abnormalities of fibrinogen is another possible cause of familial thrombophilia.

Although there are a number of possible candidate risk factors for familial thrombophilia, a genuine relationship between a genetically determined abnormality and thrombosis has been established for only a very small number of these. It cannot be overstressed that the presence of an abnormality in an individual with thrombosis does not in itself indicate an association between the two. In order to establish a causal relationship between a laboratory-based abnormality and an inherited thrombotic syndrome a number of criteria must be satisfied. Thus, it is necessary to demonstrate that:

1. The observed abnormality is also inherited
2. In the pedigree the abnormality cosegregates with the thrombotic manifestations
3. The association of thrombosis and the observed laboratory abnormality is statistically significant in a 2×2 table and that significance persists even after the proband has been eliminated from the analysis.

It is a useful exercise to apply the above criteria to inherited abnormalities of plasminogen since these are possible candidates for familial thrombophilia. There have been a number of reports which have suggested an association between thrombosis and both familial hypo- (type I) and dysplasminogenaemia (type II) (Lottenberg et al 1985, Aoki et al 1978, Gladson et al

1988). The former is characterized by a parallel reduction of functional and immunoreactive plasminogen, the latter by a disproportionately lower functional plasminogen level. Following a study of patients with venous thrombosis, Gladson et al (1988) expressed the view that inherited defects of plasminogen accounted for 2–3% of unexplained thrombosis in young adults. However, the relationship with thromboembolism seemed far from clear since in virtually all of the reported kindreds thrombosis was confined to the propositus. This led Dolan et al (1988) to express some doubt as to whether type I plasminogen deficiency is, by itself, a risk factor for thrombosis.

In an attempt to explore this further, Shigekiyo et al (1992) studied 40 members of two unrelated families with type I familial plasminogen deficiency. Of the 21 individuals who were heterozygous for the condition only three had a history of thrombosis. Moreover, there was no significant difference in the incidence of venous thrombosis amongst healthy controls and those with familial plasminogen deficiency. The results of this study strongly suggest that there is no correlation between type I plasminogen deficiency and venous thromboembolism.

Similar reservations may also be expressed about the possible relationship between thrombosis and dysplasminogenaemia. In the pedigree reported by Aoki et al (1978) there was an impressive thrombotic history in the proband but thrombosis had not occurred in any other affected member of the family. This included one female in whom the plasminogen activity level was extremely low at 10% of normal and who was therefore probably homozygous or heterozygous for the plasminogen defect. She is now 21 years of age and remains free from thrombosis (Aoki 1992). From the currently available evidence it seems clear that the case for a causal relationship between either type I or type II plasminogen deficiency and thrombosis is, at the very best, poor.

A number of groups have looked for evidence of an association between thrombosis and other genetically determined abnormalities of the fibrinolytic system but initial enthusiasm has been somewhat dampened by the lack of convincing data. For example, although one family has been described in which there appeared to be a significant association of thrombosis and impaired fibrinolytic activity of the vessel wall (Johansson et al 1978), this association has not been confirmed in more recent studies in which specific functional assays for tissue plasminogen activator (tPA) have been employed. Similarly, to date, there is no convincing evidence for an association between thrombosis and familial abnormalities of histidine-rich glycoprotein (Engesser et al 1987b). Although there are reports of families in which a thrombotic tendency has been attributed to impaired release of tPA following venous occlusion or the administration of deamino-D-arginine vasopressin (Mannucci & Tripodi 1988), there is still no firm evidence to support a causal relationship between thromboembolism and familial abnormalities of synthesis or release of tPA or plasminogen activator inhibitor.

Heparin cofactor II is a thrombin inhibitor and therefore an attractive candidate risk factor for thrombophilia. Although there are occasional reports of both arterial and venous thrombosis in kindreds with familial heparin cofactor II deficiency (Tran et al 1985, Sie et al 1985), there is no clear evidence of an association between the inherited defect and a predisposition to thromboembolism. In a more recent detailed study of the disorder Bertina et al (1987) demonstrated that hereditary heparin cofactor II deficiency is equally prevalent amongst healthy subjects and those with thrombotic disease. It would therefore seem not to be a risk factor for thrombophilia.

Another inhibitor of coagulation which could theoretically be a risk factor for thrombosis is the recently described lipoprotein-associated coagulation inhibitor (LACI) which inhibits the factor VIIa–tissue factor complex. Since plasma concentrations of LACI are unlikely to reflect its physiological activity, Reitsma (1992) attempted to detect gene mutations by sequence analysis of the exons of the LACI gene from blood samples of 30 subjects with unexplained familial thrombophilia. No mutations were detected. Similar negative results were obtained by the same group following sequence analysis of the thrombomodulin gene.

The situation in respect of dysfibrinogenaemia and thrombosis is less clear. To date, more than 100 kindreds with dysfibrinogenaemia have been described, and Gladson et al (1988) have expressed the view that the defect accounts for 1% of unexplained venous thrombosis in young adults. However, as with the inherited defects of plasminogen, thrombosis occurs in only a minority of affected subjects. It is possible that in kindreds with dysfibrino-genaemia the predisposition to thrombosis relates to the specific genetic defect. This is suggested by the observation that in some reported kindreds there appears to be a more convincing association between the presence of the defect and the development of thromboembolism. One such example is the pedigree of fibrinogen Vlissingen (Koopman et al 1991) which shares the same mutation as fibrinogen Frankfurt IV. Interestingly, in both pedigrees the defect is associated with both arterial and venous thrombosis. It is now recognized that these two families are genetically linked (unpublished data).

Several groups have suggested that familial factor XII may be a risk factor for thrombosis (Mannhalter et al 1987, Lammle et al 1991). This could relate to its role in the contact system-dependent pathway of plasminogen activation. Since there are an insufficient number of detailed family studies the relationship between inherited factor XII deficiency and thromboembolism remains unknown.

An intriguing and unresolved question is whether there is an increased risk of thromboembolism in heterozygotes for cystathione β-synthase deficiency. This rare, autosomal recessive disorder is the main cause of homocystinuria and is characterized by mental retardation, ecopia lentis, skeletal abnormal-ities and a marked tendency to thrombosis (Mudd et al 1985). By the age of 30, approximately 50% of affected individuals will have experienced at least one thrombotic event.

The mechanism whereby homocysteine induces thrombosis is not yet established and a number of possible mechanisms have been suggested. Recent evidence suggests that this could be at least partly due to inhibition of protein C activation by homocysteine at endothelial cell surfaces (Rodgers & Conn 1990). It now seems increasingly clear that homocysteinaemia is an independent risk factor for arterial vascular disease. It remains to be seen, however, whether the heterozygous state for the enzyme defect may be associated with clinically dominant venous thrombophilia.

PROTEIN C DEFICIENCY

Protein C, a vitamin K-dependent glycoprotein, is one of the major regulatory inhibitory proteins of the coagulation system. It was first isolated from plasma by Stenflo in 1976 and since it was the third protein to be eluted from the ion-exchange chromatogram it was designated protein C. In the same year Seegers et al (1976) demonstrated that activated protein C was the anticoagulant autoprothrombin IIA that they themselves had described 16 years earlier (Mammen et al 1960).

Protein C is activated to activated protein C on endothelial cell surfaces by a thrombin–thrombomodulin complex in the presence of calcium ions and phospholipid (Esmon & Owen 1981). Following activation it functions as an anticoagulant by degrading the activated forms of clotting factors V and VIII.

Familial protein C deficiency and its association with venous thromboembolism was first described by Griffin et al in 1981. This was followed by numerous other reports (Bertina et al 1982, Broekmans et al 1983, Horellou et al 1984). The mode of inheritance was found to be autosomal dominant. On the basis of phenotypic analysis two types of familial protein C deficiency can be recognized. In the more common type I deficiency there is parallel reduction of the functional and immunoassays for protein C. Type II variants are characterized by normal or near-normal immunoassay levels but reduced functional levels of protein C. DNA analysis can now be used to identify some heterozygotes. The gene for protein C, which is located on chromosome 2, consists of nine exons (Plutzky et al 1986). Since 1987, various genetic defects have been described in heterozygotes with type I and type II deficiency, in homozygotes and in compound heterozygotes (Romeo et al 1987, Grundy et al 1989, Reitsma et al 1991, Gandrille et al 1991, Bovill et al 1991, Tsuda et al 1991).

In healthy individuals protein C levels vary between approximately 0.65 U/ml and 1.45 U/ml. Although most heterozygotes have protein C levels approximately 50% of normal, they are not always easily identified since at the lower limit of the normal range there is a degree of overlap in protein C levels of heterozygotes and normal individuals. The prevalence of hereditary protein C deficiency in the general population remains the subject of considerable debate. Thus, whereas Broekmans et al (1983) and Gladson et al (1988) reported a prevalence of 1 in 16 000 and 1 in 36 000 respectively, Miletich et al (1987) in marked contrast found that 1 in 200–300 of 5000 healthy blood donors, but with no history of thrombosis, had protein C antigen levels which were consistent with type I deficiency. There are a number of possible explanations for these apparent discrepancies. The most important relates to the method of selection. Broekmans et al (1983) and Gladson et al (1988), for example, derived their figures from studies of patients with venous thrombosis, whereas Miletich et al (1987) calculated their results in healthy subjects with no history of thrombosis.

The incidence of protein C deficiency among hospital patients presenting with venous thrombosis is also confusing. In The Netherlands, Broekmans and his co-workers reported that protein C deficiency was present in 2% of 319 patients presenting with venous thromboembolism. This prevalence was higher (4.8%) in individuals less than 41 years of age and highest in young subjects with recurrent thrombosis. Similar figures were reported from West Germany by Gladson et al (1988). Here the prevalence of protein deficiency in patients with thromboembolism was 4% in adults below the age of 45 years, rising to 12% in young adults in whom thrombotic events were recurrent.

Venous thromboembolism is the main clinical manifestation of protein C deficiency (Fig. 12.1). There are no clinical differences between individuals with type I and type II deficiency and in those with type II deficiency; the clinical manifestations are not influenced by the genetic defect. In symptomatic families, thrombotic events vary from superficial thrombophlebitis to deep venous thrombosis and pulmonary embolism. Cerebral venous thrombosis (Wintzen et al 1985), splanchnic thrombosis (Green et al 1987) and axillary vein thrombosis have also been reported. Often, thromboembolism occurs at a relatively early age and recurrences may be frequent. Precipitating factors include surgery, oral contraceptives, pregnancy and prolonged periods of immobilization. Spontaneous thrombosis is also not uncommon. There are a few reports of the occurrence of arterial thrombosis in patients with protein C deficiency (Horellou et al 1984, Coller et al 1987, Israels & Seshia 1987) but it is still not clear whether protein C deficiency is a risk factor for arterial-related disease.

There have been a number of reports of coumarin-induced skin necrosis in patients with protein C deficiency (Samama et al 1984, Broekmans et al 1983, McGehee et al 1984). It seems likely that this relates to the rapid fall in protein C which occurs following the introduction of coumarin therapy. This causes a temporary dissociation between protein C levels and those of the vitamin K-dependent clotting factors. The ensuing hypercoagulable state results in thrombosis within the subcutaneous circulation, leading to interstitial bleeding and necrosis of the dermis and subcutaneous fat tissue. Coumarin-induced skin necrosis has also been reported in subjects with acquired protein C deficiency during periods of increasing intensity of therapy (Teepe et al 1986). It has also been observed in individuals with protein S deficiency (Goldberg et al 1991). Since the half-life of protein S is substantially longer than that of protein C the inducing mechanism must be

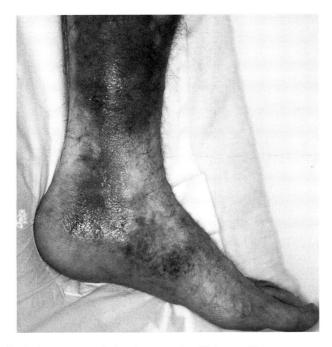

Fig. 12.1 Typical appearance of chronic venous insufficiency with venous eczema associated with protein C deficiency.

different from that proposed for protein C deficient subjects. Warfarin-induced skin necrosis has also been reported in individuals in whom there are no other detectable abnormalities of coagulation.

To date, 17 confirmed cases of severe protein C deficiency have been described in Europe and the USA. These are due either to homozygous or compound heterozygous protein C deficiency. Clinical manifestations in these children appear to relate to their level of protein C (Marlar & Neumann 1990). Infants with undetectable levels of protein C develop purpura fulminans shortly after birth (Seligsohn et al 1984, Samama et al 1984, Sills et al 1984, Peters et al 1988, Marlar et al 1989). This is characterized by disseminated intravascular coagulation and severe skin necrosis due to microvascular thrombosis of subcutaneous vessels (Marlar et al 1989, Marlar & Mastovich 1990). Cerebral and ophthalmic thrombosis has also been reported in severely affected fetuses (Marlar & Neumann 1990). In infants with very low, but detectable, protein C levels, thrombosis of large vessels may occur in the absence of associated skin necrosis (Seligsohn et al 1984).

Homozygous protein C deficiency is not invariably associated with severe neonatal thromboembolism. Tuddenham et al (1989), for example, described two children in whom thrombosis occurred in the second half of their first year of life. Even more remarkable were the two subjects described by Tripodi et al (1990). One of these, who had a low, but detectable, level of protein C, did not develop venous thrombosis until the age of 28 years whilst the other, with a similar level of protein C, remains asymptomatic at the age of 38 years.

It is of some interest that the heterozygous parents and other heterozygous relatives of the homozygous or compound heterozygous children are usually asymptomatic (Marciniak et al 1985, Sharon et al 1986). Differences in the clinical expression of heterozygous protein C deficiency do not appear to relate to specific types of genetic defect (Tsuda et al 1991). It seems likely therefore that environmental factors, which themselves may be familial in origin, may also contribute to the clinical expression of heterozygous protein C deficiency.

PROTEIN S DEFICIENCY

Protein S, arbitrarily named on account of its isolation and characterization in Seattle by DiScipio and Davie in 1979, is the non-enzymatic cofactor of activated protein C (Walker 1981). It is a vitamin K-dependent protein and is synthesized not only by the liver but also by endothelial cells (Fair et al 1986). It is also found in α-granules of platelets (Schwarz et al 1985).

In plasma, protein S exists in two forms: free protein S and a complex of protein S and C4b-binding protein (C4bBP); 60–65% of protein S is complexed with C4bBP and 35% is in the free form (Dahlback 1983). Protein S which is bound to C4bBP does not function as a cofactor for activated protein C; free protein S is thus the active moiety (Bertina et al 1985, Dahlback 1986).

Through its interaction with protein S, C4bBP exerts a regulatory role in the cofactor activity of protein S. High affinity binding between protein S and C4bBP results in low levels of free protein S when the acute phase reactant C4bBP is increased or, alternatively, when total protein S is reduced. Conversely, very high levels of free protein S cocur when plasma C4bBP concentrations are low (Griffin et al 1991, Comp et al 1990).

Three types of familial protein S deficiency have been recognized. In type I deficiency the total amount of protein S is reduced and since most of this is bound to C4bBP this results in greatly reduced levels of free protein S. In type II protein S deficiency, total plasma levels of protein S are normal as is the equilibrium between free and bound protein S. In this type of defect the abnormal molecules have reduced functional activity (Mannucci et al 1989). Type III deficiency, which is the least common, is caused by an alteration in the binding characteristics of C4bBP and protein S. The equilibrium between free and bound protein S is shifted towards the bound form resulting in low levels of free protein S (Comp et al 1986a).

There have been several attempts to establish the prevalence of inherited protein S deficiency but to date no studies have taken into account the possibility of asymptomatic protein S deficiency in the general population.

The prevalence of protein S deficiency in individuals presenting with thrombosis has been estimated to be within the range 4.8–8% (Pabinger et al

1986b, Broekmans et al 1985, Gladson et al 1988). Extrapolating their findings to the general population Gladson et al (1988) calculated that the prevalence of protein S deficiency in the general population is 1 in 29 000. As already indicated, this is likely to be an underestimate.

The identification of heterozygotes for protein S deficiency may occasionally be assisted through DNA analysis. There are two highly homologous genes for protein S and both of these are located on chromosome 3 (Ploos van Amstel et al 1987). The active gene, designated PSalpha, consists of 15 exons, whilst the pseudogene, PSbeta, contains a number of splice site, nonsense and missense mutations which makes gene expression impossible (Ploos van Amstel et al 1990). Genetic defects affecting not only the active gene but also the pseudogene have been identified in a number of kindreds with familial protein S deficiency.

In normal individuals protein S levels are within the range 0.67–1.25 U/ml for total protein S antigen and 0.23–0.49 U/ml for free protein S, with women having slightly lower levels than men (Bertina et al 1985). Reduced protein S levels occur in a number of different clinical situations and it is important therefore to exclude these possibilities before establishing a diagnosis of familial protein S deficiency (Table 12.1). Protein S becomes progressively reduced during pregnancy, the effect being most marked between weeks 18 and 28 (Comp et al 1986b, Malm et al 1988). It also falls, but to a lesser degree, in women taking oral contraceptives (Boerger et al 1987). In individuals receiving oestrogens for growth retardation, protein S levels may be markedly reduced (Huisveld et al 1987). Reduced levels of protein S are also found in subjects with renal disease (Comp et al 1985), liver disease (Bertina et al 1985, D'Angelo et al 1988), systemic lupus erythematosus (Comp et al 1985) and disseminated intravascular coagulation (Bertina et al 1985, D'Angelo et al 1988). In subjects with liver disease the reduction of both total and free protein S is less than that of the other vitamin K-dependent proteins (D'Angelo et al 1988). Male cigarette smokers also have lower protein S levels than non-smokers (Scott et al 1991). Since protein S is a

Table 12.1 Acquired deficiency of antithrombin, protein C and protein S

Antithrombin	Protein C	Protein S
Liver disease	Liver disease and	Liver disease
Protein-losing enteropathy	transplantation	Disseminated intra-vascular
Nephrotic syndrome	Disseminated intra-vascular	coagulation
Disseminated intravascular	coagulation	Warfarin therapy
coagulation	Warfarin therapy	Pregnancy
Major surgery	Cardiopulmonary bypass	Systemic lupus erythematosus
Acute thrombosis	surgery	Chemotherapy for breast
Heparin therapy	Haemodialysis	cancer
Oestrogen therapy	Asparaginase therapy	In association with
Asparaginase therapy	Chemotherapy for breast	antiphospholipid antibody
	cancer	

Reproduced with permission from Greaves & Preston (1991).

vitamin K-dependent protein it is not surprising that reduced levels are found in association with vitamin K deficiency and during treatment with coumarin derivatives (Bertina et al 1985).

The clinical manifestations of inherited protein S deficiency are indistinguishable from those associated with familial protein C deficiency. Venous thromboembolism is thus a striking feature. As with protein C deficiency, thrombophlebitis (Fig. 12.2) and deep vein thrombosis are equally common and account for approximately 60% of thrombotic events. Pulmonary embolism accounted for 23–38% of thrombotic events in the patients described by Engesser et al (1987). There are also reports of venous thromboembolism occurring in unusual sites such as axillary vein, mesenteric vein, portal vein and cerebral vein (Sas et al 1985, Engesser et al 1987). Although unusual, deep vein thrombosis has also been observed in young children (Sas et al 1985, De Stefano et al 1987).

The increased risk of thrombosis which is present in heterozygotes for protein S deficiency in symptomatic pedigrees occurs at a relatively young age. In the subjects described by Engesser et al (1987) the probability of an affected individual being thrombosis free at the age of 35 years was only 32%. As with protein C deficiency, thrombosis is frequently recurrent and may occur spontaneously or else in association with some precipitating factor such as pregnancy, oral contraceptive use, surgery or prolonged periods of immobilization.

Warfarin-induced skin necrosis has been reported in a number of patients

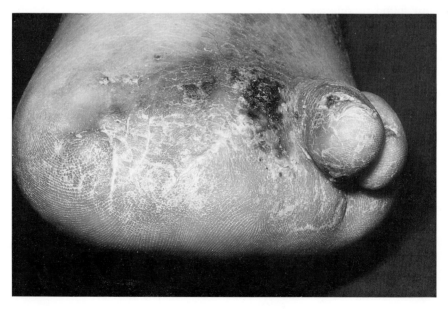

Fig. 12.2 Progressive digital loss as a consequence of recurrent thrombophlebitis and associated soft tissue infection in a man with protein S deficiency.

with protein S deficiency (Grimaudo et al 1989, Moreb & Kitchens 1989, Goldberg et al 1991), the clinical and histopathological features being indistinguishable from those described in patients with protein C deficiency. In the latter, warfarin-induced skin necrosis has been attributed to a transient hypercoagulable state consequent upon the short half-life of protein C following the introduction of the drug. This explanation is not tenable in protein S deficiency since the half-life of protein S during the introduction of coumarins is substantially longer (42.5 hours) than that of protein C.

Although there have been reports of arterial occulsive disease in subjects with protein S deficiency it cannot be concluded that this is indicative of a causal relationship and it remains to be established whether inherited protein S deficiency is a risk factor for arterial vascular disease (Coller et al 1987, Girolami et al 1989, Allaart et al 1990).

FAMILIAL ANTITHROMBIN DEFICIENCY

Antithrombin is the major physiological inhibitor of the serine proteases, inhibiting not only thrombin but also the activated clotting factors IXa, Xa, XIa and XIIa. It is a glycoprotein with a molecular weight of approximately 50 000 and is synthesized by the liver. Its function as an inhibitor is achieved through the formation of a 1:1 stoichiometric complex with the target serine protease. Complex formation occurs through an interaction involving arginine of antithrombin and serine at the active site of the serine protease. In the absence of heparin the rate of complex formation is relatively slow but this is markedly accelerated when heparin is present. The observation that heparan sulphate proteoglycans, located at endothelial cell surfaces, have a similar potentiating effect and act through an identical mechanism (Marcum et al 1984) led Rosenberg (1989) to suggest that the inhibition of serine proteases by antithrombin normally takes place at endothelial cell surfaces and that this is achieved through initial binding of a fraction of plasma antithrombin by heparan sulphate proteoglycans at the endothelial cell surface.

The association between familial antithrombin deficiency and venous thromboembolism was first established in 1965 by Egeberg. This initial observation, from Norway, has since been confirmed by a number of groups from different parts of the world (Thaler & Lechner 1981, Rosenberg 1975, Vykidal et al 1985). The pattern of inheritance of familial antithrombin deficiency is autosomal dominant. Consequently, men and women are equally affected.

A number of different groups have attempted to estimate the prevalence of familial antithrombin deficiency within the general population but, as with similar prevalence studies of protein C and protein S, selection bias continues to be a problem and the estimated prevalence of inherited antithrombin deficiency has, not surprisingly, varied widely from 1:2000 to 1:40 000

(Abildgaard 1981, Rosenberg 1975, Gladson et al 1988, Vykidal et al 1985). More recently Tait et al (1991), who studied asymptomatic blood donors, suggested that the prevalence of antithrombin deficiency in Scotland is 1:350. Although the prevalence of familial antithrombin deficiency remains uncertain it probably accounts for 2–5% of patients under 45 years of age presenting with venous thromboembolism (Thaler & Lechner 1981).

As with the inherited disorders of protein C deficiency, familial antithrombin deficiency can be classified into two groups on the basis of results of functional and immunological antithrombin assays. Type I deficiency, which accounts for 80–90% of familial antithrombin deficiencies, is characterized by parallel reductions of functional and immunological assays for antithrombin (Prochownik 1989). This usually reflects reduced synthesis of a structurally normal antithrombin molecule. In type II antithrombin deficiency a reduced concentration of functional antithrombin is associated with normal or near-normal immunoreactive antithrombin.

The cloning and characterization of the antithrombin gene has greatly facilitated our understanding of the molecular basis of inherited antithrombin disorders (Bock et al 1982, Prochownik et al 1983, Chandra et al 1983). It is now recognized that the antithrombin molecule has two important functional domains, namely a thrombin-binding domain and a heparin-binding domain (Prochownik 1989). Type I defects are usually caused by a genetic mutation producing silent antithrombin alleles whilst type II defects arise as a consequence of point mutations which modify the molecule's heparin- or thrombin-binding characteristics.

The first report of an antithrombin variant was by Sas et al in 1974. Numerous other cases have since been described (Hultin et al 1988, Lane et al 1992). The increasing complexity of antithrombin variants has prompted a number of workers to suggest new classification systems for these disorders (Finazzi et al 1987, Hultin et al 1988). More recently, Lane et al (1992) have proposed a useful new classification system for type two antithrombin variants. These are summarized as follows:

- Subtype IIa, functional abnormalities affecting both reactive site and heparin-binding site
- Subtype IIb, functional abnormalities limited to the reactive site
- Subtype IIc, functional abnormalities limited to the heparin-binding site.

The two functional antithrombin methods employed for the diagnosis of familial antithrombin deficiency are assays for heparin cofactor activity and progressive antithrombin activity. Heparin cofactor assays measure the rate of inactivation of factor Xa or thrombin by antithrombin in the presence of heparin. Consequently, reduced heparin cofactor activity is a feature of all antithrombin variants since the assay reflects both of the functional domains of the molecule (Lane & Caso 1989). The progressive antithrombin activity assay determines the proteinase inhibitory activity of antithrombin in the absence of heparin. Thus, normal results will be obtained in variants with reduced heparin binding (Lane et al 1992). Abnormalities affecting the reactive site of the molecule can be distinguished from heparin-binding site defects by performing crossed immunoelectropheresis in the presence of heparin (Lane & Caso 1989).

The distinction between variants caused by abnormalities of the heparin-binding site and those with defects of the reactive site of the molecule is of more than academic interest since there are significant differences in their associated thrombotic risk (Finazzi et al 1987, Lane & Caso 1989). Thus, the incidence of thrombosis in individuals with an abnormality affecting the reactive site of the molecule is 50–60%, which is similar to that in subjects with a type I defect. This compares with a much lower incidence (6%) in heterozygotes for a defect confined to the heparin-binding site (Finazzi et al 1987). Examples of the former are ATs Sheffield, Glasgow, Northwick Park and Hamilton (Lane & Caso 1989, Prochownik 1989).

Venous thromboembolism is the main clinical manifestation of familial antithrombin deficiency. This is most frequently manifest as deep venous thrombosis but pulmonary embolism is also not uncommon. Recurrent venous thrombosis is a feature of the disorder, as is thrombosis in unusual sites such as the inferior vena cava, renal, portal, mesenteric and cerebral veins. Although a family history may be elicited, this is not an invariable feature. Precipitating or associated factors include oral contraceptive usage, pregnancy, surgery, trauma and prolonged periods of immobilization. We have also observed the development of massive iliofemoral thrombosis in a child with an acute mycoplasma infection (Creagh et al 1991). In approximately one-third of subjects thrombosis may also occur without any obvious precipitating factor (Thaler & Lechner 1981).

Currently available evidence suggests that the risk of venous thrombosis is greater in heterozygotes for antithrombin deficiency than in those with protein C or protein S deficiency. There is a particularly strong association between the risk of venous thromboembolism and increasing age (Table 12.2). In a review of published literature, Thaler & Lechner (1981) reported that whilst thrombosis had occurred in only 10% of affected children below the age of 15 years this figure rose dramatically to 85% by the age of 55 years. It has been suggested that the relatively low incidence of thrombosis in children with antithrombin deficiency might relate to the protective effect of the high levels of α_2-macroglobulin in childhood (Hirsh et al 1989). Recently Hirsh et al (1989) have indicated that if the published data are correct then a strong case could be made for considering prophylactic anticoagulants in asymptomatic heterozygotes between the ages of 15 and 40 years.

There are suggestions that a relationship exists between arterial thrombotic disease and both high and low levels of antithrombin. A relationship between ischaemic heart disease and high levels of antithrombin was initially suggested by Yue et al (1976). Recently, Meade et al (1991), in a prospective analysis of 893 men in the Northwick Park Heart Study, reported that more

Table 12.2   AT deficiency — risk of thrombosis per decade

Age (years)	Risk of thrombosis (% per year)	Cumulative thrombosis rate
0–10	0.5	5
10–15	0.8	9
15–20	3.2	25
20–30	4.0	65
30–40	1.4	79
40–50	0.9	88
50–60	0.7	95

Reproduced with permission from Hirsh et al 1989.

deaths from arterial disease had occurred in individuals with antithrombin levels in both the low and the high thirds of antithrombin distribution than in those whose results fell in the middle third. This suggests that high and low levels of antithrombin may be associated with the risk of death from arterial disease (Meade et al 1991). It remains to be seen whether this observation is confirmed by others.

The diagnosis of a familial thrombotic disorder demands a detailed family and clinical history and appropriate laboratory investigations (Table 12.3). Before a diagnosis is established, it is necessary to exclude acquired disorders of haemostasis, especially those relating to hepatic dysfunction. It should also be appreciated that a diagnosis of familial thrombophilia cannot be established during an acute episode of venous thromboembolism when low levels of antithrombin, protein C and protein S are not unusual. Other factors which may confound a diagnosis of familial thrombophilia are pregnancy, anticoagulants and antiphospholipid antibodies.

Confirmation of familial thrombophilia is made by specific functional laboratory assays for antithrombin and protein C, and by an immunoassay for free protein S. Immunoassays for protein C and total protein S provide additional useful information on the type of genetic deficit for these inhibitors. However, these immunoassays provide no assistance in the clinical managment of affected subjects. As previously discussed, the situation is somewhat different in antithrombin deficiency, since there is clear evidence that the thrombotic risk is substantially less in individuals with a type II defect which is confined to the heparin-binding site. Consequently, if functional antithrombin deficiency is diagnosed, then immunoassays should be performed to identify subjects with type II defects.

PREGNANCY

Venous thromboembolism is an important complication of pregnancy and for more than 20 years pulmonary embolism has remained the first or second

Table 12.3   The laboratory investigation of thrombophilia

A. *Relevant screening tests*
    Full blood count
    PT
    APTT
    TT
    Reptilase time
    Fibrinogen concentration
    Liver enzymes

B. *Tests of specific diagnostic and prognostic value*
    Antithrombin assay: Functional
                                   Heparin cofactor assay
                                   Progressive antithrombin
                          Immunological
    Protein C assay: Functional
                          Immunological
    Protein S assay: Total
                          Free
    C4b-binding protein assay
    Tests for antiphospholipid antibody

C. *Tests of unproven value*
    Heparin cofactor II assay
    Euglobulin clot lysis time ($\pm$ venous occlusion)
    Assays for tissue plasminogen activator and inhibitor
    Plasminogen assay: Functional
                          Immunological

PT, prothrombin time; APTT, activated partial thromboplastin time; TT, thrombin time.
Reproduced with permission from Greaves & Preston (1991).

leading cause of maternal death in England and Wales (Bonnar 1992). Risk factors for venous thromboembolism in pregnancy and the puerperium include previous venous thromboembolism, obesity, increasing age and parity, prolonged bed rest and familial thrombophilia.

Although there are clear indications that pregnancy carries an increased risk of venous thromboembolism in women with familial thrombophilia (Conard et al 1990), the magnitude of the risk is unknown since to date there has been no formal prospective study to address this. Uncertainty about the degree of risk of venous thrombosis applies particularly to women with familial protein C or protein S deficiency. However, the growing number of reports of thrombosis complicating pregnancy in women with antithrombin III deficiency strongly suggests that the risk associated with this disorder is substantially greater than in deficiencies of either protein C or protein S (Table 12.4).

One of the first reports of the relative risk of pregnancy-associated venous thromboembolism in women with familial thrombophilia was than of Conard et al in 1987. In these women, who were not receiving prophylactic

Table 12.4 Pregnancy and thrombotic risk in familial thrombophilia

	Antithrombin	Protein S	Protein C
Pregnancies (n)	110	44	180
Thrombotic events (n)	59	10	48
Events during pregnancy (n)	33	0	11
Events in puerperium (n)	26	10	37
Overall thrombotic risk (%)	54	23	27

Cumulative data derived from: Hellgren et al (1982), Conard et al (1990), Allaart et al (1992)

anticoagulants, the incidence of thrombosis was 25% for women with protein C deficiency and 62% for those with antithrombin deficiency. In an earlier study, Hellgren et al (1982) had reported a similar risk for pregnant women with antithrombin deficiency.

More recently, Conard et al (1990) reported that the overall incidence of venous thromboembolism associated with pregnancy for women with type I antithrombin deficiency was 44%. Thrombotic events occurred during pregnancy and also during the puerperium, there being no significant difference in incidence between the two.

In the same study, Conard et al (1990) observed that, for both protein C and protein S deficiency, the risk of venous thrombosis was significantly greater in the puerperium than during pregnancy. For protein C deficiency, the incidence of venous thrombotic events during pregnancy was 7% compared with 19% following delivery. No thrombotic event was observed during 31 pregnancies in women with protein S deficiency. This compares with five episodes of thrombosis following 29 deliveries (17%) in the same group of women.

Although the magnitude of risk for pregnancy-associated thrombosis in antithrombin deficiency women is unknown, it seems likely from the volume of published reports and from the observations of Conard et al (1990) that this is substantial (Thaler & Lechner 1981, Hellgren et al 1982). In addition to the thrombotic risk, there are also suggestions that antithrombin deficiency may be associated with placental insufficiency and fetal wastage (Owen 1991).

It should be appreciated that in most of the published reports a distinction has not been drawn between the subtypes of antithrombin deficiency. This is almost certainly of clinical relevance since in the non-pregnant state the thrombotic risk is considerably greater when the molecular defect resides within the active site of the antithrombin molecule than when it is limited to its heparin-binding site (Finazzi et al 1987). If the difference in thrombotic risk is confirmed for pregnancy it will clearly have an important bearing on the strategy adopted for prophylactic anticoagulant therapy.

Since there has been no prospective study designed to assess the pregnancy-related thrombotic risk and its response to prophylactic anticoagulant therapy in women with familial thrombophilia, it is not possible to provide clear guidelines on the management of affected women. In protein C and protein S deficiency, the assessment of the thrombotic risk is particularly difficult since a history of thrombosis is frequently absent. Decisions relating to prophylactic anticoagulant therapy will be greatly influenced by the previous thrombotic and obstetric history. The clinical history of other affected family members may also provide some information about the potential thrombotic risk.

The risk of venous thromboembolism appears to be substantially greater for individuals with type I antithrombin deficiency and in the context of pregnancy it is particularly relevant that between the ages of 15 and 30 years there is a marked increase in the thrombotic risk of affected individuals (Hirsh et al 1989). Accepting the possibility of some reporting bias, Hirsh et al (1989) calculated that an asymptomatic carrier at the age of 15 years has an approximately 65% chance of developing thrombosis over the next 15 years.

There are therefore compelling reasons for recommending prophylactic anticoagulant therapy for type I antithrombin deficient women in pregnancy. Many individuals will be on long-term oral anticagulants before they become pregnant. For these women it is important that they fully understand that in the event of their becoming pregnant there is a risk of coumarin-related fetal complications. These include abnormalities of the central nervous system and warfarin embryopathy. The latter consists of nasal hypoplasia and/or stippled epiphyses and occurs as a complication of warfarin exposure during the first trimester of pregnancy (Hall et al 1980). In the only prospective study, Iturbe-Alessio et al (1986) reported the occurrence of warfarin embryopathy in 10 of 35 infants exposed to warfarin between 6 and 12 weeks' gestation. This compares with 0 of 19 infants when heparin rather than warfarin was administered during this same period.

There are a number of possible approaches to the problem of women on long-term oral anticagulants who are planning a pregnancy. One option is to substitute heparin for warfarin. A potential disadvantage is that this exposes the woman to the possible hazards of heparin-induced thrombocytopenia and osteoporosis (Gallus 1992).

A more practical approach is to monitor the woman carefully and to substitute heparin for the coumarin-related drug as soon as pregnancy is confirmed. Some clinicians choose to treat all women with type I anti-thrombin III deficiency with prophylactic anticoagulant therapy throughout pregnancy and for 3 months after delivery. During pregnancy, heparin is probably the treatment of choice since the drug does not cross the placenta and is not associated with fetal abnormalities (Ginsberg et al 1989a, b). It does, however, carry a risk of osteoporosis.

The risk of osteoporosis was highlighted in a retrospective review by Griffith et al (1965) who reported the development of severe osteoporosis accompanied by spontaneous rib and vertebral fractures in six out of 10 patients given 15 000–30 000 i.u. heparin daily for 8–60 months. These complications were not observed in 107 patients given 10 000 i.u. heparin daily or less for 1–15 years. There have been a number of case reports of heparin-induced osteopenia in pregnancy (Zimran et al 1986, Wise & Hall 1980). In addition, Howell et al (1983) and also De Swiet et al (1983) have provided evidence of significant heparin-induced osteopenia in pregnant women treated for more than approximately 20 weeks.

In order to minimize the risk of osteoporosis, an alternative approach is to administer subcutaneous heparin during the first and third trimesters of pregnancy and to use warfarin during the second trimester. During pregnancy, a suggested anticoagulant regimen is low-dose subcutaneous heparin, 5000 i.u. twice daily until the third trimester at which time the dose should be increased to prolong the APTT (activated partial thromboplastin time) a few seconds beyond the upper limit of the normal range.

Some individuals with antithrombin deficiency are difficult to anticoagulate with heparin alone. During the third trimester, therefore, an anticoagulant effect should be confirmed by means of an APTT (Hirsh et al 1989).

The management of women with antithrombin deficiency at delivery is a subject of much debate. Some workers recommend the use of antithrombin concentrates whilst others have indicated that it is possible to achieve a successful delivery without recourse to these products (Leclerc et al 1986). Since there have been no clinical trials to clarify this, it is not possible to provide clear guidelines as to whether antithrombin concentrates offer any advantage over anticoagulation with heparin alone.

The potential advantage of antithrombin concentrate is that it corrects the abnormality at a time when the risk of venous thromboembolism is high. As term approaches, basal antithrombin levels may fall even lower as a direct consequence of the increased heparin dosage. This effect, together with the reduction of heparin dosage at the time of delivery, might further increase the thromboembolic risk.

If antithrombin concentrate is given it is important to monitor the levels at regular intervals to maintain a value above the lower limit of the normal range. In non-pregnant antithrombin deficient subjects the half-life of infused material is approximately 43–77 hours (Menache et al 1990). It is important to recognize that during pregnancy it may be substantially shorter than this. As with all blood products, consideration should be given to the potential risk of viral transmission although nowadays this is substantially less than a few years ago. Following delivery, warfarin can be introduced within a day or two, dependent on the degree of trauma. If concentrates have been used to cover the delivery these can be discontinued once the target International Normalized Ratio (INR) is achieved. Warfarin should then be continued for 3 months.

KEY POINTS FOR CLINICAL PRACTICE

The clinical features of familial thrombophilia are:

- First episode at early age.
- Recurrent venous thromboembolism.
- Thrombosis may occur spontaneously.
- Family history.
- Thrombosis in unusual sites.
- Thrombophlebitis (mainly protein C and protein S deficiency).

NB Acquired disorders need to be excluded.

REFERENCES

Abildgaard U 1981 Antithrombin and related inhibitors of coagulation. In: Poller L (ed) Recent advances in blood coagulation. Churchill Livingstone, Edinburgh, 3: 151–173

Allaart C F, Aronson D C, Ruys T et al 1990 Hereditary protein S deficiency in young adults with arterial occlusive disease. Thromb Haemost 64: 206–210

Allaart R C F, Poort S R, Rosendaal F R et al 1993 Increased risk for venous thrombosis in carriers of hereditary protein C deficiency defect. Lancet 341: 134–138

Aoki N 1992 Personal communication.

Aoki N, Moroi M, Sakata Y et al 1978 Abnormal plasminogen. A hereditary molecular abnormality found in a patient with recurrent thrombosis. J Clin Invest 61: 1186–1195

Ben Tal O, Zivelin A, Seligsohn U 1989 The relative frequency of hereditary thrombotic disorders among 107 patients with thrombophilia in Israel. Thromb Haemost 61: 50–54

Bertina R M, Broekmans A W, van der Linden I K et al 1982 Protein C deficiency in a Dutch family with thrombotic disease. Thromb Haemost 48: 1–5

Bertina R M, van Wijngaarden A, Reinalda Poot J et al 1985 Determination of plasma protein S – the protein cofactor of activated protein C. Thromb Haemost 53: 268–272

Bertina R M, van der Linden I K, Engesser L et al 1987 Hereditary heparin cofactor II deficiency and the risk of development of thrombosis. Thromb Haemost 57: 196–200

Bock S C, Wion K L, Vehar G A et al 1982 Cloning and expression of the cDNA for human antithrombin III. Nucleic Acids Res 10: 8113–8125

Boerger L M, Morris P C, Thurnau G R et al 1987 Oral contraceptives and gender affect protein S status. Blood 69: 692–694

Bonnar J 1992 Epidemiology of venous thromboembolism in pregnancy and the puerperium. In: Haemostasis and thrombosis in obstetrics and gynaecology. Chapman and Hall, London, p. 257–266

Bovill E G, Tomczak J, Grant V et al 1991 Association of two novel mutations in the GLA-domain (Glu 20 to Ala and Val 34 to Met) with symptomatic type II protein C deficiency. Thromb Haemost 65: 647 (Abstract)

Broekmans A W, van der Linden I K, Veltkamp J J et al 1983 Prevalence of isolated protein C deficiency in patients with venous thrombotic disease and in the population. Thromb Haemost 50: 350 (Abstract)

Broekmans A W, Bertina R M, Reinalda-Poot J et al 1985 Hereditary Protein S deficiency and venous thromboembolism. A study in three Dutch families. Thromb Haemost 53: 273–277

Chandra T, Stackhouse R, Chidd V J et al 1983 Isolation and sequence characterisation of a DNA clone of human antithrombin III. Proc Natl Acad Sci USA 58: 1094

Coller B S, Owen J, Jesty J et al 1987 Deficiency of plasma protein S, protein C, or antithrombin III and arterial thrombosis. Arteriosclerosis 7: 456–462

Comp P C, Doray D, Patton D et al 1986a An abnormal plasma distribution of protein S occurs in function protein S deficiency. Blood 67: 504–508

Comp P C, Thurnau G R, Welsh J et al 1986b Functional and immunological Protein S levels are decreased during pregnancy. Blood 68: 881–885

Comp P C, Vigano-D'Angelo A, Thurnau G R et al 1985 Acquired protein S deficiency occurs in pregnancy, the nephrotic syndrome and systemic lupus erythematosus. Blood 66: 348a (Abstract)

Comp P C, Forristall J, West C D et al 1990 Free protein S levels are elevated in familial C4b-binding protein deficiency. Blood 76: 2527–2529

Conard J, Horellou M H, Van Dreden P et al 1987 Pregnancy and congenital deficiency in antithrombin III or protein C. Throm Haemost 58: Abstract 39

Conard J, Horellou M H, Van Dreden P et al 1990 Thrombosis and pregnancy in congenital deficiencies in AT III, protein C or protein S: study of 78 women. Thromb Haemost 63: 319–320

Creagh M D, Roberts I F, Clark D J, Preston F E 1991 Familial antithrombin III deficiency and *Mycoplasma pneumoniae* pneumonia. J Clin Pathol 44: 870–871

Dahlback B 1983 Purification of human C4b-binding protein and formation of its complex with vitamin K-dependent protein S. Biochem J 209: 847–856

Dahlback B 1986 Inhibition of protein C cofactor function of human and bovine protein S by C4b-binding protein. J Biol Chem 261: 12022–12027

D'Angelo A, Vigano-D'Angelo S, Esmon C T et al 1988 Acquired deficiencies of protein S. J Clin Invest 81: 1445–1454

De Stefano V, Leone G, Ferrelli R et al 1987 Severe deep vein thrombosis in a 2-year old child with protein S deficiency. Thromb Haemost 58: 1089

De Swiet M, Dorrington-Ward P, Fidler J et al 1983 Prolonged heparin therapy in pregnancy causes bone demineralisation. Br J Obstet Gynaecol 90: 1129–1134

DiScipio R G, Davie E W 1979 Characterisation of Protein S, a gamma carboxyglutamic acid containing protein from bovine and human plasma. Biochemistry 18: 899–904

Dolan G, Greaves M, Cooper P et al 1988 Thrombovascular disease and familial plasminogen deficiency: a report of three kindreds. Br J Haematol 70: 417–421

Egeberg O 1965 Inherited antithrombin deficiency causing thrombophilia. Thromb Diath Haemorrh 13: 516–530

Engesser L, Broekmans A W Briet E et al 1987a Hereditary protein S deficiency: clinical manifestations. Ann Intern Med 106: 677–682

Engesser L, Kluft C, Briet E et al 1987b Familial elevation of plasma histidine-rich glycoprotein in a family with thrombophilia. Br J Haematol 67: 355–358

Esmon C T, Owen W G 1981 Identification of an endothelial cell cofactor for thrombin-catalyzed activation of protein C. Proc Natl Acad Sci USA 78: 2249–2252

Fair D S, Marlar R A, Levine E G 1986 Human endotheliel cells synthesize protein S. Blood 67: 1168–1171

Finazzi G, Caccia R, Barbui T 1987 Different prevalence of thromboembolism in the subtypes of congenital antithrombin III deficiency: review of 404 cases. Thromb Haemost 58: 1094

Gallus A S 1992 Anticoagulants and the prevention and treatment of thromboembolic problems in pregnancy, including cardiac problems. In: Haemostasis and thrombosis in obstetrics and gynaecology. Chapman and Hall, London, p 319–327

Gandrille S, Vidaud M, Aiach M et al 1991 Six previously undescribed mutations in 9 families with protein C quantitative deficiency. Thromb Haemost 65: 646 (Abstract)

Ginsberg J S, Hirsh J, Turner D C et al 1989a Risks to the fetus of anticoagulant therapy during pregnancy. Thromb Haemost 61: 197–203

Ginsberg J S, Kowalchuk G, Hirsch J et al 1989b Heparin therapy during pregnancy. Arch Intern Med 149: 2233–2236

Girolami A, Simioni P, Lazzaro A R et al 1989 Severe arterial cerebral thrombosis in a patient with protein S deficiency (moderately reduced total and markedly reduced free protein S): a family study. Thromb Haemost 61: 144–147

Gladson C L, Scharrer I, Hach V et al 1988 The frequency of type I heterozygous protein S and protein C deficiency in 141 unrelated young patients with venous thrombosis. Thromb Haemost 59: 18–22

Goldberg S L, Orthner C L, Yalisove B L et al 1991 Skin necrosis following prolonged administration of coumarin in a patient with inherited protein S deficiency. Am J Hematol 38: 64–66

Greaves M, Preston F E 1991 Clinical and laboratory aspects of thrombophilia. In: Poller L (ed) Recent Advances in Blood Coagulation 5, Churchill Livingstone, Edinburgh, pp 119–140

Green D, Ganger D R, Blei A T 1987 Protein C deficiency in splanchnic venous thrombosis.

Am J Med 82: 1171–1174

Griffin J H, Evatt B, Zimmerman T S et al 1981 Deficiency of protein C in congenital thrombotic disease. J Clin Invest 68: 1370–1373

Griffin J H, Fernandez J A, Gruber A 1991 Critical reevaluation of free protein S (PS) and C4b-binding protein (C4BP) levels and implications for thrombotic risk. Thromb Haemost 65: 711 (Abstract)

Griffith G C, Nicholls G Jr, Asher J D et al 1965 Heparin osteoporosis. JAMA 193: 85–88

Grimaudo V, Gueissaz F, Hauert J et al 1989 Necrosis of skin induced by coumarin in a patient deficient in protein S. Br Med J 298: 233–234

Grundy C, Chitolic A, Talbot S et al 1989 Protein C London 1: recurrent mutation at Arg 169 (CGGGTGG) in the protein C gene causing thrombosis. Nucleic Acids Res 17: 10513

Hall J G, Pauli R M, Wilson K M 1980 Maternal and fetal sequelae of anticoagulation during pregnancy. Am J Med 68: 122–140

Heijboer H, Brandjes D P M, Buller H R et al 1990 Deficiencies of coagulation-inhibiting and fibrinolytic proteins in outpatients with deep-vein thrombosis. N Engl J Med 323: 1512–1516

Hellgren M, Tengborn L, Abildgaard U 1982 Pregnancy in women with congenital antithrombin III deficiency: experience of treatment with heparin and antithrombin. Gynecol Obstet Invest 14: 127–141

Hirsh J 1989. Congenital antithrombin III deficiency. Am J Med 87 (S3B): 37

Hirsh J, Piovella F, Pini M 1989 Congenital antithrombin III deficiency. Incidence and clinical features. Am J Med 87: 34S–38S

Horellou M H, Conard J, Bertina R M et al 1984 Congenital protein C deficiency and thrombotic disease in nine French families. Br Med J 289: 1285–1287

Howell R, Fidler J, Letsky E et al 1983 The risks of antenatal subcutaneous heparin prophylaxis: a controlled trial. Br J Obstet Gynaecol 90: 1124–1128

Huisveld I A, Greven E C G, Bouma B N 1987 Protein C and protein S levels in tall girls treated with ethinyloestradiol. Thromb Haemost 58: 406 (Abstract)

Hultin M B, McKay J, Abildgaard U 1988 Antithrombin Oslo: type 1b classification of the first reported antithrombin-deficient family with a review of hereditary antithrombin variants. Thromb Haemost 59: 468–473

Israels S J, Seshia S S 1987 Childhood stroke associated with Protein C or Protein S deficiency. Pediatr 111: 562–564

Iturbe-Alessio I, Del Carmen Fonseca M, Mutchinik O et al 1986 Risks of anticoagulant therapy in pregnant women with artificial heart valves. N Engl J Med 315: 1390–1393

Johansson L, Hedner U, Nilsson I M 1978 A family with thromboembolic disease associated with deficient fibrinolytic activity in vessel wall. Acta Med Scand 203: 477–480

Koopman J, Haverkate F, Briet E et al 1991 A congenitally abnormal fibrinogen (Vlissingen) with a 6-base deletion in the gamma-chain gene, causing defective calcium binding and impaired fibrin polymerization. J Biol Chem 266: 13456–13461

Lammle B, Wuillemin W A, Huber I et al 1991 Thromboembolism and bleeding tendency in congenital factor XII deficiency – a study on 74 subjects from 14 Swiss families. Thromb Haemost 65: 117–121

Lane D A, Caso R 1989 Antithrombin III: structure, genomic organisation, function and inherited deficiency. In: Tuddenham E G D (ed) Clinical haematology, vol 4(2). The molecular biology of coagulation, Baillière-Tindall, London, pp 961–998

Lane D A, Olds R R, Thein S-L 1992 Antithrombin III and its deficiency states. Blood Coagulat Fibrinol 3: 315–342

Leclerc J F, Geerts W, Panju A et al 1986 Management of antithrombin III deficiency during pregnancy without administration of antithrombin III. Thromb Res 41: 567–573

Lottenberg R, Dolly F R, Kitchen C S 1985 Recurring thromboembolic disease and pulmonary hypertension associated with severe hypoplasminogenaemia. Am J Hematol 19: 181–193

McGehee W G, Klotz T A, Epstein D J et al 1984 Coumarin necrosis associated with hereditary protein C deficiency. Ann Intern Med 101: 59–60

Malm J, Laurell M, Dahlback B 1988 Changes in the plasma levels of vitamin K-dependent proteins C and S and of C4B-binding proteins during pregnancy and oral contraception. Br J Haematol 68: 437–443

Mammmem E F, Thomas W R, Seegers W H 1960 Activation of purified prothrombin to authoprothrombin I or autoprothrombin II (platelet cofactor II or autoprothrombin IIa). Thromb Diath Haemorr 5: 218–249

Mannhalter C, Fischer M, Hopmeier P et al 1987 Factor XII activity and antigen concentrations in patients suffering from recurrent thrombosis. Fibrinolysis 1: 259–263

Mannucci P M, Tripodi A 1988 Inherited factors in thrombosis. Blood Rev 2: 27–35

Mannucci P M, Valsecchi C, Krachmalnicoff A et al 1989 Familial dysfunction of protein S. Thromb Haemost 62: 763–766

Marciniak E, Wilson H D, Marlar R A 1985 Neonatal purpura fulminans: a genetic disorder related to the absence of Protein C in blood. Blood 65: 15–20

Marcum J A, McKenny J B, Rosenberg R D 1984 Acceleration of thrombin–antithrombin complex formation in rat hind quarters via heparin-like molecules bound to the endothelium. J Clin Invest 74: 341–350

Marlar R A, Mastovich S 1990 Hereditary protein C deficiency: a review of the genetics, clinical presentation, diagnosis and treatment. Blood Coagul Fibrinol 1: 319–330

Marlar R A, Neumann A 1990 Neonatal purpura fulminans due to homozygous Protein C or Protein S deficiencies. Seminars in Thromb Hemost 16: 299–309

Marlar R A, Montgomery R R, Broekmans A W 1989 Report on the diagnosis and treatment of homozygous protein C deficiency. Report of the Working Party on Homozygous Protein C Deficiency of the ICTH-Subcommittee on Protein C and Protein S. Thromb Haemost 61: 529–531

Meade T W, Cooper J, Miller G J et al 1991 Antithrombin III and arterial disease. Lancet 338: 850–851

Menache D, O'Malley J P, Schorr J B et al 1990 Evaluation of the safety, recovery, half-life, and clinical efficacy of antithrombin III (human) in patients with hereditary antithrombin III deficiency. Cooperative Study Group. Blood 75: 33–39

Miletich J, Sherman L, Broze Jr G 1987 Absence of thrombosis in subjects with heterozygous protein C deficiency. N Engl J Med 317: 991–996

Moreb J, Kitchens C S 1989 Acquired functional protein S deficiency, cerebral venous thrombosis, and coumarin skin necrosis in association with antiphospholipid syndrome: report of two cases. Am J Med 87: 207–210

Mudd S H, Skovby F, Levy H L et al 1985 The natural history of homocystinuria due to cystathionine beta-synthase deficiency. Am J Hum Genet 37: 1–31

Owen J 1991 Antithrombin III replacement therapy in pregnancy. Semin Hematol 28: 46–52

Pabinger I, Bertina R M, Lechner A et al 1986a Protein S deficiency in seven Austrian families. Thromb Res (Suppl VI): 269

Pabinger I, Karnik R, Lechner K et al 1986b Coumarin induced acral skin necrosis associated with hereditary protein C deficiency. Blut 52: 365–370

Peters C, Casella J F, Marlar R A et al 1988 Homozygous protein C deficiency: observations on the nature of the molecular abnormality and the effectiveness of warfarin therapy. Pediatrics 81: 272–276

Ploos van Amstel H K, van der Zanden A L, Bakker E et al 1987 Two genes homologous with human protein S cDNA are located on chromosome 3. Thromb Haemost 58: 982–987

Ploos van Amstel H K, Huisman M V, Reitsma P H et al 1989a Partial protein S gene deletion in a family with hereditary thrombophilia. Blood 73: 479–483

Ploos van Amstel H K, Reitsma P H, Hamulyak K et al 1989b A mutation in the protein S pseudogene is linked to protein S deficiency in a thrombophilic family. Thromb Haemost 62: 897–901

Ploos van Amstel H K, Reitsma P H, van der Logt C P et al 1990 Intron–exon organization of the active human protein S gene PS alpha and its pseudogene PS beta: duplication and silencing during primate evolution. Biochemistry 29: 7853–7861

Plutzky J, Hoskins J A, Long G L et al 1986 Evolution and organization of the human protein C gene. Proc Natl Acad Sci USA 83: 546–550

Prochownik E V 1989 Molecular genetics of inherited antithrombin III deficiencies. Am J Med 87 (Suppl 3B): 15–18

Prochownik E V, Markham A F, Orkin S H 1983 Isolation of the cDNA clone for the human antithrombin III. J Biol Chem 128: 8389–8394

Reitsma P H 1992 Personal communication

Reitsma P H, Poort S R, Allaart C F et al 1991 The spectrum of genetic defects in a panel of 40 Dutch families with symptomatic protein C deficiency type I: heterogeneity and founder effects. Blood 78: 890–894

Rodgers G M, Conn M T 1990 Homocysteine, an atherogenic stimulus, reduces Protein C activation by arterial and venous endothelial cells. Blood 75: 895–901

Romeo G, Hassan H J, Staempfli S et al 1987 Hereditary thrombophilia: identification of nonsense and missense mutations in the protein C gene. Proc Natl Acad Sci USA 84: 2829–2832

Rosenberg R D 1975 Actions and interactions of antithrombin and heparin. N Engl J Med 292: 146–151

Rosenberg R D 1989 Biochemistry of heparin antithrombin interactions, and the physiologic role of the natural anticoagulant mechanism. Am J Med 97 (Suppl 3b): 2–9

Samama M, Horellou M H, Soria J et al 1984 Successful progressive anticoagulation in a severe protein C deficiency and previous skin necrosis at the initiation of oral anticoagulant treatment letter. Thromb Haemost 51: 132–133

Sas Y, Blasko G, Banhegyi D et al 1974 Abnormal antithrombin III (antithrombin III 'Budapest') as a cause of a familial thrombophilia. Thromb Diath Haemorr 32: 105–115

Sas Y, Blasko Y, Petro I et al 1985 A protein S deficient family with portal vein thrombosis. Thromb Haemost 54: 724

Scott B D, Esmon C T, Comp P C 1991 The natural anticoagulant protein S is decreased in male smokers. Am Heart J 122: 76–80

Seegers W H, Novoa E, Henry R L et al 1976 Relationship of 'new' vitamin K dependent protein C and 'old' autoprothrombin II-A. Thromb Res 8: 543–552

Seligsohn U, Berger A, Abend M et al 1984 Homozygous protein C deficiency manifested by massive venous thrombosis in the newborn. N Engl J Med 310: 559–562

Sharon C, Tirindelli M C, Mannucci P M et al 1986 Homozygous protein C deficiency with moderately severe clinical symptoms. Thromb Res 41: 483–488

Shigekiyo T, Uno Y, Tomonari A et al 1992 Type I congenital plasminogen deficiency is not a risk factor for thrombosis. Thromb Haemost 67: 189–192

Sie T, Tichou J, Dupouy D et al 1985 Constitutional heparin cofactor II deficiency associated with recurrent thrombosis. Lancet 2: 414–416

Sills R H, Marlar R A, Montgomery R R et al 1984 Severe homozygous protein C deficiency. J Pediatr 105: 409–413

Stenflo J 1976 A new vitamin K dependent protein – purification from bovine plasma and preliminary characterisation. J Biol Chem 251: 353–355

Tait R C, Walker I D, Perry D J et al 1991 Prevalence of antithrombin III deficiency subtypes in 4000 healthy blood donors. Thromb Haemost 65: 534 (Abstract)

Teepe R G, Broekmans A W, Vermeer B J et al 1986 Recurrent coumarin-induced skin necrosis in a patient with an acquired functional protein C deficiency. Arch Dermatol 122: 1408–1412

Thaler E, Lechner K 1981 Antithrombin III deficiency and thromboembolism. Clin Haematol 10: 369–390

Tran T H, Narbet G A, Duckert F 1985 Association of heparin cofactor II deficiency with thrombosis. Lancet 2: 413–414

Tripodi A, Franchi F, Krachmalnicoff A et al 1990 Asymptomatic homozygous protein C deficiency. Acta Haematol (Basel) 83: 152–155

Tsuda S, Reitsma P H, Miletich J 1991 Molecular defects causing heterozygous protein C deficiency in three asymptomatic kindreds. Thromb Haemost 65: 647 (Abstract)

Tuddenham E G, Takase T, Thomas A E et al 1989 Homozygous protein C deficiency with delayed onset of symptoms at 7 to 10 months. Thromb Res 53: 475–484

Vykidal R, Korninger C, Kyrir P A et al 1985 The prevalence of antithrombin III deficiency in patients with a history of venous thromboembolism. Thromb Haemost 54: 744–745

Walker F J 1981 Regulation of activated protein C by protein S. The role of phospholipid in factor Va inactivation. J Biol Chem 256: 11128–11131

Wintzen A R, Broekmans A W, Bertina R M et al 1985 Cerebral haemorrhagic infarction in young patients with hereditary protein C deficiency: evidence for 'spontaneous' cerebral venous thrombosis. Br Med J 290: 350–352

Wise P H, Hall A J 1980 Heparin-induced osteopenia in pregnancy. Br Med J 2: 110–111

Yue R, Gertler M, Starr T et al 1976 Alterations of plasma antithrombin III levels in ischaemic heart disease. Thromb Haemost 35: 598–606

Zimran A, Shilo S, Fisher D et al 1986 Histomorphometric evaluation of reversible heparin-induced osteoporosis in pregnancy. Arch Intern Med 146: 386–388

13

The molecular biology of factor VIII and von Willebrand factor

E. G. D. Tuddenham

The cloning of the genes for factor VIII (FVIII) and von Willebrand factor (vWF) and the establishment of their complete cDNA sequences has opened a new era in haemostasis research during the past 8 years. The search for the structure of FVIII was fuelled by the desire to produce bioengineered protein for substitution therapy. This goal has been successfully reached with the licensing of two recombinant FVIII products during 1992–1993, and is not further discussed in the present review.

Although FVIII and vWF circulate as a non-covalent complex in blood the only physiological reason for this appears to be to protect FVIII from proteolytic attack. In haemostasis, once thrombin has activated FVIII, it is released from vWF and the two proteins function completely independently. Therefore, it is convenient to consider them separately, apart from the details of the binding interaction, which have been elucidated by molecular studies, and by the discovery of specific inherited defects of the binding sites on both molecules. In this review a necessarily brief account is presented of the structure and function of each protein and of the molecular genetics of their respective disorders haemophilia A (HA) and von Willebrand disease (vWD).

Studies on the molecular genetics of human disease have advanced very rapidly indeed in the past 5 years with the introduction of PCR (polymerase chain reaction) based screening methods. Only a summary can be given here of the fast expanding databases of mutations identified in HA and vWD to which the interested reader is directed for further information (for HA: Tuddenham et al 1991; for vWD: Ginsburg & Sadler 1993).

FACTOR VIII (FVIII) AND HAEMOPHILIA A (HA)

The FVIII gene is located on Xq2.8, spanning 185 kb, with 26 exons (Fig. 13.1). The processed mRNA of nearly 9 kb encodes a protein of 2351 amino acids, of which the first 19 residues are a hydrophobic leader sequence. The overall structure contains a triplicated A domain and duplicated C domain with a unique B domain. It may be represented as A1 a1 A2 B a2 A3 C1 C2 (Fig. 13.1). The a1 and a2 domains are short acidic segments cleaved from the protein during activation (a2) and inactivation (a1) (see below).

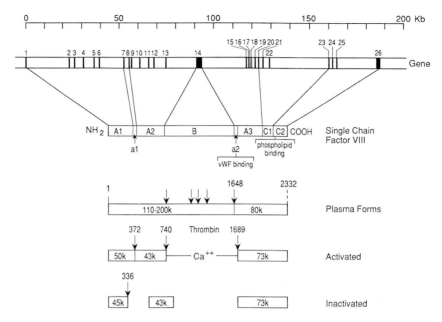

Fig. 13.1 FVIII gene and protein structure. Top line: Scale for gene map in kb pairs. 2nd line: FVIII gene, exons numbered, shaded, and connected to protein regions encoded therein. 3rd line: Domains of single chain protein and binding sites. 4th line: Arrows denote cleavages found in circulating plasma FVIII prior to activation. 5th line: The structure of activated FVIII after cleavage by thrombin. 6th line: Inactivated FVIII fragments after cleavage by activated protein C.

Structure and function of FVIII

Function of FVIII

FVIII is the protein procofactor for the serine protease FIXa. FIXa is capable of hydrolysing its substrate FX in the absence of calcium ions, phospholipid and proteolytically activated FVIII (FVIIIa) but the reaction rates are very slow indeed (Mann et al 1990). A number of groups have carried out kinetic studies of the activation of FX in the presence of FIXa and the other components of the tenase complex. In a system using bovine components Van Dieijen et al (1981) showed that the addition of calcium alone had little effect on the velocity of the reaction (V_{max}) or the affinity of the enzyme for the substrate (K_m). The addition of phospholipid, however, decreased the apparent K_m for the reaction 3000-fold. This effect is probably caused by increasing the concentration of the enzyme, FIXa, and the substrate, FX, on the phospholipid surface. The addition of FVIIIa to the reaction mixture dramatically enhanced the rate of the reaction by increasing the V_{max} 200 000-fold. Kinetic studies using human proteins suggest that the addition of FVIIIa to FIXa, FX, phospholipid and calcium alters the reaction rate by modestly decreasing the K_m and greatly increasing V_{max} (Griffith et al 1982,

Hultin 1981). Thus, phospholipid acts to increase the local concentration of the enzyme and the substrate, whereas FVIIIa binds to the enzyme and/or the substrate increasing the forward rate constant. One possible explanation for this effect would be that FVIIIa binds to FIXa and induces a conformational change in the enzyme, increasing its activity towards the scissile bond in FX. Recently, evidence for this, based on fluorescein-labelled FIXa, and the effect of adding FVIIIa, has been presented by Mutucumarana et al (1992). Alternatively, or in addition, FVIIIa might induce increased susceptibility of the substrate to cleavage. There is evidence that FVIII is capable of directly interacting with both FIXa (Rick 1982, Lollar et al 1984, O'Brien et al 1992) and FX (Vehar & Davie 1980).

The requirement for the preactivation of FVIII prior to participation in tenase is absolute. FVIII is activated through selective proteolysis by thrombin and FXa and, as will be discussed later, variant molecules with cleavage site mutations have reduced or absent function. When unactivated procofactor VIII is used in kinetic analyses there is a considerable lag phase prior to maximal rates of FXa generation. This reflects the back-activation of FVIII by FXa in the reaction mixture. The initial generation of FXa in vivo probably occurs as a FVIIIa-independent process whereby tissue factor (TF) and FVIIa generate FXa directly before that pathway is damped by TF pathway inhibitor (Rapaport 1991). Trace amounts of thrombin and FXa are capable of proteolytically activating FVIII and so the model in which the TF/FVIIa pathway generates sufficient FXa and thrombin for subsequent full activation of the FVIII is plausible.

Interaction of FVIII with vWF

FVIII and vWF circulate in plasma in a non-covalent complex that can be dissociated with reducing agents or by high ionic strength buffers. vWF is a multimeric glycoprotein with a role in platelet adhesion in primary haemostasis. vWF is also required to stabilize FVIII in plasma as evidenced by the near absence of FVIII in plasma of patients suffering from severe homozygous vWD. The $t_{1/2}$ of purified FVIII relatively free of vWF administered to a patient with severe vWD was 2.5 hours, compared to 10–12 hours observed in HA patients, who have endogenous vWF capable of binding to, and stabilizing, infused purified FVIII (Tuddenham et al 1982). vWF therefore acts as a carrier protein, protecting FVIII from proteolysis in vivo. It would appear that each vWF protomer has a single FVIII binding site (Lollar & Parker 1987). FVIII binds to vWF through the N-terminal region of the 80 kDa light chain.

Foster et al (1987) mapped the epitope of a monoclonal antibody to FVIII which inhibited the binding of the cofactor to vWF. Residues 1670–1684 of FVIII bound to the monoclonal antibody — a region which incorporates the highly acidic a_2 segment at the N-terminus of the A3C1C2 polypeptide (Fig. 13.1). Leyte et al (1991) produced a series of site-directed mutants of recombinant FVIII with deletions in the B domain and the second acidic segment. Deletion of the entire B domain from positions 741 to 1648 had no effect on FVIII–vWF binding. Further truncation of the molecule from positions 741 to 1668 retained vWF binding. A third mutant, with a deletion of the B domain extending into the second acidic segment from positions 740 to 1689 was no longer able to bind vWF. This confirmed the results of the monoclonal antibody epitope mapping indicating a role for residues within the sequence 1669–1689 in the formation of a vWF binding site. Site-directed mutants of FVIII, with conservative substitution of Tyr residues at positions 1664 and 1680 by Phe, bound poorly to vWF (Pittman et al 1987). These two Tyr residues, which lie in the second acidic segment, are sulphated (Pittman et al 1992). The recombinant mutant FVIII des 741–1668 produced by Leyte et al (1991) lacked the Tyr at position 1664, but bound vWF efficiently and so the Tyr at position 1680 is probably directly involved in the vWF interaction. This was further confirmed by the lack of vWF binding by the recombinant FVIII mutant 1680 Tyr to Phe. A naturally occurring dysfunctional FVIII molecule with replacement of Tyr 1680 by Phe is associated with mild HA, presumably reflecting the lack of binding to, and stabilization, by vWF (Higuchi et al 1991). Thus the charged second acidic segment, and specifically the highly charged tyrosine sulphate at position 1680, most probably forms the vWF binding site on FVIII.

Tyrosine sulphation also occurs at residues 346 and 1664, as well as at three positions (probably 718, 719 and 723) in the A2 domain (Pittman et al 1992). Total inhibition of sulphation with chlorate ions in vitro reduces the procoagulant activity of desulphate FVIII five-fold (Pittman et al 1992). Fay & Smudzin (1990) investigated the physical topography of the FVIII–vWF complex using fluorescence quenching. Isolated FVIII subunits labelled with the fluorescence donor were used to label fluorescence acceptor vWF SPIII homodimers. Modified FVIII light chain showed an interfluorophore distance of 28Å. Heavy chains did not interact with vWF, consistent with the observation that removal of the light chain a2 domain releases the whole FVIII molecule from its carrier.

Activation and inactivation of FVIII

A number of blood coagulation serine proteases modulate the activity of FVIII by specific limited proteolysis. The interactions between FVIII and thrombin, FXa, FIXa and activated protein C have all been studied in detail.

By studying both the effects of site-directed mutagenesis and the properties of certain naturally occurring dysfunctional FVIII molecules, critical activation and inactivation cleavages have been determined. Transiently expressed mutants with radical substitutions at positions Arg 740 and 1648 were resistant to cleavage at these sites but were still activated following thrombin cleavage at positions 372 and 1689 (Pittman & Kaufman 1988). The removal of the B domain from the A1A2 polypeptide is therefore not a prerequisite for

FVIII activation. Mutation of Arg 372 or Arg 1689 to Ile resulted in the expression of recombinant FVIII that was not activated by thrombin. Naturally occurring dysfunctional FVIII molecules isolated from the plasma of haemophiliacs have also been studied. A mutation in a mildly affected haemophiliac's FVIII gene lead to the expression of a molecule with an Arg to Cys substitution at position 372 (O'Brien et al 1990). This molecule was only three-fold activated by thrombin following cleavage at positions 740 and 1689 but not 372 (Fig. 13.1). A patient with an Arg to His substitution had a similar phenotype (Arai et al 1989).

Bihoreau et al (1989) have presented evidence for two-stage activation of FVIII, the first stage resulting from cleavage at positions 1689 and 740 to generate a two chain complex (A_1 a_1 A_2/A_3 C_1 C_2) resulting in a five-fold activation of FVIII. In the second stage full activation is concomitant with the cleavage at position 372. This is in keeping with the finding that the variant FVIII 372 Arg to Cys molecule was partially activatable, therefore causing only a mild bleeding phenotype. Another patient was shown to have a circulating variant molecule with substitution of Arg 1689 by Cys (O'Brien & Tuddenham 1989). This molecule was completely inactive even though it was cleaved efficiently at positions 372 and 740. Gel permeation chromatography studies showed that this abnormal molecule was not released from vWF following incubation with thrombin, indicating that at least one of the functions of this cleavage is to effect the release of the cofactor from the carrier molecule. Interestingly, other cases with the same mutation sometimes have residual FVIII activity (Tuddenham et al 1991). Activation of porcine FVIII in the absence of vWF by a snake venom protease which cleaved the (homologous) 372 and not the 1689 site suggested the function of the latter cleavage is simply to release FVIII from vWF (Hill-Eubanks et al 1989). In contrast, the variant molecule 1689 Arg to Cys was not activated by thrombin following purification from vWF (O'Brien & Tuddenham 1989), and vWF-free recombinant FVIII 1689 Arg to Ile was also inactive (Pittman & Kaufman 1988). It is possible that the lack of activity in these molecules is the result of non-conservative amino acid substitutions at this site, sterically inhibiting the activated form of the cofactor.

Nesheim et al (1991) using a mutant FVIII lacking the vWF binding domain concluded that FVIII will bind directly to thrombin-activated platelets but in normal plasma it is prevented from doing so by competitive binding to vWF. Thrombin is therefore essential to release FVIII from vWF as well as to make the other activation cleavage in the heavy chain.

Structure of activated FVIII

Several studies have shown that activation of FVIII by thrombin is followed by a first-order decay with no apparent alteration in the polypeptides resolved by sodium dodecyl sulphate polyacrylamide-gel electrophoresis (SDS-PAGE) (Fulcher et al 1983, Rotblat et al 1985, Lollar et al 1984). The maximally activated form of the cofactor and the inactive species resolved as polypeptides at 70, 50 and 40 kDa on SDS-PAGE. It was not clear from these studies which polypeptide, or combination of polypeptides, represented the active moiety. When porcine FVIIIa was subjected to cation exchange high-performance liquid chromatography by Lollar & Parker (1989), the coagulant activity was isolated as a single peak containing three polypeptides, A1, A2 and A3C1C2. This material remained stably activated for several weeks at pH 6.0. All three FVIII fragments were shown to be associated by analytical ultracentrifugation. Thus porcine FVIIIa was shown to be a complex of the A1, the A2 and the A3C1C2 domains. The stability of the active form of porcine FVIII was found to be markedly pH- and concentration-dependent (Lollar & Parker 1991) being stable at pH 6.0 but irreversibly inactivated by elevation of the pH to 8.0 which caused FVIIIa to elute from cation exchange columns as a complex of the A1 and A3C1C2 fragments, with loss of the A2 domain by adsorption to the column. The stability of the active species was also markedly improved by increasing the concentration of FVIII in reaction mixtures. These data indicated that the inactivation of FVIIIa was associated with the dissociation of the A2 domain from the active moiety, and suggested a mechanism for the pH dependence of FVIIIa stability. Since the loss of activity and dissociation of FVIIIa occurs over a narrow pH band it seems that deprotonation leads to disruption of the quaternary structure of the active complex.

Molecular genetics of HA

Table 13.1 summarizes the total number of missense and nonsense mutations located in each exon of the FVIII gene (extracted from tables in Tuddenham et al 1991). The data are somewhat skewed by the fact that, until recently, selective screening procedures were used, biased towards mutations in CG dinucleotides. Latterly, general screening methods based on denaturing gradient gel electrophoresis, chemical cleavage or single-strand conformation have been employed. The most rapid and powerful approach has been devised by Naylor et al (1991) in which 'ectopic' FVIII mRNA in lymphocytes is reverse transcribed, then PCR amplified. Mutations were detected by chemical cleavage and sequenced. An exciting result from this approach has been that up to half the mutations causing severe HA cannot be located within exons or flanking sequences. In these cases there is failure of proper mRNA processing across intron 22, such that exons 22 and 23 are not contiguous in mRNA (Naylor et al 1992). The molecular basis for this tantalizing result has not yet been elucidated. Intron 22 is the largest in FVIII, spanning nearly 40 kb and containing two genes of unknown function (Gitschier et al 1991), so the possibilities are legion.

A large and diverse group of deletions ranging in size from one nucleotide to the entire FVIII gene has also been detected. A significant association exists between deletion genotype and inhibitor development, although not as strong as that noted for haemophilia B. As regards point mutations and development of inhibitors, although only a limited number of cases have been

Table 13.1 Unique mutations in the FVIII gene in HA

Exon	Nonsense	Missense	Splice junction*	
			5′	3′
1	1	1		
2				
3		2		
4		3		
5		1		
6			1	
7	1	5	1	
8	1	4		
9	1	2		
10		3		
11		6		
12	1	5		
13		1		
14	3	7		
15		1		
16		5		
17		1		
18	2	4		
19		1		
20				
21				
22	1	4		
23	1	3		
24	1	2		
25		1		
26	1	4		

*Only mutations affecting the canonical gt or ag donor and acceptor sequences are listed.

successfully analysed an interesting discrepancy was noted. Inhibitor frequency with genotype R336 Stop was low (six cases, no inhibitors) and with R2147 Stop it was high (five cases, three inhibitors). A possible explanation for this is that exon 8 containing 336 Stop, when containing this mutation is excluded giving rise to an in-frame transcript bridging exons 7 and 9 and such transcripts have indeed been observed (Giannelli F, 1992, personal communication). Hence factor VIII peptides corresponding to most of the full length protein could be produced at levels sufficient to induce tolerance. Whereas exon 23 containing 2147 Stop, if excluded would not give rise to an in-frame transcript, and the premature stop codon would terminate translation with perhaps a less stable truncated protein in amounts too low to induce tolerance.

Linkage analysis in HA

Direct gene defect analysis is the method of choice in family studies for genetic counselling. However, in those instances where the mutation causing

HA in a given kindred cannot be identified by currently available screening strategies, it is still worth attempting classical linkage analysis. This approach has been greatly strengthened recently by the discovery of a highly polymorphic $(CA)_n$ repeat within intron 13 of the FVIII gene (Lalloz et al 1991). With more than eight alleles over 90% of females are informative (heterozygous), making this the preferred linkage marker for initial studies (Figs. 13.2 and 13.3). Detailed recommendations on the methods for prevention of haemophilia are contained in a report of the World Health Organization (Peake et al 1993).

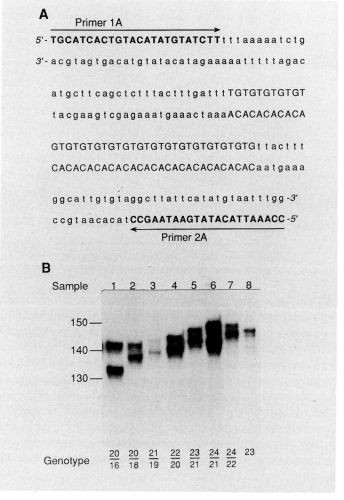

Fig. 13.2 FVIII intron 13 $(CA)_n$ polymorphic repeat. **A.** Primers 1A and 2A are used to amplify repeat segment. **B.** Pattern of repeats obtained by PCR amplification of DNA with polymorphic repeat lengths. Lane 1: DNA containing two alleles with $(CA)_{20}$ and $(CA)_{16}$ respectively. Lane 2: $(CA)_{20}$ and $(CA)_{18}$; and so on. Reproduced with permission from Lalloz et al (1991).

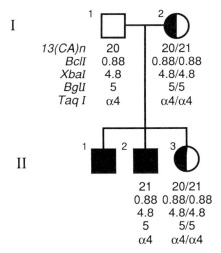

Fig. 13.3 Linkage analysis in family segregating HA using four intragenic and one extragenic marker (*Taq*I). The obligate carrier female (I2) is only informative (heterozygous) for intron 13 $(CA)_n$. Based on the segregation of this marker's $(CA)_{21}$ allele with haemophilia (shaded boxes = affected males) it is clear that the daughter (II3) is a carrier (half-shaded circle). She can also be offered antenatal diagnosis in future using the $(CA)_{21}$ marker as she is herself heterozygous.

VON WILLEBRAND FACTOR (vWF)

Structure and function of vWF

Recently an excellent review on this topic has appeared which is strongly recommended to the interested reader (Ruggeri & Ware 1992). Therefore only an abbreviated overview is given here, mainly to serve as an introduction to the molecular genetics of vWD.

vWF is synthesized in megakaryocytes and endothelial cells as a primary translation product of 2813 amino acids. After cleavage of a 22-residue signal peptide, this undergoes dimerization through specific C-terminal Cys residues to yield a pro-vWF dimer. The dimers then undergo multimerization through disulphide linkage at the N-termini — a process catalysed by the large 741-residue propeptide acting as an endodisulphide isomerase within the environment of the trans golgi. The propeptide is excised and the mature protein consisting now of extremely long multimers is either packaged in alpha granules (platelets), Weibel–Palade bodies (endothelial cells) or directly secreted in plasma or subendothelial matrix (by endothelial cells). The forms present in the storage organelles are released as the largest multimers upon activation of platelets or stimulation of endothelial cells (e.g. after infusion of DDAVP (deamino-D-arginine vasopressin)). The variable length of multimers gives rise to a complex pattern upon immunoelectrophoresis in acrylamide gels. The complexity of the pattern is increased by the presence of partially proteolysed forms due to the presence of a scissile bond, Tyr

842 – Met 843 which is partially cleaved in the circulation. Increased or, in rare cases, decreased susceptibility to cleavage of this bond gives rise to some of the aberrant multimer distributions seen in type II vWD.

Figure 13.4 shows the functional domains that have been mapped onto the vWF protomer by a variety of methods including protein fragmentation, peptidyl mimicry and antibody epitope analysis. Of note is that the FVIII binding site is clearly localized to the N-terminus while the glycoprotein Ib (GPIb) binding site – the essential functional ligand involved in vWF-dependent platelet adhesion – is localized to a region from residues 449 to 728. The protein functional localizations have been amply confirmed by studies of dysfunctional molecules (see below).

Molecular genetics of vWF

The gene for vWF is located at 12p12, spanning 178 kb and divided into 52 exons (Fig. 13.4). A pseudogene including homologues of the central portion of the gene occurs on chromosome 22. Mutations causing several subtypes of vWD have now been localized. A database summarizing these mutations has very recently been published (Ginsburg & Sadler 1993). Analysis of primary sequence shows that four types of internal repeat occur. The A type repeats

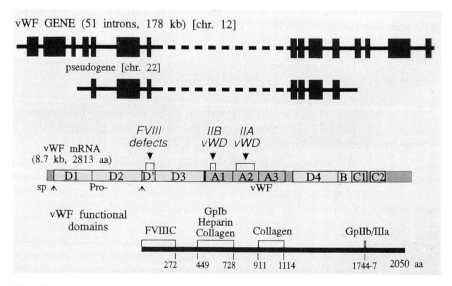

Fig. 13.4 vWF gene, pseudogene and protein structure. Top line: vWF gene (not to scale). Wide shaded bars = exons. 2nd line: Pseudogene. 3rd line: Domain structure of vWF mRNA indicating: above the line, region of specific defects; below the line, post-translational processing event sites. Sp = signal peptide; Pro = propeptide, also called vW antigen II; vWF = mature protomer. 4th line: Ligand binding domains of vWF protein. (Figure kindly provided by Dr. D. Ginsburg.)

Table 13.2   Type IIA vWD mutations

Amino acid substitution	Nucleotide substitution	Affected individuals	Independent families	Group*
Cys 509 Arg	T3814C	1	1	–
Val 551 Phe	G3940T	1	1	–
Gly 742 Arg	G4513C	1	1	I
Gly 742 Glu	G4514A	5	2	II
Ser 743 Leu	C4517T	3	3	I
Leu 777 Pro	T4619C	1	1	I
Leu 799 Pro	T4685C	1	1	–
Arg 834 Trp	C4789T	13	9	II
Arg 834 Gln	G4790A	3	3	–
Val 844 Asp	T4820A	1	1	I
Ser 850 Pro	T4837C	1	1	–
Ile 865 Thr	T4883C	8	1	II
Gln 875 Lys	G4912A	1	1	–

*Group I = defective intracellular transport; group II = normal secretion ?proteolysis in plasma; – = not determined.

occur in several other proteins, and mutations within these domains give rise to most cases of variant type IIB and IIA vWD. FVIII binding defects (Mazurier 1992) occur predictably in the N-terminal region of the mature subunit, which lies within a partial D type domain.

Tables 13.2–13.5 summarize the reported mutations identified in these subtypes of vWD (full details with references are available in the database). In relation to type IIA vWD, a variant in which only lower multimers are present, two subdivisions have been made on the basis of in vitro synthesis studies. The primary defect is either in secretion or is presumed to be due to enhanced susceptibility to proteolysis in plasma (Fig. 13.5). The mutations associated with type IIB vWD all occur within a single disulphide loop Cys 509 to Cys 695 (Fig. 13.6). Evidently these mutants affect local structure such that the mutant vWF has increased avidity for the platelet GPIb receptor, causing loss of the highest MW multimers from plasma together with platelet aggregates. Sufferers usually have moderate thrombocytopenia as well as

Table 13.3   Type IIB vWD mutations

Amino acid substitution	Nucleotide substitution	Affected individuals	Independent families	Functional studies*
540 Ins Met	3910 Ins ATG	3	1	–
Arg 543 Trp	C 3916 T	13	10	+
Arg 545 Cys	C 3922 T	17	10	–
Trp 550 Cys	G 3939 C	1	1	+
Val 551 Leu	G 3940 C	1	1	–
Val 553 Met	G 3946 A	13	8	+
Pro 547 Leu	C 4010 T	1	1	+
Arg 578 Gln	G 4022 A	10	9	+

Table 13.4   Type III (null) vWD mutations

Amino acid substitution	Nucleotide substitution	Affected individuals	Independent families
Arg 365 ter	C1093T	4	1
Arg 1772 ter	C7603T	3	3
Arg 896 ter	C4975T	3	3
Deletions		8	5
mRNA expression defect		7	5

Table 13.5   Miscellaneous mutations in vWD

Amino acid substitution	Nucleotide substitution	Affected individuals	Independent families	Clinical phenotype
Arg 19 Trp and His 54 Gln	C 2344 T and T 2451 A	1	1	FVIII binding defect
Arg 53 Trp	C 2466 T	4	2	"
Thr 28 Met	C 2372 T	3	2	"
Arg 91 Gln	G 2561 A	5	4	"
Gene deletion	(exons 26–34)	1	1	Type II variant
Gly 561 Ser	G 3970 A	1	1	Type B
Phe 606 Ile	T 4105 A	2	1	Normal multimers decreased RiCoF activity

RiCoF = Ristocetin cofactor.

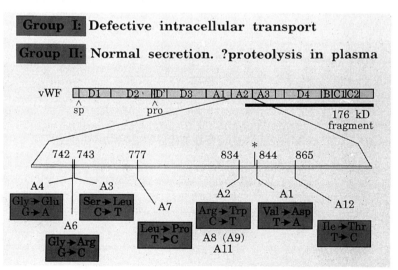

Fig. 13.5   Location of mutations in type IIA vWD. All cases of this variant lack high and intermediate molecular weight vWF multimers and usually have an aberrant subunit structure visualized on high-resolution immunoelectrophoresis. Group I mutants reproduce this defect when expressed in vitro. Group II mutants direct synthesis of normally multimerized vWF in vitro, and it is presumed that the variant vWF is proteolysed excessively in vivo. 176 kDa fragment represents the peptide produced by proteolysis of vWF at scissile bond, I*. (Figure kindly provided by Dr. D. Ginsburg).

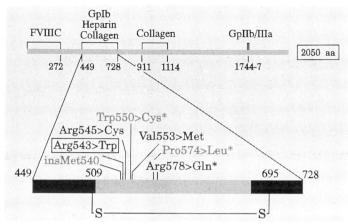

Fig. 13.6   Mutations in type IIB vWD. All described missense mutants found in this variant lie within the disulphide loop C509 to C695. Type IIB vWF shows enhanced binding to platelet membrane GPIb, which has been independently mapped to this region of vWF. In normal vWF an 'activation' step is required before the binding site is available. (Figure kindly provided by Dr. D. Ginsburg.)

platelet adhesion defect as a consequence. Only a few mutations causing type I or type III vWD have been identified so far. Historically of great interest is the finding that a single cytosine deletion in exon 18 of the vWF gene, causing frame shift and premature termination at residue 48 of the mature subunit, is present in half the cases of type III vWD in Sweden and in the original family described by von Willebrand (Zhang et al 1992).

Still undetected are the mutations in the majority of cases (75%) with type I disease.

Based on the above a pathophysiological classification of vWD is emerging to complement the previously used descriptive and functional classifications (Table 13.6).

KEY POINTS FOR CLINICAL PRACTICE

Haemophilia A

- Methods now exist to detect the causative mutation in virtually all cases of mild haemophilia A and about half the cases of severe haemophilia A.
- Direct mutation detection can be used for gene tracking in many families segregating haemophilia A.
- Linkage analysis for gene tracking using intragenic markers is possible in most families requesting genetic counselling.

von Willebrand disease

- The causative mutation can be identified in von Willebrand disease types IIA and IIB.
- Few mutations have yet been identified in von Willebrand disease type I.

Table 13.6 Classification of von Willebrand's disease (deficient and/or defective vWF)

Descriptive	Functional	Pathophysiological	EXAMPLES
Type I (all multimers present)	*Quantitative*	*Molecular genetics*	
A	Type IA	Deletion	III
B	Platelet normal	Nonsense	III
C	Type III	Missense	IIA, IIB, VIII, Type B
		Promoter	
		RNA processing	III
Platelet: Normal	*Qualitative*	*Cell biology*	
Low	Loss of function: IB	Synthesis	III
Discordant	IC	Processing	Some IIA
	IIA	Assembly	Some IIA
'Normandy'	IIC→H	Secretion	Some IIA
'New York'	'Type B'		
'Type B'		*Protein function*	
	Gain of function: IIB	Stability:	Some IIA
	'New York'	Binding sites for:	GPIb–IIB
			FVIII 'Normandy'
Type II (some multimers missing)	FVIII binding defect: 'Normandy'		
A			
B			
C→			
H			
Type III (all multimers absent)			

REFERENCES

Arai M, Inaba H, Higuchi M et al 1989 Direct characterization of factor VIII in plasma: detection of a mutation altering a thrombin cleavage site (arginine-372→histidine). Proc Natl Acad Sci USA 86: 4277–4281

Bihoreau N, Sanger A, Yon J M et al 1989 Isolation and characterization of different activated forms of factor VIII, the human antihemophilic A factor. Eur J Biochem 185: 111–118

Fay P J, Smudzin T M 1990 Topography of the human factor VIII–von Willebrand factor complex. J Biol Chem 265: 6197–6202

Foster P A, Fulcher C A, Marti T et al 1987 A major factor VIII binding domain resides within the amino-terminal 272 residues of von Willebrand factor. J Biol Chem 262: 8443–8446

Fulcher C A, Roberts J R, Zimmerman T S 1983 Thrombin proteolysis of purified factor VIII procoagulant protein: correlation of activation with generation of specific polypeptide. Blood 61: 807–811

Ginsburg D, Sadler J E 1993 von Willebrand's disease: a database of point mutations, insertions and deletions. Thromb Haemost 69: 177–184

Gitschier J, Kogan S, Diamond C et al 1991 Genetic basis of haemophilia A. Thromb Haemost 66: 37–39

Griffith M J, Reisner H M, Lundblad R L et al 1982 Measurement of human factor IXa activity in an isolated factor X activation system. Thromb Res 27: 289–301

Higuchi M, Antonarakis S E, Kasch L et al 1991 Towards complete characterization of mild-to-moderate hemophilia A: detection of the molecular defect in 25 of 29 patients by denaturing gradient gel electrophoresis. Proc Natl Acad Sci USA 88: 8307–8311

Hill-Eubanks D C, Parker C G, Lollar P 1989 Differential proteolytic activation of factor VIII – von Willebrand factor complex by thrombin. Proc Natl Acad Sci USA 86: 6508–6512

Hultin M B 1981 Role of human factor VIII in factor X activation J Clin Invest 69: 950–958

Lalloz M R A, McVey J H, Pattinson J K et al 1991 Haemophilia A diagnosis by analysis of a hypervariable dinucleotide repeat within the factor VIII gene. Lancet 338: 207–211

Leyte A, van Schijndel H, Niehrs C et al 1991 Sulphation of Tyr 1680 of human blood coagulation factor VIII is essential for the interaction of factor VIII with von Willebrand factor. J Biol Chem 266: 740–746

Lollar P, Parker C G 1987 Stoichiometry of the porcine factor VIII – von Willebrand factor association. J Biol Chem 262: 17572–17576

Lollar P, Parker C G 1989 Subunit structure of thrombin-activated porcine factor VIII. Biochemistry 28: 666–674

Lollar P, Parker E T 1991 Structural basis for the decreased procoagulant activity of human factor VIII compared to the porcine homolog. J Biol Chem 266: 12481–12486

Lollar P, Knutson G J, Fass D N 1984 Stabilization of thrombin-activated porcine factor VIII:C by factor IXa and phospholipid. Blood 63: 1303–1308

Mann K G, Nesheim M E, Church W R et al 1990 Surface dependent reactions of the vitamin K-dependent enzyme complexes. Blood 76: 1–16

Mazurier C 1992 von Willebrand's disease masquerading as haemophilia A. Thromb Haemost 67: 391–396

Mutucumarana V P, Duffy E J, Lollar P et al 1992 The active site of factor IXa is located far above the membrane surface and its conformation is altered upon association with factor VIIIa. A fluorescence study. J Biol Chem 267: 17012–17021

Naylor J A, Green P M, Montandon A J et al 1991 Detection of three novel mutations in two haemophilia A patients by rapid screening of whole essential region of factor VIII gene. Lancet 337: 635–639

Naylor J A, Green P M, Rizza C R et al 1992 Factor VIII gene explains all cases of haemophilia A. Lancet 340: 1066–1067

Nesheim M, Pittman D D, Giles A R et al 1991 The effect of plasma von Willebrand factor on the binding of human factor VIII to thrombin-activated human platelets. J Biol Chem 266: 17815–17820

O'Brien D P, Tuddenham E G D 1989 Purification and characterization of factor VIII 1689 Cys: a non-functional cofactor occurring in a patient with severe haemophilia A. Blood 73: 2117–2122

O'Brien D P, Pattinson J K, Tuddenham E G D 1990 Purification and characterization of factor VIII 372-Cys: a hypofunctional cofactor from a patient with moderately severe haemophilia A. Blood 75: 1664–1672

O'Brien D P, Johnson D, Byfield P et al 1992 Inactivation of factor VIII by factor IXa. Biochemistry 31: 2805–2812

Peake I R, Lillicrap D P, Boulyjenkov V et al 1993 Report of a joint WHO/WFH meeting on the control of haemophilia: carrier detection and prenatal diagnosis. Blood Coag Fibrinol 4: 313–344

Pittman D D, Kaufman R J 1988 Proteolytic requirements for thrombin activation of anti-hemophilic factor (factor VIII). Proc Natl Acad Sci USA 85: 2429–2433

Pittman D D, Wasley L C, Murray B L et al 1987 Analysis of structural requirements for factor VIII function using site-directed mutagenesis. Thromb Haemost 58: 804a (Abstract)

Pittman D D, Wang J H, Kaufman R J 1992 Identification and functional importance of tyrosine sulfate reisudes within recombinant factor VIII. Biochemistry 31: 3315–3325

Rapaport S I 1991 The extrinsic pathway inhibitor: a regulator of tissue factor-dependent blood coagulation. Thromb Haemost 66: 6–15

Rick M E 1982 Activation of factor VIII by factor IXa. Blood 60: 744–751

Rotblat F, O'Brien D P, O'Brien F et al 1985 Purification of factor VIII:C and its characterization by Western blotting using monoclonal antibodies. Biochemistry 24: 4294–4300

Ruggeri Z M, Ware J 1992 The structure and function of von Willebrand factor. Thromb Haemost 67: 594–599

Tuddenham E G D, Lane R S, Rotblat F et al 1982 Response to infusions of polyelectrolyte fractionated human factor VIII in human haemophilia A and von Willebrand's disease. Br J Haematol 52: 259–267

Tuddenham E G D, Cooper D N, Gitschier J et al 1991 Haemophilia A: database of nucleotide substitutions, deletions, insertions and re-arrangements of the factor VIII gene. Nucleic Acids Res 19: 4821–4833

Van Dieijen G, Tans G, Rosing J et al 1981 The role of phospholipid and factor VIIIa in the activation of bovine factor X. J Biol Chem 256: 3433–3441

Vehar G A, Davie E W 1980 Preparation and properties of bovine factor VIII (antihemophilic factor). Biochemistry 19: 401–410

World Health Organization 1992 Report of a joint WHO/WFH meeting on control of haemophilia. WHO/HDP/WFH 92.4.

Zhang Z P, Falk G, Blomback M et al 1992 A single cytosine deletion in exon 18 of the von Willebrand factor gene is the most common mutation in Swedish vWD type III patients. Hum Mol Gene 1: 767–768

Index

257